DATE DUE

	JUN 1 8 2010	

GAYLORD   #3523PI   Printed in USA

HEALTH PROMOTION IN COMMUNITIES

Holistic and Wellness Approaches

Carolyn Chambers Clark, EdD, ARNP, FAAN, HNC, DABFN, FAAIM, is on the Health Services Doctoral Faculty at Walden University and has been on the graduate and undergraduate nursing faculty at several other universities. Dr. Clark is founder, The Wellness Institute, and Founding Editor, *Alternative Health Practitioner: The Journal of Complementary and Natural Care* (now called *Complementary Health Practice Review*). Her book, *Wellness Practitioner: Concepts, Research, and Strategies*, 2nd edition (Springer, 1996) won an American Journal of Nursing Book-of-the-Year Award, and *The Nurse as Group Leader* is now in its third edition (Springer, 1994) and has been published in German and Swedish. She has published widely on complementary and holistic topics for both academic and consumer audiences and is Editor-in-Chief of the *Encyclopedia of Complementary Health Practice* (Springer, 1999) and author of *Integrating Complementary Health Procedures into Practice* (Springer, 2000), both of which received *AJN* Book-of-the-Year Awards. Dr. Clark is certified as an holistic nurse by the American Holistic Nurses' Certification Corporation, is a Diplomate of the American Board of Forensic Nursing, an Advisory Board member and Fellow of the American Association of Integrative Medicine, and has been a Fellow of the American Academy of Nursing since 1980. She serves as a research grant reviewer for Sigma Theta Tau International, has maintained a wellness/holistic private practice since 1976 and has provided community health and wellness consultation since 1973.

HEALTH PROMOTION IN COMMUNITIES

Holistic and Wellness Approaches

Carolyn Chambers Clark, *EdD, RN,*
ARNP, FAAN, HNC, DABFN, Editor

 Springer Publishing Company

WA
546
AA1
H42
2002

Copyright © 2002 by Springer Publishing Company, Inc.

Springer Publishing Company, Inc.
536 Broadway
New York, NY 10012-3955

Acquisitions Editor: Ruth Chasek
Production Editor: J. Hurkin-Torres
Cover design by Susan Hauley

03 04 05 06 / 5 4 3 2

Library of Congress Cataloging-in-Publication Data

Clark, Carolyn Chambers.
   Health promotion in communities : holistic and wellness approaches / editor Carolyn Chambers Clark.
      p. ; cm.
   Includes bibliographical references and index.
   ISBN 0-8261-1407-5
   1. Community health services.   2. Holistic medicine.   3. Health promotion.
   4. Medicine, Preventive.   I. Title.
   [DNLM: 1. Community Health Services—organization & administration—United States.   2. Health Promotion—methods—United States.   3. Holistic Health—United States.
WA 546 AA1 C592h 2001]
RA427 .C54 2001
362.1'2—dc21   00-067911
                                                                                              CIP

Printed in the United States of America by Sheridan Press.

This book is dedicated to my granddaughter, Morgaine,
whose first word was "book."

Contents

List of Tables

List of Boxes

List of Figures

Contributors

Julia W. Aucoin, DNS, RN, C
Associate Professor
School of Nursing
Tennessee Technological University
Cookeville, TN

Kitty Corbett, PhD, MPH
Associate Professor of Anthropology
University of Colorado
Denver, CO

**Janice Unruh Davidson, PhD, RN, CS,
  CNAA, ARNP-FNP**
Professor
Department of Nursing
Fort Hays State University
Hays, KS

Pamela P. DiNapoli, RN, MSN, PhD
Assistant Professor
Department of Nursing
University of New Hampshire
School of Health and Human Services
Durham, NH

Margo Drohan, MSN, RN, CS, PNP
Clinical Assistant Professor
School of Nursing
University of Massachusetts, Amherst
Amherst, MA

Susan MacLeod Dyess, RN, MS
Director, Nursing through Faith Communities
Christine E. Lynn Center for Caring
College of Nursing
Florida Atlantic University
Boca Raton, FL
and
Coordinator, Health Ministry
Parish Nurse Program
St. Mary's and Good Samaritan Medical
  Centers
West Palm Beach, FL

**Grace Erickson, EdD, MPH, MSN,
  RN, BC**
University of South Florida
College of Nursing
Tampa, FL

Elizabeth Erkel, PhD, RN
Associate Professor
Medical University of South Carolina
College of Nursing/FNP Program
Charleston, SC

Douglas Fernald, MA
Department of Family Medicine
University of Colorado Health Sciences
  Center
Denver, CO

Carl Helvie, RN, DrPH
Professor Emeritus
Old Dominion University
School of Nursing
Norfolk, VA

Sandra Hopper, RN, MSN
Associate Director & Adjunct Faculty to
    Department of Nursing
Blue Ridge Area Health Education
    Center
James Madison University
Harrisonburg, VA

Jennifer Horton, DO
Department of Family Medicine
University of Colorado Health Sciences
    Center
Denver, CO

Cynthia G. Johnson, MSN, EdD, RN
Associate Professor
Division of Nursing
California State University, Dominguez
    Hills
Carson, CA

Kathryn Allen Judge
OMNI Research and Training & OMNI
    Institute
Denver, CO

Beth Keely, MSN, PhD, RN
Director, Undergraduate Nursing
    Programs
California State University, Long Beach
Long Beach, CA

Charlene Long, PhD, RN
Professor Emerita
College of Nursing
University of South Florida
St. Petersburg, FL

Sandra MacDonald, RN, BN, MN, PhD
Assistant Professor
Memorial University of Newfoundland
School of Nursing
St. John's, Newfoundland
Canada

Deborah S. Main, PhD
Department of Family Medicine
University of Colorado Health Sciences
    Center
Denver, CO

Nancy R. Oliver, PhD, RN, HNC
Associate Professor
California State University
Department of Nursing
Long Beach, CA

Jill Parker, MPH
Special Projects Coordinator
for the Community Health Plan
of the Rockies
Denver, CO

Marva Mizell Price, DrPh, MPH, RN, CS(FNP)
School of Nursing
Duke University
Durham, NC

Barbara Resnick, PhD, CRNP
Assistant Professor
University of Maryland
School of Nursing
Baltimore, MD

Sheilda G. Rodgers, PhD, RN
Associate Professor
North Carolina Central University
Durham, NC

Judy L. Sheehan, RN
Faculty, University of Rhode Island
Educational Consultant, E.B. Tech, Inc.
Educator, Westwood Pembroke Health
    Systems
Rehoboth, MA

Robert W. Strack, PhD, MBA
Center for Adolescent Health
Johns Hopkins University
Baltimore, MD

Carolyn Tressler, MPH
Department of Family Medicine
University of Colorado Health Sciences
    Center
Denver, CO

Chen-Yen Wang, PhD, APRN
Assistant Professor
University of Hawaii at Manoa
School of Nursing
Honolulu, HI

Preface

As hospital stays shrink and community residents demand more say in their health and wellness, new models for community practice emerge. This book is the culmination of an effort to provide one of those models.

After working as a community health practitioner in many settings and striving to teach community health students at various levels, I have come to this book. It is a practical manual for the community practitioner. Although there is a strong conceptual framework and research studies are presented, the basic mission of this book is to help community practitioners practice.

This book uses a unique holistic/wellness view of community practice with clients as full partners. Clients are viewed as whole persons and experts in their own wellness who collaborate with community practitioners to set goals, promote health, enhance wellness, and evaluate progress toward their goals. Although *Healthy 2010* goals are provided, it is clients, not practitioners, who must decide which goals they wish to pursue. It is the practitioners' role to facilitate client dreams and goals. Giving up the expert role to work on one's own wellness is also unique. To role model wellness for clients, and to allow clients to make their own informed decisions (even when we disagree) is challenging.

This book speaks directly to you, the reader, providing specific suggestions for working with clients, be they individuals, families, groups or communities. Ways to mobilize communities, and develop effective community health materials and programs as well as principles for effective community health program marketing and program evaluation are provided.

This book is organized into six parts. Part I presents theory and concepts and a model for health promotion in communities. Part II is devoted to skills needed to assist communities to assess, plan, mobilize, market, and evaluate programs. You will also find information about developing programs in rural settings and on the Internet.

Although strategies for practice are presented in other sections, Part III specifically focuses on strategies for wellness, providing more specific approaches for nutrition, fitness and flexible movement, the environment, stress management, smoking cessation, holistic and complementary practices, and violence prevention.

Part IV provides advanced interaction skills with individuals, groups, and families. Part V focuses on health promotion in cultural contexts and Part VI provides lessons learned from sample health promotion programs: youth service, schools, small community-based initiatives, and a homeless center.

The goal of this book will be met if you develop a sense of what to do and how to do it when working as a community practitioner. Best wishes in your work with clients.

Carolyn Chambers Clark
Carolyn Chambers Clark
Englewood, Florida

PART I

Theory and Concepts

CHAPTER 1

A Model for Health and Wellness Promotion in Communities

Carolyn Chambers Clark

HOLISM, WELLNESS, AND COMMUNITY

When you look at the community from a holistic point of view, patterns and processes begin to emerge and combine to form a unified whole. This whole is greater than the sum of its parts, and consciousness of self and others is an important factor in wellness (Dossey, 1997).

From this view, health and disease are seen as a part of the total human experience. Both provide exceptional opportunities for learning and growth (Dossey, 1997). Box 1.1 lists the primary assumptions underlying holistic health promotion.

Wellness is another part of the health promotion model you will be using for practice. Dunn (1961) coined the term "high-level wellness." He described wellness not as an end or static goal but as an ongoing journey of self-creation, leading to ever higher levels of functioning. Key elements of his high-level wellness vision include:

- having direction and purpose in life
- meeting the challenges of the environment

- maximizing potential
- looking beyond the needs of self to the needs of society
- having a joy or zest for living

Using this definition, you can see the difference between a community that is well and one that is not. Members of communities that strive for wellness look beyond themselves and can experience joy or zest for certain aspects of living.

Using a *holistic wellness model* means to avoid focusing on risks and disease. Instead, community strengths and resilience become the focus. Community strengths can be physiological, psychological, social, or spiritual. They include such factors as education, coping skills, support systems, knowledge, communication skills, positive nutrition, coherent belief systems, problem-solving abilities, spirituality, fitness, ability to develop a supportive environment, and self-care skills.

Resilience is the ability to avoid negative outcomes by doing well in the face of adversity. Using a wellness model, you can provide crucial information, energy, and

---

Box 1.1   Holistic Health Promotion Assumptions

- Patterns and causes of illness and wellness can be determined
- The whole community-as-client is the focus of concern
- Human values are important to wellness and illness
- Caring is an important component of healing
- Pain and disease are signals from our inner selves to change our lifestyles
- Noninvasive, self-care strategies (diet, exercise, movement, spiritual actions, environmentally sensitive actions, enhanced communication and support skills, and calming procedures) are combined to move toward wellness
- Individuals, composed of body-mind-spirit and electromagnetic energy, live in dynamic interaction with one another and with the environment, family, groups, and community
- Disease or disability is a process that can be perceived as a life lesson
- Increasing well-being and wellness is the focus of care
- The client is capable of self-assessment, wellness action, and self-evaluation
- The professional forms an alliance with the client to provide assistance in meeting wellness goals
- The mind is part of all illness and the province of all health care practice
- The placebo effect is evidence that the mind is a powerful element in disease and healing
- The client's subjective reports are of primary importance in assessment and evaluation
- Wellness involves wholeness in all things: work, relationships, goals, body-mind-spirit

---

materials to help raise communities to higher levels of wellness while promoting their resilience.

Healing is a term that will come to have great importance in your repertoire if doesn't already. *Healing* in community terms includes a process of balancing and integrating community members by using a deep level of inner knowledge. The word heal comes from the Anglo-Saxon *haelan* meaning to be whole or to become whole. During the healing process, the physical, social, emotional, and spiritual aspects of both individuals and the community are as a whole given equal value and importance (Dossey, 1997).

Dunn (1961) believed that high-level wellness is movement toward self-actualiza-

tion by means of reintegrating oneself with the social environment. This reintegration involves bringing together parts of the whole. Self-reintegration is really a creative process in which individuals develop new capabilities to reorganize the self and the environment so that there is meaning and purpose that transcends stress or suffering (Rosenow, 1997).

In a community model, *wellness* is conceptualized as the process of achieving a greater awareness and deriving satisfaction from activities that move the community toward its goals for fitness, positive nutrition, positive relationships, peace, clear life purpose, consistent belief systems, commitment to self-care, and environmental sensitivity and comfort. From this perspective, you and the community-as-client are dynamic systems that interact to exchange information, matter, and energy.

Chaos can ensue when you or the community is greatly out of balance. A higher, more adaptive level of wellness can follow when wellness and health promotion interventions occur after such an imbalance. This change can lead to a new and often improved balance.

In this model, *environment* refers to a changing field that is continuous and contiguous with communities. Environment can be modified by community and can modify the people within it.

Self-care is defined as those activities and programs that the community performs for itself. In this model, you are involved in community self-care activities at times, but the decisions about goals, actions, and evaluation are the community's.

Self-responsibility is a state of choosing to act in one's own behalf (Gaydos, 1997). Self-awareness comes first, opening the path and enabling a person to alter lifestyle patterns that will lead to wellness.

Figure 1.1 exemplifies practitioner-community interactions from a wellness perspective. In this model, both you and the community move forward in your journey toward wellness.

Communities are believed to evolve toward wellness by learning to do the following:

- manage life experiences
- seek out challenges
- self-assess level of wellness
- identify wellness self-care goals
- relate to others in a flexible, differentiated, assertive manner
- use self-care strategies
- examine and readjust beliefs and practices into an integrated whole
- develop successful coping procedures

During the evolutionary process of moving toward wellness, communities interact with stressors more rationally and more efficiently by perceiving and managing situations differently. Although biological, historical, social, and cultural factors may be established, they can be readjusted. For example, perceptions or traumatic situations can be readjusted, and the immune system (a genetic given) can be strengthened by using self-care strategies. Table 1.1 shows a model of community wellness.

Some assumptions underlying this model are that communities are capable of the following:

- self-assessing their own wellness needs
- setting their own wellness goals
- setting up a process for moving toward wellness
- taking action to meet their wellness goals
- evaluating their progress toward wellness
- displaying characteristics of wellness even when stressed
- activating the self-healing process to enhance wellness
- learning to move to a higher level of wellness
- learning from peers and using clearly structured goals and constructive means to meet those goals.

In this model for practice, *motivation* is intrinsic because the community chooses a goal that has meaning. Compliance becomes irrelevant because the community takes control over decision-making. The process of moving toward wellness assumes top priority over the outcome: wellness.

HEALTH PROMOTION ROLES

As a whole person, you will be in a state of flux between the dimensions of wellness.

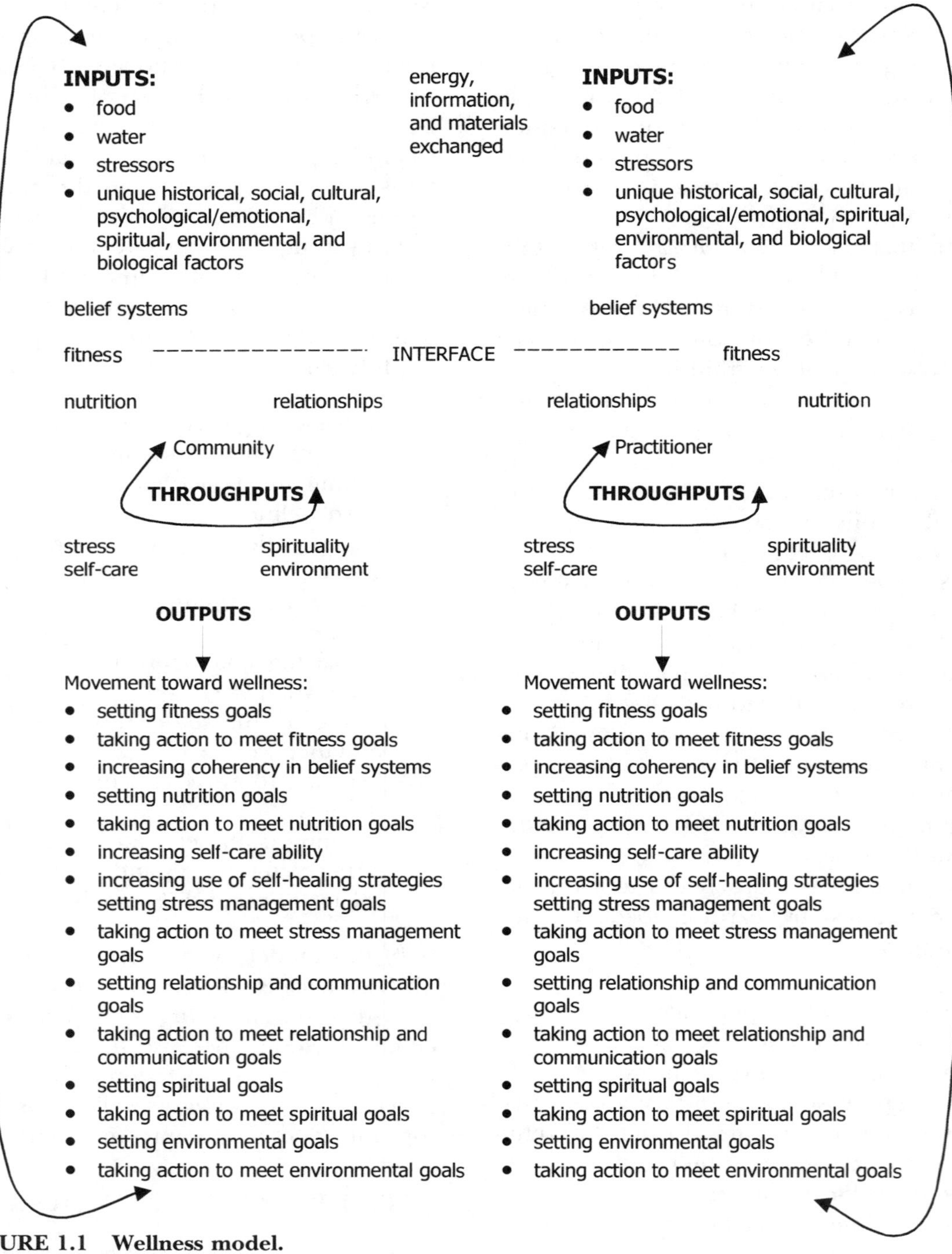

INPUTS:

- food
- water
- stressors
- unique historical, social, cultural, psychological/emotional, spiritual, environmental, and biological factors

energy,
information,
and materials
exchanged

INPUTS:

- food
- water
- stressors
- unique historical, social, cultural, psychological/emotional, spiritual, environmental, and biological factors

belief systems

belief systems

fitness   – – – – – – – – – – – –   INTERFACE   – – – – – – – – – –   fitness

nutrition   relationships   relationships   nutrition

Community   Practitioner

THROUGHPUTS   **THROUGHPUTS**

stress   spirituality   stress   spirituality
self-care   environment   self-care   environment

OUTPUTS   **OUTPUTS**

Movement toward wellness:

- setting fitness goals
- taking action to meet fitness goals
- increasing coherency in belief systems
- setting nutrition goals
- taking action to meet nutrition goals
- increasing self-care ability
- increasing use of self-healing strategies setting stress management goals
- taking action to meet stress management goals
- setting relationship and communication goals
- taking action to meet relationship and communication goals
- setting spiritual goals
- taking action to meet spiritual goals
- setting environmental goals
- taking action to meet environmental goals

Movement toward wellness:

- setting fitness goals
- taking action to meet fitness goals
- increasing coherency in belief systems
- setting nutrition goals
- taking action to meet nutrition goals
- increasing self-care ability
- increasing use of self-healing strategies setting stress management goals
- taking action to meet stress management goals
- setting relationship and communication goals
- taking action to meet relationship and communication goals
- setting spiritual goals
- taking action to meet spiritual goals
- setting environmental goals
- taking action to meet environmental goals

FIGURE 1.1   Wellness model.

Note: Adapted from: Intersystems "Wellness Practitioner Model." Copyright 1996 by Carolyn Chambers Clark.

TABLE 1.1 Community Wellness

Biological, Historical, Social, and Cultural Factors	Community Wellness	Stressors
Childhood experiences Cultural expectations Socioeconomic status and role expectations Genetic factors (immunological strength, charm, beauty, plasticity of body systems)	Increases perceptions of the world and individual experiences as manageable crises Seeks access to materials, resources, and other elements that promote a comfortable environment Uses problem-solving creatively to solve life problems Builds coherent, consistent, integrated, stable, flexible, assertive selves Readjusts beliefs to makes a consistent, whole, rich network of social supports and ties Interrelates energy fields of individual, family and community Maintains open communication with others Gains skill in working and getting along with others Uses energy efficiently in a goal-directed way Shows commitment to patterns of community behavior Increases use of values to guide behavior toward coherence Functions effectively in family and work or learner roles Develops flexible, reasonable, farsighted, and successful coping strategies	Situational/developmental/changes/illness/chance disabilities Interpersonal conflict Internal conflict Daily hassles Community/world change Physical and biochemical interactions Gaps and means to meet goals

Note: From *Wellness Practitioner: Concepts, Research and Strategies* (p. 5), © Carolyn Chambers Clark, 1996, New York: Springer. (Suggested by the works of Ahmed and Coehlo [*Toward a Definition of Health*, 1979, New York, Plenum]; Antonovsky [*Health, Stress and Coping*, 1979, San Francisco, Jossey-Bass]; and Dunn [*High Level Wellness*, 1961, Arlington, VA: Beatty]. Reprinted with permission.

Your role in assisting communities toward wellness includes:

- being an effective role model for wellness
- facilitating consistent community involvement in assessing, implementing, and evaluating wellness and wellness goals
- teaching communities to perceive life experiences as manageable and meaningful

- increasing community responsibility and commitment to self-care
- teaching self-care strategies to enhance fitness, nutritional status, and environment; to manage stress, build positive relationships, and develop coherent belief systems (including spiritual beliefs)
- teaching creative problem solving
- facilitating self-assertion
- teaching communication skills

- facilitating richness of community social supports
- teaching effective learner, family, and work role behaviors to communities

In a health promotion and wellness approach, you are a *facilitator*. Your task is to aid in the removal of obstacles that impede energy flow in the community, resulting in enhanced well-being and self-actualization.

In this model, you are also a *master teacher* who provides self-assessments and shows communities how to assess their wellness, decide on wellness goals, plan self-healing and self-care actions to meet their goals, and evaluate success. You focus on the whole community, helping to determine what is interrupting the smooth flow of energy and action.

You may also play the role of *Creator of Sacred Space* (McKivergin, 1997). In this role, you devise a sacred space in which healing work can occur. You may shape the physical environment or provide a relationship-focused environment to evoke healing. Natural light, plants, fresh air, pleasant sounds or music, comforting smells, and comfortable surroundings are some of the elements of creating sacred space.

Another health and wellness promotion role is that of the *collaborator*. Together you agree on ways to remove obstacles, and you support the community in rechannelling energy flow. As balance is approached, the result is enhanced well-being and self-actualization.

Another part of your wellness function is that of *role model*. Providing information about suggested change is often insufficient. From a very early age, human beings watch the behavior of others and often mimic it. For this reason, being a positive role model is an extremely important role for community health practitioners.

Before becoming a role model for communities, you will be setting goals for your own wellness behavior and taking action to meet these goals. Assessing your own wellness may involve finding a supportive peer to assist you in this role.

Because of the holistic nature of the model used in this book, you will be challenged in your efforts to produce useful findings. Chapter 11 provides issues and methods involved in measuring effectiveness of health and wellness promotion.

HEALTHY PEOPLE INITIATIVE

Healthy People is a national prevention initiative that identifies opportunities for improving the health of Americans. For two decades, the U.S. Department of Health and Human Services (DHHS) has used health promotion objectives for this purpose. Similar initiatives in Canada focus on the role of individual lifestyle rather than on the role of work, income distribution, control over the environment, or the conventional medical establishment.

Healthy People 2000 built upon the lessons of the first Surgeon General's report and is the product of an unprecedented collaboration among government, voluntary and professional organizations, businesses, and individuals. Three broad goals underlie Healthy People 2000: to increase the span of healthy life for Americans; to reduce health disparities among Americans; and to achieve access to preventive services for all Americans.

The context for *Healthy People 2010* differs from *Healthy People 2000* as new relationships are defined between public health departments and health care–delivery organizations. There are four main areas of interest: to promote healthy behaviors; to promote healthy and safe communities; to improve systems for personal and public health; and to prevent and reduce diseases and disorders.

Note that although public opinion input is requested, the objectives are based primarily on a medical model. Table 1.2 shows *Healthy People 2010* objectives.

CHANGING COMMUNITY PRIORITIES

Community disillusionment with medical care has led to the use of complementary practices that are wellness-oriented, holistic, less intrusive, and have fewer side effects (Eisenberg et al., 1993; Clark, 1996). Following consumer interest the U.S. govern-

ment established the Office of Alternative Medicine (OAM)—now called the Center for Alternative and Complementary Medicine—within the National Institutes of Health. Part III discusses complementary interventions in detail.

CULTURAL FACTORS AFFECT HEALTH PROMOTION

Health beliefs and wellness are affected by the forces of culture. Efforts to promote health and wellness must identify cultural factors and consider them when working with communities. Three important actions are: (a) attempt to enter the community's world to enhance your understanding; (b) suspend your personal biases and judge-

TABLE 1.2 Healthy People 2010 Objectives

Promote Healthy Behaviors	Promote Healthy and Safe Communities	Improve Systems for Personal and Public Health	Prevent and Reduce Diseases and Disorders
Physical activity and fitness • Nutrition • Tobacco use	Educational and community-based programs • Environmental health • Food safety • Injury, violence prevention • Occupational safety and health • Oral health	Access to Quality Health Services • Preventive care • Primary care • Emergency services • Long-term care • Family planning • Maternal, infant, and child health • Medical product safety • Public health infrastructure • Health communication	• Arthritis, osteoporosis, and chronic back conditions • Cancer • Diabetes • Disability and secondary conditions • Heart disease and stroke • HIV • Immunization and infectious diseases • Mental health and mental disorders • Respiratory diseases • Sexually transmitted diseases • Substance abuse

Note: Adapted from *Healthy People 2010 Objectives: Draft for Public Comment*, http://web.health.gov/healthypeople/2010/Draft/objectives, 2/17/99.

ments about community beliefs; (c) observe and talk to members of the cultural group until you have sufficient data to verify your impressions. Table 1.3 provides information about the possible meaning of health and wellness to various cultural groups. Bear in mind that even within cultural groups there is diversity.

THE AGING OF AMERICA AFFECTS HEALTH PROMOTION

According to the U.S. Department of Health and Human Services, about 22% of the population will be 65 or older by the year 2030. Up to 80% of these older adults will be healthy, engaging in everyday activities, and only about 5% of older adults will live in nursing homes. Those who live in the community may be quite active, engaging in self-care activities (Clark, 1998).

DISEASE FACTORS AFFECT HEALTH PROMOTION

The major cause of death is chronic illness, including cardiovascular disease and cancer, both of which can be mitigated and in some cases eliminated by changes in lifestyle. As a community health promoter, your biggest task is to find ways to convince your targeted community to take action to modify their lifestyles and environment, and put pressure on their government to reduce the incidence and symptoms of chronic illness. A first step in that direction is to assess progress toward wellness.

WELLNESS SELF-ASSESSMENT

Take a look at Table 1.4. You'll be using this self-assessment later on with targeted communities. Before you do, it is important that you assess your own level of wellness, choose some wellness goals, and take action to meet them. Not only will these actions allow you to better understand what community members will be going through, but they will also enhance your level of wellness and assist you in becoming a more effective role model.

Facilitating movement toward community-chosen goals may require a change in your beliefs. The model also suggests that you, as a whole person, examine your beliefs for consistency, choose wellness goals,

TABLE 1.3   Cultural Beliefs About Health and Wellness

Cultural Group	Beliefs
African American	Mind and body inseparable
Latino	"Hot" illnesses (e.g., tonsillitis) treated with "cold" remedies (e.g., cold tomatoes)
South Asian	Tao: harmony between heaven and earth
	Yin and Yang: opposite ends of a complementary and interacting system
Hmong	Mild illness due to organic causes; serious illness due to supernatural forces
Vietnamese	Magic, ancestors, natural spirits, and natural organic causes as agents of illness
Native American	Health linked to spirituality; focus on behavior and lifestyle
Pacific Islander	Illness as a consequence of breaking rules; little control over destiny

Note: Summarized from "Cross-cultural Concepts of Health and Disease" by R. M. Huff (pp. 23–39). In R. M. Huff and M. V. Kline (Eds.), *Promoting Health in Multicultural Populations*, 1999, Thousand Oaks, CA: Sage.

TABLE 1.4   Wellness Self-Assessment

DIRECTIONS: Read the statements for each dimension of wellness. Circle the number that most appropriately resembles the importance of each statement to you and your well-being, as well as you current interest in changing your lifestyle as follows:

1. I am already doing this. (Congratulate yourself!)
2. This is very important to me and I want to change this behavior now.
3. This is important to me, but I'm not ready to change my behavior right now.
4. This is not important in my life right now.

NUTRITIONAL WELLNESS

I include plenty of local fresh fruits and uncooked vegetables in my eating plan.	1	2	3	4
I limit the use of candy, sweets, and sugars.	1	2	3	4
I eat whole foods rather than processed ones.	1	2	3	4
I read labels and avoid foods that have artificial color, flavor, or added preservatives.	1	2	3	4
I avoid coffee, tea, cola drinks, or other substances that are high in caffeine or other stimulants or depressants.	1	2	3	4
I eat high-fiber foods daily.	1	2	3	4
I have a good appetite, but I eat sensible amounts of food.	1	2	3	4
I avoid crash diets.	1	2	3	4
I eat only when I am hungry and relaxed.	1	2	3	4
I drink 8–10 (or more) glasses of water daily.	1	2	3	4
I avoid foods high in saturated fat such as beef, pork, lamb, soft cheeses, gravies, bakery items, and fried foods.	1	2	3	4
I obtain sufficient minerals from my food or supplement my nutrition so that my muscles do not spasm or ache.	1	2	3	4
I drink distilled water or use a reverse osmosis filtration system to insure that my drinking water is safe.	1	2	3	4
I use muscle testing, food rotation methods, or the pulse test to make sure I don't eat foods I am sensitive to.	1	2	3	4

FITNESS AND WELLNESS

I weigh within 10% of my desired weight.	1	2	3	4
I walk, swim, garden, dance, or engage in some form of exercise I enjoy daily.	1	2	3	4
I digest my food well (no gas, bloating, diarrhea, constipation, irregular bowel movements, etc.).	1	2	3	4
I urinate or have a bowel movement when my body tells me it is time and never hold back from using the toilet.	1	2	3	4
I take steps to maintain healthy organs (liver, intestines, heart, etc.).	1	2	3	4
I wear clothes that do not leave marks on my skin or inhibit my breathing (no push-up or tight bras, tight jeans or pants, girdles, etc.).	1	2	3	4

(continued)

TABLE 1.4   *(continued)*

I breathe easily from my abdomen most of the time.	1	2	3	4
I take regular breaks (at least every hour) from strenuous or repetitive movements.	1	2	3	4
I do flexibility or stretching exercises daily and always prior to and following vigorous exercise.	1	2	3	4
I am satisfied with my sexual activities.	1	2	3	4
I obtain sufficient daily touch (massage, hugs, sex, hand holding, etc.)	1	2	3	4
When I am ill, I am resilient and recover easily.	1	2	3	4
I have a good memory.	1	2	3	4
When I look at myself nude I feel good about what I see.	1	2	3	4
I use imagery daily to picture myself well and healthy.	1	2	3	4
I use affirmations and other self-healing measures when ill, injured, or to enhance my fitness.	1	2	3	4
I avoid smoking and smoke-filled places.	1	2	3	4
My balance is good.	1	2	3	4
I rarely experience pain and when I do I know how to reduce it without taking drugs or alcohol.	1	2	3	4
STRESS AND WELLNESS				
I sleep well.	1	2	3	4
I live relatively free from disabling stress or painful, repetitive thoughts.	1	2	3	4
I laugh at myself occasionally and I have a good sense of humor.	1	2	3	4
I use constructive ways to release my frustration and anger.	1	2	3	4
I feel good about myself and my accomplishments.	1	2	3	4
I assert myself to get what I want instead of feeling resentful toward others for taking advantage of or intimidating me.	1	2	3	4
I can relax my body and mind at will.	1	2	3	4
I feel accepting and calm about people and about people things I have lost through separation.	1	2	3	4
I live with a sense of joy and a zest for life.	1	2	3	4
I have a peaceful expectation about my death.	1	2	3	4
WELLNESS RELATIONSHIPS				
I have at least one other person with whom I can discuss my innermost thoughts and feelings.	1	2	3	4
I can ask people for help when I need it.	1	2	3	4
I keep myself open to new experiences.	1	2	3	4
I listen to others' words and the feelings behind the words.	1	2	3	4
I can give and accept love.	1	2	3	4

TABLE 1.4   *(continued)*

What I believe, feel, and do are consistent.	1	2	3	4
I allow others to be themselves and to take responsibility for their thoughts, feelings, and actions.	1	2	3	4
I allow myself to be me.	1	2	3	4
I live with a sense of purpose.	1	2	3	4
I believe in something or someone.	1	2	3	4
I can forgive myself and others.	1	2	3	4
My life has meaning.	1	2	3	4

WELLNESS AND THE ENVIRONMENT

I have designed a wellness support network of friends, family and peers.	1	2	3	4
I have designed my personal living, playing, and working environments to suit me.	1	2	3	4
I work in a place that provides adequate personal space, comfort, safety, direct sunlight, fresh air; limited air, water, or material pollutants; or I use nutrition, exercise, and stress-reduction measures to minimize negative results.	1	2	3	4
I avoid cosmetics and hair dyes that contain harmful chemicals.	1	2	3	4
I avoid pesticides and the use of harmful household chemicals.	1	2	3	4
I use muscle or pulse testing to make sure I use safe household and lawn products.	1	2	3	4
I avoid x-rays except in cases of serious disease or injury, and I have dental x-rays for diagnostic purposes only every 3 to 5 years.	1	2	3	4
I keep up with the latest research and follow a safe course related to sunscreen use and other environmental protections.	1	2	3	4
I use the earth's resources wisely.	1	2	3	4
I meet the challenges of my environment.	1	2	3	4

COMMITMENT TO WELLNESS

I examine my values and actions to see than I am moving toward wellness.	1	2	3	4
I take responsibility for my thoughts, feelings, and actions.	1	2	3	4
I keep informed of the latest health and wellness developments rather than relying on experts to decide what is best for me.	1	2	3	4
I wear seatbelts when driving and insist that others who ride with me do so also.	1	2	3	4
I ask pertinent questions and seek second opinions whenever someone suggests surgery, medication, or other treatment.	1	2	3	4
I know which chronic illnesses are prominent in my family and I take steps to avoid incurring them.	1	2	3	4

(continued)

TABLE 1.4 *(continued)*

I work toward achieving a balance in all wellness dimensions (nutrition, fitness, stress, relationships, environment, and commitment).	1	2	3	4
I look beyond my needs to the needs of society.	1	2	3	4

facilitate movement toward those goals, and evaluate your success.

When mind, body, and spirit are in harmonious balance, a high level of wellness evolves. The *collaborative process* enables you to assist communities in assuming ownership of the dynamic health-illness interchange.

The scope of health promotion encompasses you and the community no matter what the targeted settings are. This book encourages you to serve as a wellness role model for communities, taking care to cherish your own well-being while celebrating your ability to help others. The quality of the relationship is enhanced by the processes of communication, education, participation, research, and self-responsibility.

REFERENCES

Clark, C. C. (1996). *Wellness Practitioner: Concepts, Research and Strategies.* New York: Springer.

Clark, C. C. (1998). Wellness self-care by healthy older adults. *Image: Journal of Nursing Scholarship, 30*(4), 351–355.

Dossey, B. M. (1997). Holistic nursing practice. In Barbara Montgomery Dossey (Ed.), *The American Holistic Nurses' Association (AHNA) Core Curriculum for Holistic Nursing* (pp. 4–12). Gaithersburg, MD: Aspen.

Dunn, H. (1961). *High Level Wellness.* Arlington, VA: Beatty Press.

Eisenberg, D., Kessler, R., Foster, C., Norlock, F., Culkins, D., & Delbanco, R. (1993). Unconventional medicine in the United States: Prevalence, costs and patterns of use. *New England Journal of Medicine, 328,* 246–252.

Evans, R. G., Barer, M. L., & Marmor, T. R. (1994). The determinants of a population's health. In R. G. Evan, M. L. Barer, & T. R. Marmor (Eds.), *Why Are Some People Healthy and Others Not? The Determinants of Health of Populations* (pp. 219–230). New York: Aldine De Gruyter.

Gaydos, H. L. B. Concepts of Health—Wellness—Disease—Illness. In M. McKivergin (Ed.), *Core Curriculum for Holistic Nursing* (pp. 28–33). Gaithersburg, MD: Aspen.

McKivergin, M. (1997). The nurse as an instrument of healing. In M. McKivergin (Ed.), *Core Curriculum for Holistic Nursing* (pp. 17–25). Gaithersburg, MD: Aspen.

Rosenow, D. J. (1997). Some core components of healing: A theory of self-reintegration: A journey within oneself. In P. B. Kritek (Ed.), *Reflections on Healing: A Central Nursing Construct* (pp. 500–518). New York: NLN Press.

CHAPTER 2

Health Promotion with Changing and Vulnerable Populations

Grace Erickson

Why are some people more vulnerable to illness and injury than others? Is a health promotion and wellness approach relevant to people whose priorities stem from various physical, psychological, social, economic, or environmental needs? And if so, what do you need to know and understand in order to promote health and wellness among changing and vulnerable population groups?

In response to these questions, this chapter will discuss the relationship between vulnerability, resilience, and change. It will identify a variety of causative factors and consequences associated with vulnerability and consider resources that prompt movement from vulnerability to resilience. While there are many vulnerable populations, this chapter will focus on three whose vulnerability has increased and changed due to the impact of a complexity of interacting physical, psychological, social, and environmental factors. These three populations are adolescents, overweight and obese chil-

dren, and homeless families. Causative factors and consequences of vulnerability for each population will be identified and discussed to provide the basis for exploring resources and strategies that can prompt resilience and foster readiness for making behavioral changes necessary to promoting health. The chapter will conclude by explaining why promoting health and wellness is a responsibility of individuals, families, and communities.

VULNERABILITY, RESILIENCE, AND CHANGE

As you start to think about promoting health and wellness among changing and vulnerable populations, it is important to understand what it means to be vulnerable or resilient and why some people are more vulnerable and resilient than others. *Vulnerability* is a condition of being open to something undesirable or harmful (Aday, 1993).

Of course, all human beings are vulnerable to threats to their health and most actually do experience adverse health at one time or another. But some population groups are less likely than others to develop health problems (physical, psychological, environmental, or social) because they have *resilience*. Members of populations groups who have personal and environmental resources (assets, strengths, protective mechanisms) experience fewer adverse health events, are able to cope more effectively with actual and potential threats to their health, and recover faster because they have the capacity to bounce back from adversity when it does occur (Stewart, Reid, & Mangham, 1997).

Conversely, *vulnerable populations* are more sensitive to threats to their health and are more likely to experience poor health with more serious outcomes. As those events combine and accumulate over time, resources diminish and vulnerability becomes multidimensional (Aday, 1993; Nichols, Wright, & Murphy, 1986). For example, many older people live alone on limited resources and suffer from accumulated chronic illnesses. In addition, they may experience multiple, interacting threats to their health such as adverse sensory and cognitive losses (physical) that make them vulnerable to falls (environmental); depression (psychological); and diminished or lost socialization and support systems (social).

If you have ever seen homeless people searching for discarded food in a refuse container or sleeping in a doorway, you have observed members of a more obvious vulnerable population. People who are homeless have much greater sensitivity to physical, psychological, social, and environmental factors and are without the basic resources that most other people take for granted. Therefore they experience com-

plex adverse health events that multiply, recur, and increase their vulnerability.

Pregnant teenagers also comprise a vulnerable population. They are more likely to experience complications of pregnancy and poor birth outcomes due to multiple and cumulative factors of age, immaturity, poor nutrition, knowledge deficits, interrupted education, low socioeconomic status, substance abuse, and inadequate prenatal care. And when pregnant teenagers also lack self-esteem, a support system, and prenatal care, they are quite likely to develop complications of pregnancy, to deliver premature, low birthweight infants, and to have more difficulty adjusting to the challenges of parenthood. Then, as infant- and child-care demands increase and opportunities for teenage activities decrease, behavioral and educational problems arise for both mother and child and the probability of child neglect or abuse escalates (U.S. Preventive Services Task Force, 1996). See Table 2.1 for a comparison of factors that prompt resilience and vulnerability.

Everyone experiences *change*; it is inevitable. As human beings we have a great capacity for change but we also have a tendency to resist it. The process of change is something you need to consider as you begin thinking of ways to help people become less vulnerable and move toward resilience. Understanding change enables you to help people move through the necessary process, to develop the resources that enable them to deter or cope more effectively with adverse outcomes, and to take responsibility for promoting their health.

Lewin (as cited in French, Bell, & Zawacki, 1989) identified *three phases of change:* unfreezing, moving, and refreezing. His theory outlines a sequence for thinking and taking action that influences whether and how change will occur. Picturing ice as it melts and refreezes into another form is

TABLE 2.1   **Factors Associated with Resilience and Vulnerability**

FACTORS	RESILIENCE	VULNERABILITY
Health status	Generally healthy	Frequently unhealthy
Socioeconomic status	High-low to high	Poverty to low-low
	Independent	Dependent
Socialization	Interactive	Noninteractive
Support systems	Strong	Weak
Family life	Functional	Dysfunctional
Developmental tasks	Accomplished	Missed or delayed
Spirituality	Strong belief system	Weak or no belief system
Self-awareness	High	Low
Stress	Low	High
Hope	Hopeful	Hopeless
Power	Empowered	Powerless
Community	Integral	Diffuse

one way to envision the process. Applying this process to a personal desire for change is a realistic ways of understanding the essential features of change.

Unfreezing is the phase in which there is dissatisfaction with the status quo; a desired need for change develops; a better way to recover, protect, and promote health is recognized; and resistance to change is diminished. Unfreezing must be as complete as possible because incomplete unfreezing can compromise the efforts of moving toward change.

Moving is the second phrase. Based on desired outcomes, work begins to modify (adapt, adjust, transform) attitudes, knowledge, skills, and behaviors and move toward the desired change.

Refreezing occurs in response to positive reinforcement as planned modifications are implemented and potential results can be forecast. During this third phrase, evaluation must take place while there is time to make other modifications that will support the desired outcomes. If refreezing occurs too quickly, the modifications may be less than optimal and efforts to maintain change may be abandoned.

Let's take a look at this three-phase theory and see how it applies to weight loss diets. The initial desire for change was probably weakened by inadequate planning or inertia (incomplete unfreezing). Actions to modify dietary or activity behaviors therefore were weak and ineffective because of resistance to moving away from past behaviors. That resulted in premature refreezing and a failure to achieve desired outcomes because the weight reduction plan was rejected.

FACTORS ASSOCIATED WITH VULNERABILITY

As with population groups, the vulnerability of individuals, families, and communities also emanates from their greater sensitivity to an array of factors that combine and accumulate in the absence of resilience and resources to deter or diminish their vulnerability. *Vulnerable individuals* experience adverse health events that stem from a mix of personal characteristics and poor physical, psychological, social, and spiritual health as well as high risk behaviors such as substance abuse and acts of violence (Aday, 1993). *Vulnerable families* are likely to have a low tolerance for stress, a tendency to blame others for problems, nonacceptance of differences of opinion, and negative conflict resolution. In addition, patterns of interaction among family members are fixed and rigid, and dependence and emotional immaturity are encouraged (Heiney, 1993). Complex events and circumstances contribute to the vulnerability of communities when they fail to take responsibility and invest resources to create healthy environments for all their citizens. Factors associated with *vulnerable communities* include inadequate health and human services, inflation, unemployment, overcrowded schools, inadequate housing, growing populations of economically disadvantaged and uninsured persons, inadequate recreational facilities for youth, media portrayals of violence and sex without consequences, and a resurgence of communicable diseases.

RESOURCES NECESSARY FOR MOVING FROM VULNERABILITY TO WELLNESS

Possession of *resources* (assets, strengths, protective mechanisms) that prompt resilience is predictive of the difference between resiliency and vulnerability and between good and poor health. So it is not surprising that resources are often the opposite of the factors associated with vulnerability and that change—for individuals, families, and communities—is essential for growth toward wellness.

Think about the population examples presented earlier in this chapter. Consider how the addition of resources would shift the factors associated with vulnerability to factors that would prompt resilience in

older people, empowering them to move toward wellness. Instead of living alone with limited resources, senior residences and adult day centers could solve the problems associated with living alone on limited resources. These living centers provide aids for safety and stability (environmental) as well as socialization and support systems (social) that can reduce the probability of depression (psychosocial). And health and wellness education would prompt behaviors and processes for reducing unnecessary cognitive loss and for fostering optimal management of chronic diseases and sensory impairments (physical).

Also suppose that resources for pregnant teenagers were available such as prenatal care at a school health clinic or a teen clinic, school classes for pregnant teens, age-appropriate instruction for healthy pregnancy and infant care, and family and peer support systems. The result of combining such resources could result in the development of resilience among teenagers that would empower them to adhere to prenatal care and healthy behaviors. That would go a long way in deterring or eliminating complications of pregnancy, enabling delivery of healthy full-term infants of appropriate birthweight, and promoting positive adaptation to parenthood.

CHANGING AND VULNERABLE POPULATIONS

The three populations discussed next have experienced changes that have increased their vulnerability to adverse health and social consequences: adolescents, overweight and obese children, and homeless families. It is important to understand the factors and consequences associated with their vulnerability in order to comprehend the challenges associated with their transition from vulnerability to resilience and healthier behaviors and lifestyles.

Adolescents

Vulnerability to an array of risks accompanies the physiological and psychosocial changes that occur during the preteen and teenage years. This a time of profound change and mixed emotions and of a tendency to live for today without thought of tomorrow. Everyone can probably recall experiencing changes in body growth and appearance and early sexuality with a mix of excitement and apprehension. New social roles are tinged with doubt and challenges to self-esteem, and the striving for independence from parents alternates with the need to depend on them. And who has not experienced peer pressure or tried to emulate the teen role models of the day? These are not new phenomena. But in recent years, the increasing complexity of biological, personal, environmental, and societal factors have resulted in an alarming rise among adolescents of pregnancy, sexually transmitted diseases (STDs) including HIV and AIDS, substance abuse, violent and abusive behaviors, eating disorders, homelessness, and suicide (Roberson-Beckley & Schubert, 1999).

Causative Factors for Adolescent Vulnerability

Because adolescence involves rapid change and an orientation to the present that prompts high-risk behaviors, it is important to understand the interaction of several factors that contribute to adolescent vulnerability. There is abundant evidence that a shift in value systems has changed the character of interpersonal behaviors and relationships and has increased societal tolerance for substance abuse, sexual intercourse, and premature childbearing out-

side of marriage. This is reflected in media presentations that convey explicit and implicit sexual messages and portray high-risk behaviors without consequence. Another factor is earlier biological maturity as evidenced by a lowering in the average age for menarche from 15 years to 12.5 years. At the same time, technological and social complexity in the United States now requires more educational preparation for responsible work (Foster, 1997). Can you see how all the messages here influence adolescent vulnerability?

Consequences of Adolescent Vulnerability

The high-risk behaviors of adolescents result in life-changing consequences, particularly premature pregnancy and parenthood, inadequate parenting, and infection with one or more sexually transmitted diseases. Although a decline in teen pregnancies has been noted in some states, 1 million American teenage pregnancies still occur every year, more than 80% of which are unintended (Foster, 1997); and one in six pregnant teens becomes pregnant again within a year (Morgan, Chapar, & Fisher, 1995). In another study, Singh and Darroch (1999) found that the proportion of low-income and Black teenagers having sexual intercourse remained stable while there was an increase among higher income and non-Hispanic teenagers and among Hispanic girls under the age of 15. Because adolescent sexual encounters are frequently unplanned and may involve different partners, communication about safe sex rarely takes place and condoms frequently are not used. Therefore, in addition to 1 million pregnancies each year, about 3 million adolescents contract an STD (Whitaker, Miller, May, & Levin, 1999).

Clearly, the changes in adolescent sexual activity and its consequences are an urgent concern. A list of personal and developmental, educational, and social factors that increase adolescent vulnerability for pregnancy and STDs is found on Table 2.2.

As you reflect on this list, look at Box 2.1. See how many factors you can identify that suggest alternative behaviors or interventions that could reduce vulnerability and promote more positive consequences.

Resources and Strategies for Prompting Resilience and Promoting Health in Adolescents

The natural need for sexual expression involves responsible personal and social behaviors based on accurate information and reasoned goals for adolescent health and maturational development that can lead to

self-responsibility and wellness. Moreover, interventions need to be culturally relevant and multifaceted. For example, the Children's Aid Society's program in Harlem focused on career awareness, family and sex education, medical and mental health services, academic assessments and homework help, and self-esteem programs through the performing arts and sports activities. Outcomes were positive. The teen participants had higher educational aspirations, lower alcohol consumption, less sexual activity, increased use of contraceptives within sexual activity, and better outcomes following high school graduation (Cockey, 1997).

Let's see how Lewin's three stages of change (as cited in French, Bell, & Zawacki, 1989) apply to this program. The multifac-

TABLE 2.2   Factors That Increase Vulnerability for Adolescent Pregnancy and STDs

Personal/Developmental	Educational	Social
Early onset of menarche	Poor access to quality education	Low socioeconomic status
Knowledge deficits about sexuality	Poor school performance	Single-parent family
Non-use of contraceptives	School dropout	Inadequate parenting
Lack of knowledge or belief in consequences of adolescent pregnancy and STDs	No academic or career role models	Poor or dysfunctional family
Role modeling of contemporary teen idols	Lack of parental expectations for school performance	Lack of access to contraceptives
Low perception of career or other future options		Sexual and other high-risk behavior messages in the media
Peer pressures		Peer or sibling role models who engage in intercourse or are perceived as doing so
Need to conform and be popular among peers		Inconsistent or no rules or supervision of dating or other activities

---

Box 2.1   Try This: Reflect on Factors to Lower Vulnerability

Review the list of factors that increase vulnerability for adolescent pregnancy and STDs displayed in Table 2.2. Which ones suggest alternative factors that could decrease vulnerability to adolescent pregnancy? How could these positive correlates of negative behaviors be developed?

(This box developed by Grace Erickson.)

eted approach apparently facilitated the unfreezing of adolescent vulnerability for actual or potential negative behaviors and assisted the participants in moving toward positive change through collaboration between adolescents and parents and the development of adolescent strengths. Based on reported outcomes, refreezing included new knowledge and skills, capacity for resilience, intrinsic motivation for higher achievements, protective mechanisms for health and wellness (contraceptive use and decreased alcohol consumption), and the potential for greater self-responsibility and beginning self-actualization.

Parents Too Soon, a teen prevention program in Illinois, focused on helping adolescents make healthy choices. Using a multifaceted approach, this program incorporated family and peer support, adult mentors, role modeling, and special education. Improvements in teen confidence and self-control, which are components of resilience, and other more healthy behaviors were reported as well (Randolph and Bogdanovich [as cited in Stewart, Reid, & Mangham, 1997]).

Another multifaceted approach for promoting health has been successful in Kansas (Paine-Andrews et al., 1999). This was accomplished through a 4-year comprehensive school and community program in three localities.

This exploration of factors associated with adolescent vulnerability and resilience and the outcomes of these three programs show that multifaceted interventions to promote healthy adolescent sexuality include much more than advocating a "just say no" policy and dispensing condoms. Decreases in adolescent risks for pregnancy and STDs require a holistic approach to adolescent health and self-efficacy with interventions geared to each community population. See Box 2.2 for a list of strategies that promote adolescent health and wellness.

Overweight and Obese Children

During the past two decades, the number of overweight children in the United States has increased by 50% (U.S. Department of Health and Human Services [DHHS], 1997). A dramatic increase in excess body mass in relation to the height of children and adolescents has been well documented (Bouchard, 1997), and a large study of school-age children and adolescents found that those who were overweight already had one or two cardiovascular risk factors (Freedman, Dietz, Srinivasan, & Berenson, 1999). Moreover, many studies suggest an association between child and adolescent overweight and obesity and adult obesity and chronic health problems (Koplan & Dietz, 1997; Must et al., 1999; Mokdad, Serdula, Dietz, Marks, & Koplan, 1999).

Psychological problems also arise from the social pressures overweight and obese children and adolescents experience when peers and even parents tease or ridicule them and call them fat, ugly, lazy, or clumsy. Being overweight and obese is much more than cosmetic or something to be outgrown. Overweight and obese children and adolescents are vulnerable to deviations in health that compromise normal childhood and adolescent activities and precipitate health problems that continue throughout their adult lives.

Causative Factors Associated With Overweight and Obesity in Children

Obesity tends to run in families and many children become overweight during their preschool years (Christoffel & Ariza, 1998). Although genetic factors do influence body mass in some people, most researchers agree that the major determinant of overweight and obesity is high energy intake with low energy expenditure (Bouchard, 1997; Christoffel & Ariza, 1998; DHHS,

---

Box 2.2   Resources and Strategies to Promote Adolescent Health and Wellness

- Develop healthy self-esteem
- Encourage and enable participation in arts, sciences, sports, and other youth development activities
- Urge postponement of sexual activity, staying in school, and preparing for responsible work
- Present future options and enable preparation for access to them
- Strengthen families
- Parent-adolescent discussions and listening to adolescent interests and concerns, including sexuality
- Parents establish clear rules and boundaries
- Parental role-modeling of responsibility and appropriate behaviors
- Provide clear, accurate information on sexuality, pregnancy, and STDs
- Establish school health services, including clinics, for health education, physical examinations, and promotion of pregnancy and STD prevention
- Recognize that many adolescents will become sexually active and urging condom use for pregnancy and STD prevention

---

1997; Koplan & Dietz, 1999). Can you see the link between physiology and behavior? It is the combination of high-fat and high-calorie dietary patterns and minimal physical activity—which often begins in early childhood and is influenced by parental modeling and later by factors in the community—that leads to overweight and obesity.

The home is where children's eating patterns are established. Parents make the first decisions about what food is purchased and consumed, and children soon copy the eating habits of family members. Economics also play a part. For example, The Federal Interagency Forum on Child and Family Statistics (1999) reported that in poor families 19% of children ages 2 to 5 have a diet that is rated good compared to 28% of children in nonpoor families. The Forum also indicated that most American children ages 2 to 12 have a diet that is poor or in need of improvement. Community influences also affect children's food con-

sumption and eating patterns. These influences include the content of school lunch menus, choices available in vending machines (e.g., soda instead of milk), and media advertising which tends to promote taste, appearance, and packaging rather than nutritional value. Below is a list of factors that influence childhood overweight and obesity.

Home: Parent and Family

- Parental knowledge deficits regarding healthy nutrition
- Parental overfeeding of infants
- Family members who are overweight or obese

Community

- Media advertisements that target children and promote foods high in fat and cholesterol and low in complex carbohydrates and fiber

- Frequent fast-food meals
- High-calorie beverages including whole milk
- Junk food
- Lack of regular mealtimes
- Children preparing own meals due to parent work schedules
- Frequent sedentary activity (TV, video games)
- Being driven, rather than walking, short distances

- School lunches, as above
- Vending machine choices, as above
- Curtailment of school physical education and sports programs
- Lack of community recreation and exercise facilities for children

tween 1973 and 1994. Data were collected to identify adverse levels of low density lipoprotein, triglycerides, insulin, and diastolic and systolic blood pressure. Of 813 overweight children and adolescents, 58% had at least one adverse level and 50% had two or more. Even 7- and 8-year-olds had several factors predictive of cardiovascular disease. The researchers concluded that successful prevention and treatment of obesity in childhood could reduce the frequency of cardiovascular disease in adults, and they suggested that overweight be used as an initial screening tool.

Overweight and obese children and adolescents also experience social pressures that lead to a negative body image, low self-esteem, and stigmatization from name-calling and derogatory comments directed at them. Feeling unaccepted and embarrassed about their weight, they avoid participating in sports and beach or pool activities. Instead they tend to stay home, watch television, and consume snacks, which results in further weight gain and unhealthy eating patterns. And as children enter adolescence, the accumulation of negative experiences may result in a series of fad diets or in eating disorders such as anorexia nervosa and bulimia (American Obesity Association, 1999; Lechky & Rafuse, 1994).

Consequences Associated With Overweight and Obesity in Children

Overweight and obese children are subject to current and future adverse health consequences. Overweight children and adolescents experience moderate to severe asthma more often than their peers of normal weight and may develop orthopedic complications such as bowing and overgrowth of leg bones (American Obesity Association, 1999). Moreover, childhood overweight and obesity can lead to obesity in adulthood and associated chronic health problems (Must et al., 1999; Mokdad et al., 1999).

To study the correlation between childhood overweight and obesity and cardiovascular disease, Freedman et al. (1999) examined seven studies that were conducted among 9,167 children and adolescents ages 5 to 17, who where enrolled in the Bogalusa Heart Study in Louisiana be-

Resources and Strategies for Moving Children Away From Overweight and Obesity and Toward Health and Wellness

Strategies to unfreeze unhealthy patterns in children and encourage movement toward health-promoting patterns require interventions directed to children, parents, and community programs and services. It is essential to teach parents how to implement weight reduction and control strategies for their overweight or obese children. But they must also understand healthy nutrition and the serious consequences their children may experience due to poor eating habits and physical inactivity. This is often a challenge since the parents may be overweight or obese also.

The same information is essential for the community decision-makers who are responsible for food services and media presentations directed to children. Can you guess what the challenge is here? You were right if you chose cost—the bottom line—since budgets and profit margins rather than nutritional guidelines too often drive such decisions. Box 2.3 lists several actions for achieving a balance between energy intake and energy expenditure.

Take a minute now to reflect on the causative factors and consequences of childhood overweight and obesity and the resources and strategies for balancing energy intake and energy expenditure. Do you see how patterns of good nutrition and physical activity become essential protective mechanisms for moving to health and wellness? The challenge then is to help parents and children comprehend the consequences of overweight and obesity in a way that will empower them to turn away from the seductive and pervasive contemporary influences that result in unhealthy eating and physical inactivity: that is, to assist them in unfreezing negative patterns, moving toward resilience and behavioral change, and establishing (refreezing) healthful eating and activity patterns. Box 2.4 provides suggestions on how to help parents promote healthier eating habits and regular physical activities for their children.

After studying the strategies suggested, read the case study in Box 2.5 and choose the strategies that you would use to help Joey's parents.

Homeless Families

The face of homelessness in the U.S. has changed. Over the past 10 to 15 years, the number of families with children has

---

Box 2.3 Resources and Strategies to Balance Energy Intake and Energy Expenditure

Home: Parent and Family

- Parental education during prenatal visits and childbirth classes
  - during child health clinic and medical office visits
  - during parent-teacher meetings
  - by school nurse
- Restrict time for TV, video games
- Parent role-modeling of healthy eating and exercise
- Family sharing in sports, walking, or other exercise
- Parental support of children's participation in physical activities

Communities

- Seek media presentations on healthy nutrition, e.g., milk mustache commercials
- In-school nutrition at each grade level
- Promote healthy snacks in vending machines
- Upgrade school lunch menus
- Restore regular physical education and sports programs
- Support development and maintenance of children's recreational facilities

---

Box 2.4   Teaching Parents How to Help Their Overweight and Obese Children

Supporting Your Child

- Let your child know you accept him/her "as is"
- Be sensitive to his/her needs
- Don't institute a restrictive diet unless medically ordered
- Don't set the child apart
- Be a role model for your child
- Limit time for TV, video games
- Guide your child into an age- and ability sport or other physical activity

(DHHS, 1997)

Focus on the Family

- Healthier eating patterns will help all family members
- Learn about healthier foods and snacks for balanced nutrition
- Gradually introduce new foods to promote healthier family eating patterns
- Develop family exercise habits
- Initiate family walks for exercise and relationship-building

---

Box 2.5   Case Study: Teaching Parents of an Overweight Child

Joey is a 5-year-old boy whose body mass index in 40% higher than that recommended for his age and gender. (According to Leading Health Indicators for *Healthy People 2010* [Chrvala & Bulger, 1999], body mass index should be no greater than 20% higher.) Joey's mother and father are also overweight. By reviewing the family's eating patterns, you have learned that, because both parents work, Joey's breakfast is usually sweetened cereal and whole milk, lunch is at day care (nutritional content not yet identified), and fast foods are often the dinner meal. What would you need to consider in providing nutritional counseling to help these parents recognize the need to make dietary changes to promote weight loss and improved nutrition for their son (and for themselves)?

---

grown, and they now comprise 40% of that population (Bassuk et al., 1997; Committee on Community Health Services, 1996). Older men on "skid row" are no longer the only people who are homeless. A survey by the U.S. Conference of Mayors (as cited in National Coalition for the Homeless, 1999) confirmed the growth of the number of homeless families with children and found that in 30 cities children accounted for 25% of the homeless population. In addition, Vissing (1996) found increasing numbers of homeless families, single mothers, and children in rural areas. In order to care for homeless families, it is important to gain knowledge and understanding of their unique health problems and the social and environmental factors that influence their daily lives.

Causative Factors for Vulnerability in Homeless Families

The root causes of homelessness are multiple and diverse: lack of affordable housing, unemployment, scarcity of education and job training to meet the demands of employment in contemporary society; lack of reasonable income, unsafe communities, unstable environments in which to raise children; insufficient accessible and affordable preventive, curative, and restorative health care services. Cutbacks in public welfare and the continuing effects of deinstitutionalization also contribute to homelessness. And intertwined with all these causes are personal and parental characteristics and crises that are both cause and consequence. Psychological disorders and physical health problems, single parenthood, lack of supportive social networks, limited job skills, variable educational levels, and alcohol and substance abuse are among the characteristics of homeless parents. Divorce and domestic violence often tip a delicate balance and the result is family homelessness (Bassuk et al., 1997; Committee on Community Health Services, 1996; Davidhizar & Frank, 1992; National Coalition for the Homeless, 1999; Sebastian, 1985; U.S. Conference of Mayors [as cited in National Coalition for the Homeless, 1999]).

Consequences of Family Homelessness

Homelessness is a disruptive and devastating experience for families. It affects the physical and psychological health of all family members. According to Murata, Mace, Strehlow, and Shuler (1992), homelessness is an extreme case of poverty and, because most poor families are headed by women, poverty has become feminized. That may explain why information on homeless parents is centered around mothers.

The average homeless mother is single with two children, has gynecological problems, and may have an STD. Prior to becoming homeless, many of these women have experienced physical and sexual abuse and depressive disorders, resulting in social instability and low self-esteem. When homeless, they struggle to provide the basic necessities for their children under extremely difficult conditions and other stressors including fatigue and sleep deprivation. Overwhelmed and distracted, homeless mothers often become unable to provide for the physical and emotional needs of their children (National Coalition for the Homeless, 1999; Coll, Buckner, Brooks, Weinreb, & Bassuk, 1998; Herth, 1996; Davidhizar & Frank, 1992).

As a consequence, the effects of homelessness on children are all-encompassing and interfere with their normal growth and development. An array of physical and psychological stressors result from living in unhygienic conditions and experiencing constant change and mobility. Lacking traditional toys, homeless children often sustain injuries from unsupervised play in busy streets, abandoned buildings, and refuse-ridden areas. Hunger and erratic eating patterns are common, and excessive consumption of carbohydrates and fats results in undernutrition, growth delays, and obesity. Health care is erratic, is obtained from multiple providers in several places, and is sought primarily for acute problems. Consequently, immunizations are not up-to-date, preventive care is rare, and continuity of care, which would benefit homeless families the most, is practically nonexistent (Committee on Community Health Services, 1996; Davidhizar & Frank, 1992; Murata et al., 1992). A list of common acute, chronic, and communicable disease among homeless children is displayed in Table 2.3.

A variety of psychosocial and mental health problems also affect homeless children. Problems range from sleep disturbances and unhealthy eating patterns to overactivity, aggression, and emotional problems such as depression, anxiety, and self-harm (Vostanis, Gratten, & Cumella,

TABLE 2.3   Acute, Chronic, and Communicable Disease Associated with Childhood Homelessness

Acute	Chronic	Communicable
infections of ear, eye, skin, upper respiratory, and urinary tract	sinusitis	pediculosis
diaper rash	enuresis	scabies
lacerations	bowel dysfunction	impetigo
trauma-related injuries	neurological deficits	influenza
failure to thrive	anemia	pharyngitis
	asthma	tuberculosis
	dental disease & decay	
	visual disturbances	
	inadequate nutrition	
	obesity	
	developmental delays	
	behavioral problems	

1998; Davidhizar & Frank, 1992). Developmental problems have been found to be 2 to 3 times more frequent in homeless children than in other poor children who are not homeless (Bassuk et al., 1997). Coll et al. (1998) studied developmental patterns of homeless and low-income housed infants and toddlers and found little difference in cognitive and motor skills up to 18 months of age. Older children, however, scored lower on most measures of developmental status. This suggested that the cumulative effects of impoverished environments may increase with time. Similarly, Vostanis et al. (1998) found that even after re-housing, children remained vulnerable to mental disorders, developmental delays, and loss of peer relationships due to the psychosocial problems and instability of their families.

Homeless children of school age face problems with both school entry and grade progression. Residency requirements, the inability to obtain previous school records, transportation problems, and lack of clothing and school supplies often result in delayed enrollment. But homeless children also have sporadic attendance which, along with developmental delays, often results in below-average school performance and grade repetition (National Coalition for the Homeless, 1999; Davidhizar & Frank, 1992).

Resources and Strategies for Promoting Health Among Homeless Families

Despite their vulnerability and the daily need to determine how and where to obtain the basic necessities for life, homeless people are not without hope. Herth (1996) explored the meaning of hope among homeless families. Findings included the delineation of six categories of hope-engendering strategies with definitions based on behaviors and verbal responses that were gleaned from interviews with adult family members. These strategies provide useful guides to working with homeless families. Moreover, the pragmatic definitions give evidence of resilience and offer insight into the assets, strengths, and protective mechanisms of homeless families. These categories, with brief, pragmatic defining phrases, are presented at Box 2.6.

After reading Box 2.6, can you see how an understanding of the perspectives of homeless families can provide a foundation

---

Box 2.6   Categories of Hope-Engendering Strategies
with Brief Pragmatic Definitions

Strategy	*Definition*
Connectedness with others	Meaningful relationships with others; trust, respect, "being there"
Personal attributes	Attributes that facilitate hope: perseverance, endurance, being tough, not giving up
Cognitive strategies	Purposeful use of thought processes to manage negative thoughts and use positive self-talk; envisioning hopeful events and images
Attainable stepwise goals	Having possible goals within sight, being able to reset or redefine goals in ever-changing situations
Energizing moments	Special times within daily life when everything else is forgotten in the enjoyment of a celebration or favorite activity
Affirmation of worth	Being accepted, acknowledged, valued, understood; being treated as a worthwhile person in spite of difficult circumstances

(Adapted from Herth, 1996)

---

for establishing therapeutic relationships with them? For example, "being there" enables you to communicate respect and genuine interest in them as valuable people. And the use of active listening strategies—"I can see you are very worried about your child and his injury"—can encourage families to verbalize their very real needs and concerns. These strategies help to establish connectedness and will enable you to understand their perspectives and discover their personal attributes (e.g., courage, perseverance, resilience) and goals. Then you have the opportunity, and obligation, to guide and support them in accessing the health, socioeconomic, educational, and other resources they need to cope with their situations and move toward improved health (Herth, 1996; Davidhizar & Frank, 1992).

The following health care resources are representative of some of the services for homeless families that are available in many American cities. New York City's Children's Health Project brings pediatric primary care to family shelters and welfare hotels. In addition to immunizations and care of chronic conditions such as asthma and anemia, the unit provides regular physical examinations, screening tests, and developmental assessments that frequently uncover conditions that would otherwise remain undetected and untreated (Redlener, 1994). In Los Angeles, the Union Rescue Mission, which is managed by nurses, provides primary care services to severely impoverished homeless children and families. Besides caring for an array of acute, chronic, and communicable diseases similar to those listed on Table 2.3, preventive and health-promoting interventions include contraception, prenatal and postpartum care, tuberculosis screening, and the teaching of nutrition as well as well child care and immunizations (Murata et al., 1992).

INDIVIDUAL, FAMILY, AND COMMUNITY RESPONSIBILITY FOR PROMOTING HEALTH AND WELLNESS

The potential for health and wellness is within everyone, even though it may be hidden by the causes and consequences of vulnerability. But as discussions of these three changing and vulnerable populations indicate, vulnerability does not exist in a vacuum. Some people are more vulnerable to deviations from health and wellness than others due to complex negative factors that interact to influence behaviors, lifestyles, and living conditions. Yet with the exception of genetic endowments, which are unique to each individual and are not subject to modification, other factors arise from family and community influences that can be modified. When the need for change is understood and responsibility is shared, wellness strategies can be implemented. A shift from vulnerability to resilience and a movement toward health-promoting behaviors and living conditions to support healthy lifestyles can then become a reality.

The importance of shared individual, family, and community responsibility is evident in relation to promoting health and wellness among adolescents and overweight and obese children. Recall the multifaceted components implemented by the three pregnancy prevention programs for adolescents that were discussed earlier. Reductions in adolescent vulnerability were prompted by challenging individual teenagers to take responsibility for unfreezing negative behaviors. Several strategies were used to provide assistance and support as adolescents moved toward more health-promoting behaviors. Peers provided mentoring and families took responsibility by supporting their adolescent's participation in the programs. Connections were established with health, religious, business, and media resources in the communities, and their participation was instrumental in providing adult mentors, career awareness, homework help, family and sex education, medical and mental health services, and sports and performing arts programs to build self-esteem. This was shared responsibility in action. A strong collaborative and caring message was provided that led to empowering adolescents to modify their behaviors and gain new knowledge and skills that could open pathways to self-actualization they had probably never considered before.

The vulnerability of overweight and obese children demonstrates how essential shared family and community responsibility is in promoting healthy behaviors in youngsters, behaviors that will continue into their adult years. Family lifestyles related to social and economic pressures are implicated as causative factors. Read the resources and strategies in Box 2.3. Where and how can health-promoting educational programs be provided to help parents, children, and adolescents unfreeze some of the factors associated with overweight and obesity? Parental education and age-appropriate instruction to children and adolescents about eating patterns are essential strategies for fostering individual and shared responsibility for healthier behavior and lifestyles.

There are local, regional, and national aspects to community responsibility. Individuals and families can challenge local community leaders to mandate healthy foods for school lunches and to fund community recreation programs for citizens of all ages. Community groups can work together to influence food advertisements in local and regional sites and TV programming and band together with other community groups to challenge the messages in national advertising. But the strongest and most effective health-promoting strategies will be those that change individual and family food choices and purchases.

Homelessness is a prime example of what happens even when there is shared responsibility. More than 20 years ago, the Stewart B. McKinney Homeless Assistance Act (Public Law 100-77) legislated much-needed funding as an initial step to providing programs and resources for health care, housing, emergency food and shelter, job training, and education for children and youth. Community providers and organizations responded by developing the health and social services that are now in place. The marked increase in homeless families is evidence that the problem has not gone away but has actually increased and changed in character. Existing primary care and social services, no matter how appropriate, supportive, and exemplary, are insufficient to respond to all the physical, psychological, social, economic, and environmental needs of the current population of homeless families. And, as the causes and consequences indicate, individual and family behaviors are not the major reasons for homelessness. The root causes of homelessness remain: That is where community and societal responsibility comes in. People who understand the needs and problems of homeless families have a responsibility to advocate for social and political action that will continue and expand the work initiated by the McKinney Act. Everyone can be helped to understand that to reduce homelessness and promote health for homeless families, the fundamental re-

quirements for healthy living (which are the opposite of the root causes) must be recognized and addressed. Only then can families build on the resilience they have gained by coping with the demands of homelessness and become empowered to move toward health and wellness.

While there is much to learn about promoting health and wellness in vulnerable and changing populations, you will be off to a good start if you remember that relationship-building is the first step. Learning the concerns of people creates opportunities to help, and understanding the three phases of change enables you to recognize why behavioral change is often slow. Always remember that shared responsibility is essential for effective interventions. It requires you to be resilient and to promote resilience in vulnerable populations.

REFERENCES

Aday, L. A. (1993). *At risk in America: The health and health care needs of vulnerable populations in the United States.* San Francisco: Jossey-Bass.

American Obesity Association. (1999). *Facts about obesity in youth: 9/99 conference outcomes.* [Online]. Available: http://www.obesity.org

Bassuk, E. L., Buckner, J. C., Weinreb, L. F., Browne, A., Bassuk, S. S., Dawson, R., & Perloff, J. N. (1997). Homelessness in female-headed families: Childhood and adult risk factors and protective factors. *American Journal of Public Health, 87*(2), 241–248.

Bouchard, C. (1997). Obesity in adulthood—the importance of childhood and parental obesity. *New England Journal of Medicine, 337*(13), 926–927.

Christoffel, K. K., & Ariza, A. (1998). The epidemiology of overweight in children: Relevance for clinical care. *Pediatrics, 101*(1), 103–105.

Chrvala, C. A., & Bylger, R. J. (Eds.). (1999). *Leading health indicators for Healthy People*

2010. Washington, DC: National Academy Press.

Cockey, C. D. (1997). Preventing teen pregnancy: It's time to stop kidding around. *AWHONN Lifelines, 1*(3), 32–40.

Coll, C. G., Buckner, J. C., Brooks, M. G., Weinreb, L. F., & Bassuk, E. L. (1998). The developmental status and adaptive behavior of homeless and low-income housed infants and toddlers. *American Journal of Public Health, 88*(9), 1371–1374.

Committee on Community Health Services. (1996). Health needs of homeless children and families. *Pediatrics, 98*(4), 789–791.

Davidhizar, R., & Frank, B. (1992). Understanding the physical and psychological stressors of the child who is homeless. *Pediatric Nursing, 18*(6), 559–562.

Federal Interagency Forum on Child and Family Statistics. (1999). *Healthy eating index shows most children and adolescents have a diet that is poor or needs improvement.* [On-line]. Available: http://childstats.gov/ac1999/heirel.asp

Foster, H. W. (1997). The national campaign to prevent teen pregnancy. *Journal of Pediatric Nursing, 12*(2), 120–121.

Freedman, D. S., Dietz, W. H., Srinivasan, S. R., & Berenson, G. S. (1999). The relationship of overweight to cardiovascular risk factors among children and adolescents: The Bogalusa Heart Study. *Pediatrics, 103*(6), 1175–1182.

French, W. L., Bell, C. H., & Zawacki, R. A. (Eds.). *Organizational development: Theory, practice, and research.* Homewood, IL: BPI Irwin.

Heiney, S. P. (1993). Assessing and intervening with dysfunctional families. In G. D. Wagner & R. J. Alexander (Eds.), *Readings in family nursing.* Philadelphia: Lippincott.

Herth, K. (1996). Hope from the perspective of homeless families. *Journal of Advanced Nursing, 24*(4), 743–753.

Koplan, J. P., & Dietz, W. H. (1999). Caloric balance and public health policy. *Journal of the American Medical Association, 282*(16), 1579–1581.

Lechky, O., & Rafuse, J. (1994). Epidemic of childhood obesity may cause major public health problems, doctor warns. *Canadian Medical Association Journal, 150*(1), 78–81.

Mokdad, A. H., Serdula, M. K., Dietz, W. H., Marks, H. S., & Koplan, J. P. (1999). The spread of the obesity epidemic. *Journal of the American Medical Association, 282*(16), 1519–1522.

Morgan, C., Chapar, N. B., & Fisher, M. (1995). Psychosocial variables associated with teen pregnancy. *Adolescence, 30*(118), 277.

Murata, J., Mace, J. P., Strehlow, A., & Shuler, P. (1992). Disease patterns in homeless children: A comparison with national data. *Journal of Pediatric Nursing, 7*(3), 196–203.

Must, A., Spadano, J., Coakley, E. H., Field, A. E., Colditz, G., & Dietz, W. H. (1999). The disease burden associated with overweight and obesity. *Journal of the American Medical Association, 282*(16), 1523–1529.

National Coalition for the Homeless. (1999). *Homeless families with children.* Fact Sheet #7. [on-line]. Available: http://nch.ari.net/families.html

Nichols, J., Wright, L. K., & Murphy, J. F. (1986). A proposal for tracking health care for the homeless. *Journal of Community Health, 11*(3), 204–209.

Paine-Andrews, A., Harris, K. J., Fisher, J. L., Lewis, R. K., Williams, E. L., Fawcett, S. B., & Vincent, M. L. (1999). Effects of a replication of a multicomponent model for preventing adolescent pregnancy in three Kansas communities. *Family Planning Perspectives, 31*(4), 182–189.

Redlener, I. (1994). Health care for the homeless: Lessons from the front line. *New England Journal Of Medicine, 331*(5), 327–328.

Robertson-Beckley, R., & Schubert, P. E. (1999). Care of infants, children, and adolescents. In J. E. Hitchcock, P. E. Schubert, & S. A. Thomas (Eds.), *Community health nursing: Caring in action* (pp. 372–377). Albany, NY: Delmar.

Sebastian, J. B. (1985). Homelessness: A state of vulnerability. *Family and Community Health, 8*(3), 11–24.

Singh, S., & Daroch, J. E. (1999). Trends in sexual activity among adolescent women: 1982–1995. *Family Planning Perspectives, 31*(5), 212–219.

Stewart, M., Reid, G., & Mangham, C. (1997). Fostering children's resilience. *Journal of Pediatric Nursing, 12*(1), 21–29.

U.S. Department of Health and Human Services. (1997). *Helping your overweight child* (#NIH 97-4096, Public Health Service). Rockville, MD: Author.

U.S. Preventive Services Task Force. (1996). *Guide to clinical preventive services (2nd ed.).* Baltimore: Williams & Wilkins.

Vissing, Y. (1996). *Out of sight, out of mind: Homeless children and families in small town America.* Lexington: University Press of Kentucky.

Vostanis, P., Grattan, E., & Cumella, S. (1998). Mental health problems of homeless children and families: Longitudinal study. *British Medical Journal, 316*(7135), 899–902.

Whitaker, D. J., Miller, K. S., May, D. C., & Levin, M. L. (1999). Teenage partners' communication about sexual risk and condom use: The importance of parent-teenage discussions. *Family Planning Perspectives, 31*(3), 117–121.

PART II

Developing Programs in the Community

CHAPTER 3

Community Self-Assessment

Carolyn Chambers Clark

In developing programs in the community, the first step is to assess the needs and characteristics of a community. This book holds firm to the idea that communities must be involved in their own assessment. Thus, this chapter describes the assessment process from this perspective. This self-assessment process can help community members grow while obtaining valuable information about wellness program needs. Once an assessment has been done, program planning and implementation can begin in earnest, and these tasks are described in the chapters following this one.

USING A COMMUNITY DEVELOPMENT APPROACH

A *community development approach* to assessment views health and wellness within the broader context of social and economic improvement, and it views resident empowerment as a vital element in achieving health and wellness. When using a community development approach, set your sights on the current social and education levels, and help the community assess their control of health care services, including self-care measures (Bracht, 1999).

If you are working with a large community, you may wish to collaborate with academic and health department partners, drawing upon their expertise and using census data and vital statistics to define priority areas. It may be wise also to collaborate with *key informants*, those individuals who are knowledgeable about the community and respected within it. These key people can help you identify other individuals or groups with a history of effective community-level collaboration. The larger the community, the more individuals you may need to bring on board as key informants. Within a small community, you may be the sole working practitioner.

Among the many questions you may have when seeking to enhance health and wellness in a community are: (a) Whom do I work with to collect needed information? (b) How can I work most effectively with the identified community representatives? (c) How can I understand the processes that affect health and wellness in this community?

DEFINING A COMMUNITY

Your defined community may entail any of the following or a combination thereof:

- a geographical area
- a group that shares a common history, interest, identity or values, and norms
- a group with mutual influences among members
- a group that shares common symbols

A community may define itself and come to you for assistance in gathering information. Perhaps you are the person in an organization or school who is assigned to work with a community. In this case, you may be the one to define who is part of that community.

USING A COMMUNITY-BASED PARTICIPATORY RESEARCH PROCESS

Community-based participatory action research is a useful tool no matter how your community is defined. In this model, community participants who represent a variety of perspectives and experiences contribute and learn from each other. The building process is connected to planned change. This change occurs after community members collaborate to define and critically analyze community concerns and then plan, implement, and evaluate their concern-based actions.

Such a model focuses on community strengths and issues, engaging residents in the data collection process. Participants' insights will enhance and enrich your understanding, so be sure to seek out key community people in your collaborations. It will also strengthen the data collection and planned-change skills of community

members who participate (Schulz et al., 1998).

If you are working with a large community, you may wish to collaborate with academic and/or health department partners, drawing upon their expertise and using census data and vital statistics to define priority areas. See Box 3.1, Guidelines for Establishing Community Partnerships.

It may be wise also to collaborate with *key informants*, those individuals who are knowledgeable about the community and respected within it. These key people can help you identify other individuals or groups with a history of effective community-level collaboration. The larger the community, the more individuals you may need to bring on board. Examples of key informants are town government officials, school personnel, student leaders, community service leaders, health care workers, business and church leaders, and local artisans (Smith & Barton, 1992). You might also want to work with *primary informants* or randomly identified individuals who represent all population segments in the community. Examples of primary informants include students, shop owners, store clerks, and residents from every age and socioeconomic group (Smith & Barton, 1992).

DIVIDING THE WORK

Once you have a number of committed people who agree to work on the community assessment, you need to divvy up the tasks. Table 3.1 provides a timeline of tasks for conducting a participatory community survey.

Regardless of the size of your steering committee, it needs to develop and administer a survey. Its work may also include determining the boundaries of the community that will be part of the survey. For exam-

---

Box 3.1 Guidelines for Establishing Community Partnerships

ORGANIZE

1. Think about potential new partners to enhance your existing efforts and broaden your scope.
2. Send a letter asking partners if they would be part of your effort. Include a fact sheet, a contact phone number, and any other persuasive material you have.
3. Confirm participation partners through follow-up phone calls or letters.

COORDINATE

1. Send an information packet to participating partners.
2. Ask partners to use their own press office to create a media advisory and press release regarding a press event announcing their partnership.
3. Ask partners to include survey or health information in their existing advertising.
4. Get public service announcements and artwork from an Ad Council if partners are willing to use it.
5. Use event checklists and contact sheets to help organize.

PROMOTE

1. Work closely with participant partners' press offices when possible.
2. Distribute a media advisory for local media to learn about any survey or forum events.
3. Distribute a press release describing partner involvement.
4. Make follow-up calls to the press to confirm that they have received and will use the information.

FOLLOW UP

1. Send thank you letters to partners.
2. Ask new partners to continue their relationship after the survey or forum.
3. Clip articles that appear in the paper and use them to promote your upcoming efforts.

Note: Revised from *Seven Days of Immunizations: National Infant Immunization Week,* U.S. Department of Health and Human Services (1995). Public Health Service Centers for Disease Control and Prevention (CDC). Atlanta, GA.

TABLE 3.1   Tasks and Timeline for a Participatory Community Survey

Define the survey population	1–4 weeks
Set up a steering committee	2–4 weeks
Identify survey items	3 weeks
Develop and pretest the questionnaire	2–6 weeks
Block listing	1–4 weeks
Draw the sample	1–4 weeks
Train community interviewers	1–8 weeks
Administer survey	3–12 weeks
Monitor survey administration	3–12 weeks
Analyze data	1–10 weeks
Share findings with community	1–3 weeks
Write up report	1–4 weeks

Box 3.2   Services Available in One Community

Transportation
Homemaker
Home Health Care
Hospitals
Legal
Health department
Chamber of Commerce
Respite
Hospice
Colleges and universities
Local department of highway safety
Police Department
Juvenile Welfare Board
Meals on Wheels
Congregate meals
Home repairs
Information and referral
Counseling
Case management
Housing assistance
Small Business Administration
Employment referral
Red Cross
American Lung Association
Recreation
Multiple Sclerosis Association
YWCA

ple, if the community is a university, are students being surveyed only or will administrators, faculty, and staff also be included? The steering committee can also help define the most effective strategies for administering the survey. Using the university example, will the survey be published in the student newspaper?; will students interview other students?; will it be handed out at the cafeteria or in dorms? Which would provide the most reliable answers and why?

Developing the Survey

One or more members of the steering committee may survey the literature for ideas about survey items. Other members may ask key informants for local knowledge of the community to guide question development. You may want to conduct a telephone interview with existing agencies to see what services they are already providing in the community. Box 3.2 provides a list of some agencies and services you might want to interview.

If you decide to conduct an interview, make sure that everyone is using words in the same way or your answers won't be reli-

able or valid. For example, what is each agency's meaning of the term "counseling"? You may need to ask each agency what they mean by the terms they are using to ensure that there is no misunderstanding.

The steering committee may also draw upon personal experience to provide items for the survey, and it is also useful to leave plenty of space for community input: What community services are residents aware of? What do residents think the problems, strengths, resiliencies and needs of their community are? These questions will provide information about what needs to be targeted and what barriers (financial, physical, or attitudinal) exist in the community. When needs and barriers have been identified, they will provide information about the various support services that should be put in place (transportation, outreach, education, advocacy). Data gathered can also serve to legitimize change and marshal support for that change (see Box 3.3) (Kettner, Moroney, & Martin, 1999).

When planning, keep in mind the time and financial resources you have, because surveys take time and effort. Despite these limitations, it is one of the most powerful methods available for assessing community needs (Kettner, Moroney, & Martin, 1999) and provides original data tailored specifically to the needs of that community.

Students or community members who are in training as interviewers can pretest the survey. Their comments about the readability, clarity, and any omissions or duplications can be used to make revisions. To be reliable and valid, questions must be understandable and elicit the kind of information you need.

Preparing to Conduct the Survey

When preparing to conduct the survey, you may want to use one or more methods of sampling the community, especially if the community is large. *Block listing* involves listing every housing or organizational unit on a block. Steering committee members may pair with university or organizational staff to prepare folders for each block within the survey area. If you can, get community members involved in this process. They can help you locate hard to find or vacant units, access specialized buildings or entrances, and find residents who have moved.

Random sampling is another method of finding participants for you community survey. You can use a table of random numbers or choose to interview every 4th or 10th person you meet. Remember that the more information and variables on which you collect data, the more respondents you will need in the survey to make it representative of the total community. It may not matter which method you use as long as you are consistent and random in your approach.

If you have time, announce that your team will be surveying community members. This approach brings credibility to your effort and alerts potential participants to your presence. Depending on the community, you may wish to alert the police or other community groups that interviewers affiliated with your survey will be in the area.

Members of your steering committee may wish to develop a unique cover sheet that introduces the survey, establishes eligibility for participation, and randomly selects one eligible respondent by household, class, or other relevant unit. Your cover ma-

---

Box 3.3 Data Sources for Your Community Assessment

Bureau of the Census (demographics)
U.S. Postal Service (for zip codes)

Vital statistics (talk to the department of health)

Health care personnel (local American Medical Association and American Nurses' Association)

Inventory of primary care services (consult a local information and referral service inventory or, if not available, contact the state department of health)

Medicaid and Aid to Dependent Children

terial may also document informed consent and recontact information and record attempted contacts with that unit and the final outcome—completed survey, refusal, and other.

Training Yourselves to Conduct the Survey

Even if you are all familiar with administering surveys, it is a good idea to train together. This will reduce the chance of misunderstandings, especially with the use of the cover sheet information. Training can also provide additional or refreshed experience via role-playing, group discussion, and feedback. Your survey may or may not contain information you wish to hold confidential and anonymous. Depending on what type of information you are soliciting, you may not want to use nurses, educators, or social workers whose license requires them to report illegal behaviors such as child abuse (Schulz et al., 1998).

Conducting a Public Forum

If you have neither the time nor the funds to conduct a survey, you can opt for a public forum. Some funding and regulatory agencies (such as the Office of Economic Opportunity) require that hearings be conducted through neighborhood meetings. It is hoped that those attending your forum will articulate their needs and concerns as well as those of their neighbors. Community forums are highly compatible with democratic decision-making. Still, you must ask whether those who attend are really representative of the community. Ensure that all interested groups have a way to attend, e.g., the poorer community residents may not have transportation. Be aware that the more vocal community members may attend. Also, anticipate possible problems, including how to advertise the forum. If radio and television is the mode of advertising, will a cross-section of the community attend? You may have to outreach to churches, shopping centers, social service organizations, and schools to ensure that a broadly representative group attends your forum. Don't assume that attendance means equal participation. Use a process technique such as nominal group process to ensure that all voices are heard (Van de Ven & Delbecq, 1972).

Ethnographic Interviewing

If you decide to conduct interviews with community leaders and representative residents, ethnographic interviewing may be more in line. It also produces rich, descriptive quotes that can put a human face on data. In this case, use some of the following questions to obtain information: What is it like to live in your community? How do people get along in your community? Other questions are generated and emerge from the interview data. For more information on this approach, see Smith and Barton (1992).

Key Components of a Community Assessment

You may have already gathered information about the community. Maybe you live in the community and know many of the residents and agencies. Box 3.4 provides questions that can be used obtain information about a community.

IDENTIFYING WELLNESS PROGRAM NEEDS

All communities, schools, companies, and agencies can benefit from wellness pro-

Box 3.4   Community Assessment

Who and What Is the Community?

1. How is space distributed and used? (Buildings, crowded areas, natural and physical barriers to social interaction, parks, playgrounds?)
2. How safe and healthful are work and school environments? (Are smokers and non smokers segregated? Are junk food and cigarette vending machines highly accessible? Are alternatives offered? Is the use of stairways promoted? Are they accessible? Well lit? Is car-pooling encouraged? Is flex time used to allow employees time to engage in wellness activities before work or during lunch? Are high-quality child care services available for residents? Are buildings well ventilated and do they have adequate natural light and sufficient work/learning space?)
3. What are the cultural mix and stability of the population? (Are there one or more cultural groups living in harmony or in conflict, and how much acculturation and stress occur due to people who move in or out of the area?)
4. What are the age, sex, and family groupings? (Older population, single-occupancy commuter group, young marrieds with children, singles, a mix?)
5. What income levels are represented and to what extent? (Wealthy? Middle class? Poor people receiving governmental or charitable assistance for health care? Or a mix?)
6. What are the occupational levels? (Hard-driving executives who leave the family's health concerns to their wives? Action-oriented population that learns by doing? A mix? What does the occupational level tell you about the population's education, health problems, problem-solving patterns, and methods of learning?)
7. What community resources are available and where are they? (Where are the schools, hospitals, shopping areas, and clinics located in relation to available transportation? What self-help or supportive groups and services exist in the community? What facilities are there for wellness programs? What space could be developed to provide further wellness services? What skills or resources do the residents have that could be shared through a wellness program exchange? Is there any way to trade unused sick leave for a well day? Could unused sick leave be converted to cash? Do faculty, bosses, or town legislators support personal health promotion objectives? Can additional rewards or incentives be built into the current health/illness insurance programs without taking away existing benefits? If there are company or school-subsidized cafeterias, could wellness-promoting foods be subsidized more than junk foods?)

How Are Needs Met?

1. Are needs met or prevented from being met by space, culture, age, sex, family, income, occupational level, or community resource factors?

(continued)

Box 3.4   *(continued)*

2. What do the community's clergy, health care practitioners, welfare agencies, and clients know about what needs are not being met?
3. What do records of health services, worker's compensation claims, and accident and safety records tell you about how needs are met and what wellness needs are not being met?
4. What do questionnaire or survey methods tell you about what community residents say are the types of wellness activities they would participate in if offered?
5. What specific risk factors exist in this population and how are they being addressed or not?
6. How can family members of community residents be considered in planning wellness programs and used to provide needed support systems?

How Are Deviance and Disturbance Handled?

1. Are those with psychiatric/mental health difficulties rejected by the community? In what way?
2. How are delinquents or those who abuse alcohol, drugs, or food treated by community members?
3. What political, educational, or social views lead to rejection or those who deviate from the norm?
4. Are there humane or highly institutionalized agencies available in the community to help deal with deviate members? What are they?
5. Does the community reject the idea of placing treatment facilities for its deviants within the community? How?
6. Is there a prevailing view that people who deviate from accepted behavioral patterns should be punished? How is this belief put into practice?

How Are Identities Developed?

1. How do families, faculty, administrators, etc. teach their members to act?
2. What kinds of religious/spiritual organizations or groups exist in the community and what is their prevailing view of human motivation?
3. What youth agencies/helpers are there and how do young people relate to them?
4. What kind of formal and special education programs are available and how are they used by the community?
5. How could already existing agencies or groups be used more effectively?

How Are Community Functions Accomplished?

1. Are community decisions made before adequate information has been obtained? What possible effect(s) might this have?

Box 3.4 *(continued)*

2. Are decisions made by default, based on the personal concerns of a few, or made by consensus? What are the consequences of this type of decision making?
3. Is communication fragmented and inefficient? How does such communication seem to affect the community?
4. Are communication messages based on a sense of community ("We're all in this together") or on stereotypes and the establishment of distance between groups ("It's us against them")? What are the effects of both types of communication messages?
5. How accurately do the local media convey information to the community?
6. Are there informal (rumor) communication channels?
7. Are problems solved informally with board and committee meetings used only to record earlier decisions? How might this affect the community or the decision-making process?
8. How are ad hoc, neighborhood, or block associations used in decision making?
9. How readily are newcomers accepted by the community?
10. Is leadership concentrated among a few groups or is it widely distributed in the community?
11. Are there wide vacillations in power or frequent changes in the power base that could affect health planning or treatment?
12. Where is power located, how is it perceived, and how is it used?
13. What overlapping areas and missing links are there in wellness services?
14. What segments in the community are receptive and hostile to outside influence?
15. Is there a sense of trust between community members and leaders?
16. Is there community disintegration? (Has a recent disaster, widespread ill health, extensive poverty, confusion of cultural values, weakening of religious affiliations, extensive migration of new groups, or rapid social change radically affected the community?)

What Are the Resistances to Change in This Community?

1. What factors in the system will be affected as a result of a change toward wellness?
2. What forces are operating to inhibit change toward wellness?
3. What information or experiences must precede the change toward wellness?
4. What new procedures or experiences will need to be developed as a result of a movement toward wellness?
5. Who is likely to suffer from the change?
6. How aware of the need for change are community residents?
7. Are community residents sufficiently involved in planning for the change?
8. What is the relationship between the change agent and community residents?

(continued)

Box 3.4 *(continued)*

9. What past relationship between the change agent and the client might be influencing resistance to change now?

10. How open have community residents been to the introduction of change in the past?

11. How can free and open communications, administrative support of and reward for problem-solving efforts, shared decision making, sufficient time to problem solve, written statements of what the change goals will be, professionalism, concern for long-term planning, cohesiveness among change agents, feelings of security among residents, timing, and resident confidence in ability to change be enhanced to lower resistance to change?

Copyright Carolyn Chambers Clark, 1996.

---

grams. Many have developed programs, but they may be based on what planners believe to be important. A wellness perspective demands that the client be involved in the planning process. Some questions to ask that will help communities assess their wellness program needs are listed below:

- What are the sociodemographic characteristics of your community? (This includes determining the age, sex, ethnic origin, occupation, employment status, and education levels of the selected population.)
- What are the costs of health care and disability? (Include insurance claims and average the rate by the number of people. Determine the number, frequency, duration, and costs of incidental and disability absences.)
- What are the patterns of health care use now? (Determine what kinds of preventive and wellness issues are brought to health care providers. Find out what kind of chronic and acute conditions are being treated. Talk with health care providers and obtain summaries of use patterns if possible.)
- What conditions or diseases are present or potential in the community?

(Randomly sample the population or obtain a representative sample and use written questionnaires, phone interviews, or one-on-one interviews to obtain information. Determine blood pressure, height, weight, lipids, blood sugar, and other information indicative of wellness states. What are current resident lifestyle habits regarding nutrition, exercise and movement, stress management, parenting, communication, knowledge of how to obtain wellness information, self-care skills, smoking, drinking, and the use of drugs and medications?

- What wellness and health promotion programs are currently available? Talk with providers of these programs and participants or use a questionnaire to obtain the information you need. If the media publicizes these programs, obtain information from their public relations departments.
- How well are wellness and health promotion programs working? Obtain evaluation information from program providers and interview or survey participants.
- What kinds of health and wellness programs does the community think

should be included? Interview or survey the population or obtain a representative sample.

- What is the need? Use the information you've collected to make a determination of need.

REFERENCES

Bracht, N. (1999). *Health Promotion at the Community Level.* Thousand Oaks, CA: Sage Publications.

Kettner, P. M., Moroney, R. M., & Martin, L. L. (1999). Needs assessment: Approaches to measurement. *Designing and Managing Programs, An Effectiveness-Based Approach* (pp. 49–70). Thousand Oaks, CA: Sage.

Schulz, A. J., Parker, E. A., Israel, B. A., Becker, A. B., Maciak, B. J., & Hollis, R. (1998). Conducting a participatory community-based survey. *Journal of Health Management Practice, 4*(2), 10–24.

Smith, M. C., & Barton, J. A. (1992). Technologic enrichment of a community needs assessment. *Nursing Outlook, 40*(1), 33–37.

Van de Ven, A., & Delbecq, A. (1972). The nominal group as a research instrument for conducting health studies. *American Journal of Public Health, 62,* 337–342.

CHAPTER 4

Principles of Planning Effective Community Programs

Elizabeth Erkel

PROGRAM PLANNING: WHAT? WHY? WHO? WHO ME?

Broadly defined, *program planning* includes community assessment and diagnosis, problem and goal analysis, program design, marketing, implementation (policy-making, administration, and operations), and program evaluation. This chapter will discuss and provide you with tools for selecting the focus of a health promotion program and for decision-making in program design. It focuses on the portion of program planning that follows community assessment and diagnosis and precedes marketing, implementation, and evaluation.

Design-planning is the determination of specific methods, activities, and tasks to be accomplished by whom, how, when, and at what cost for a package of services intended to achieve particular objectives. The elements of a program design include the program's focus, objectives, intervention strategies (usually called methods), timeline for implementation, and budget.

Why plan? You plan to solve a problem, to reach a goal, to do something and have it turn out right; in short, you plan to create a better future. In developing a health promotion program, you plan so that the program will be effective. An *effective health promotion program* produces changes in client knowledge, beliefs, behavior, and environmental conditions, which in turn facilitates achievement of the community's desired health outcomes. If you plan the program in collaboration with potential clients, the providers who will implement the program, and the decision makers who will allocate resources for the program, it is more likely that the program will obtain sufficient resources, be implemented according to design, and be accepted by the community, thus assuring program effectiveness and empowering the community. Research has shown that empowered communities experience better health, for whatever reason (Rissel, 1994).

In reading this chapter, assume that you are working with a coalition of potential clients, health care providers, and key decision makers from a community agency. Following a needs assessment, participants in the coalition have collectively identified a desired health outcome, which will enable the community to increase control over its health, assist the community in reaching a higher level of wellness, and promote community resilience. Your role is to facilitate the coalition's reaching its goal by collectively designing a health promotion program. In your partnership with the coalition, you have mutually agreed that you will do the necessary detail work to get a plan down on paper. In periodic meetings the remaining members of the coalition will provide you with direction and feedback on all plan decisions.

ENSURING PROGRAM EFFECTIVENESS

You can ensure that your health promotion program will be effective by making it part of a community partnership, by focusing on changeable behavioral and environmental causes of health and their determinants, and by making it culturally congruent. Community partnerships are built over time through early and continued involvement of participants, collective action, collaboration, and networking, all guided by client-focused goals. In this section you will learn to use the PRECEDE-PROCEED Model for Health-Promotion Planning and Evaluation to choose the appropriate focus for a health-promotion program; then you will learn to plan a culturally congruent health-promotion program by practicing the principles of the *Six Steps Toward Cultural Competence* (Minnesota Public Health Association [MPHA], 1996).

Choosing an Appropriate Focus for a Health Promotion Program

The PRECEDE-PROCEED Model for Health Promotion Planning and Evaluation

The basic premise of this PRECEDE-PROCEED Model is that while there are multiple behavioral and environmental causes of a community's health and quality of life, an effective health promotion program focuses on a particular subset of influencing factors which, if modified, are likely to result in position health-directed behaviors and environmental living conditions (Green & Kreuter, 1999). See Figure 4.1 for a visual display of the PRECEDE-PROCEED Model and see below for an explanation of the PRECEDE-PROCEED acronym.

PRECEDE

Predisposing
Reinforcing
Enabling
Constructs in
Educational/ecological
Diagnosis and
Evaluation

PROCEED

Policy
Regulatory
Organizational
Constructs in
Educational and
Environmental
Development

Source: Green & Kreuter, 1999

The predisposing, reinforcing, and enabling factors are central to the model in that, with few exceptions, they all must be operating together for a health-directed behavior to occur and continue over time. Thus, your health promotion intervention must address all three types of behavioral determinants if is to be effective. *Predisposing factors* such as knowledge, beliefs, values, attitudes, and perceptions incline individuals toward particular health-related behavior patterns. Although demographic, socioeconomic, and personality factors also predispose individual behavioral health patterns, health promotion programs are unlikely to modify these factors. *Enabling factors* include skills, accessibility to resources, and community commitment to

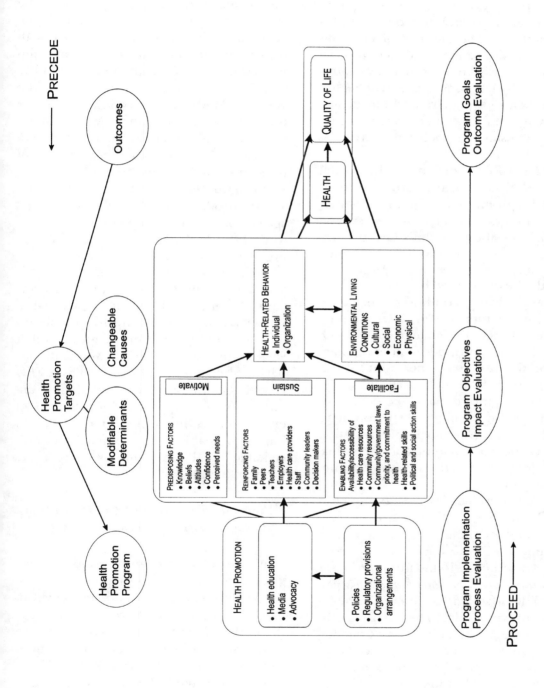

FIGURE 4.1 The PRECEDE-PROCEED model for health promotion planning and evaluation.

Note: Adapted by permission of L. W. Green.

health (laws, policies, regulatory provisions, and organizational arrangements) which, if present, facilitate desired health-directed behaviors and environmental living conditions. The absence of enabling factors may act as a barrier to action. *Reinforcing factors* are the positive and negative social and physical consequences of health-directed behavior (e.g., rewards, feedback, relief of discomfort), which provide the incentive to sustain the behavior (Green & Kreuter, 1999).

The PRECEDE portion of the model guides the selection of an appropriate focus for a health promotion program and generates the program objectives—the criteria used to judge the program's effectiveness in the PROCEED portion of the model. The *focus of a health promotion program* includes the health-related behaviors and environmental living conditions and their influencing factors (called determinants) that are selected for change. The PROCEED portion of the model guides (a) planning for the resources (personnel, time, budget) needed for the program in the context of organizational policies and arrangements and the political environment; (b) monitoring program implementation through process evaluation; and (c) evaluation of program effectiveness through impact evaluation.

A more in-depth description of the PRECEDE-PROCEED Model with its theoretical base and examples of applications in community, occupational, school, and health care settings is found in *Health Promotion Planning: An Educational and Ecological Approach* by Green and Kreuter (1999), developers of the model. The Web page of the Institute of Health Promotion Research, University of British Columbia (1999) has a searchable bibliography of hundreds of publications in which the model has been applied, adapted, or extended.

The PRECEDE-PROCEED Model is an analytical, decision-making model for planning health promotion programs and the Wellness Model described in chapter 1 conceptualizes your dynamic interaction with the community-as-client in program-planning and health promotion. The PRECEDE-PROCEED Model is a tool, the Wellness Model a perspective. Both share the purpose of community health promotion, which is to enable the community to increase control over the determinants of its health in order to improve it (First International Conference on Health Promotion, 1986, Introduction). The Wellness Model speaks of the commitment to self-care, while PRECEDE-PROCEED addresses the organizational and social supports left in place by health promotion efforts that enable the community to continue to exert control over the determinants of its health. In the Wellness Model, health promotion is linked to a higher, more adaptive level of wellness through a community-practitioner partnership; in the PRECEDE-PROCEED Model, health promotion maintains, enhances, or interrupts behavior patterns and environmental living conditions linked to improved health or increased risks for preventable health conditions (Green & Kreuter, 1999).

Using the PRECEDE-PROCEED Model to Choose Health Promotion Targets

The focus of your health promotion program is reached first through selection of the health-related behaviors and environmental conditions that are likely to cause the desired health outcomes and that are changeable through health promotion. Next you will select *determinants of health*, those factors that influence a community's health by predisposing, enabling, and reinforcing its lifestyle and shaping its environmental living conditions (Green & Kreuter, 1999). The selected behavioral and environmental causes of health and their determinants are the *targets of change* or focus of your health promotion program. You will design a health promotion intervention to modify specific determinants likely to maintain, enhance, or interrupt the behavioral and environmental causes of the desired health outcome.

Green and Kreuter (1999) suggest choosing the targets of change based on their *importance* and *changeability*. The following example illustrates how this was done for "Shedding Pounds . . . Adding Years," a wellness program to improve cardiovascular health through physical fitness and positive nutrition. Following a community assessment in Clarendon County, South Carolina, which had been facilitated and funded by the local United Way, a community activist spearheaded a group of volunteers to plan a wellness program for the community. The group included potential clients and representatives from the local health department, hospital, and agricultural extension program. The idea came from qualitative data from the community assessment. During neighborhood focus groups led by the volunteer coordinator of the United Way community-assessment task force, low-income residents had stated that they wanted affordable ways to "get fit and watch what we eat and look slim." One resident said, "So many people I know have heart trouble or high blood or sugar and I want to stay healthy. Did you know we live in the stroke belt?" Another resident stated that she had tried walking in her neighborhood, but that the dogs had scared her. Local health care providers who had been interviewed wanted a wellness program for their overweight clients and others with limited financial resources who were at risk for preventable health conditions such as heart

disease, diabetes, hypertension, and stroke (Bilodeau, Collins, & Hussey, 1999).

To determine the focus of the health-promotion program, the members of the group asked the community activist to study community input along with statistical indicators of health for the county and bring suggestions back to the them. Epidemiological data confirmed a high rate of heart disease in Clarendon County. For example, 56% of hospitalizations in the county over the past 10 years were related to heart disease (United Way, 1996).

Using *importance* and *changeability* as criteria, the community activist rated the following behavioral and environmental causes of heart disease found in the literature: smoking, high-fat foods, lack of exercise, inconsistent medication patterns, inconsistent monitoring of blood pressure, stressful living conditions, and inaccessibility to medical care. Nutritional and physical fitness patterns were selected as the *changeable* health-related behaviors ranked most *important*, i.e., those occurring most frequently in their community and strongly linked to preventing heart disease. Among Clarendon County residents, nearly 25% were obese, and physical inactivity was extraordinarily high: 71% reported no leisure physical activity compared to a median of 29% for the nation (Powell-Griner, Anderson, & Murphy, 1997; United Way, 1996).

In analyzing nutritional and exercise patterns in Clarendon County, importance (frequency linked to behavioral and environmental cause) and changeability were again used as criteria to select modifiable determinants. These can also be thought of as community capacities to be strengthened through health promotion. Data showed that 43% of residents had less than a high school education, which *predisposed* residents to a knowledge deficit regarding positive nutrition and fitness and low self-confidence in community self-care. South-

ern food preferences for high-fat, high carbohydrate foods (fried chicken, corn
bread) were *reinforced* through family gath-
erings with extended kin, church socials,
and get-togethers with friends. *Enabling factors* hindering access to primary health care,
preventive services, and community resources for many rural African-American
residents included poverty among 29% of
the population and lack of transportation,
which was reported by key informants to
be a major barrier. Nutritional counseling
in the county was limited to those enrolled
in the Special Supplemental Food Program
for Women, Infants, and Children (WIC)
seeking food vouchers. There were no satel-
lite WIC centers in rural areas of the community. Many residents could not afford
the privately owned, for-profit fitness center in the community. Finally, residents
need skill training for aerobic exercise,
weightlifting, reading food labels, and measuring food portions (Bilodeau, Collins, &
Hussey, 1999; United Way, 1996).

Given this information, the coalition
concluded that in order to meet the needs
of the low-income, largely African-American community for an accessible, affordable wellness program, a culturally
congruent, multidimensional package of
services would be developed. Health promotion efforts would focus on (a) increasing residents' knowledge and skills for
positive nutrition and physical fitness and
(b) facilitating access to the wellness program by overcoming the transportation
and cost barriers (Bilodeau et al., 1999).

Practicing Cultural Competence

Using the PRECEDE-PROCEED Model will
assist you in choosing *appropriate* health promotion targets. If the focus of the program
meets the community's needs, the changes

in health-related behavior and environmental living conditions are likely to result
in the desired health outcomes. For clients
to participate in the program and make the
desired behavioral changes, the program
must also be acceptable or culturally congruent to them. *Culturally congruent* health
promotion means providing health promotion that is meaningful and that fits the
cultural beliefs and lifestyles of participants
(Leininger, 1999). A *culturally competent* person is one who is sensitive to the cultural
differences and responses of individuals,
avoids stereotyping, and interacts respect-
fully with people of all cultures in a way
that recognizes their worth and supports
their dignity (Meleis, 1999; MPHA, 1996).

Your cultural competence will continually evolve because cultures are dynamic.
Realize that it is impossible to be completely
familiar with the health beliefs and lifestyles
of all of your clients. However, by practicing
the following principles adapted from *Six
Steps Toward Cultural Competence* (MPHA,
1996), you can ensure that your program
will be acceptable to your clients:

1. *Involve clients in their own care.* Teaching self-care practices for physical fitness,
positive nutrition, stress management, environmental health, and other healthful patterns is a major role in health promotion
programs. Fostering environmental supports (e.g., smoke-free facilities) and social
supports (skilled parents, concerned teachers, understanding employers, informed officials) in conjunction with client health
promotion will facilitate and sustain individual health-directed behaviors following
program intervention (Green & Kreuter,
1999).

2. *Learn more about cultures, starting with
your own.* Read about the language, customs, and health beliefs of participants in
your program, keeping in mind that cul-

tural lifestyles are constantly influenced by contemporary events, the media, and interaction with other cultures. It is important to observe the health beliefs and lifestyles of your clients through conversation and participation in community daily life and attendance at their cultural events. When I was a public-health nurse on Guam, I learned that accepting invitations to family weddings and birthday parties and attending village religious celebrations built trust between us, increasing my stature as a source of health information and thus my ability to influence health-directed behavior.

3. *Speak the language or use a trained interpreter.* All health promotion strategies involve communication, either directly or indirectly. Communication is hindered when you and your clients or community speak different languages or converse in the same language but different dialects (regional, social, or age-related). You can overcome dialectical differences through close observation and feedback. Using trained interpreters is recommended, however, to overcome language differences when learning the language is impractical. Use of family members or other untrained interpreters may result in misinterpretation and misunderstanding. Helpful materials related to using interpreters include: "Guidelines for Working with Interpreters," by B. T. Downing (n.d.); "A Proposed Code of Ethics for Community Interpreters," by University of Minnesota (n.d.); and "Professional Interpreter Standards, Training, and Skill Assessment," by the Advisory Committee on Interpreter Standards (1998). Resources for translated health-education materials include: "Translated Health Education Resources: A Listing of Distributors of Translated Materials" by the Minnesota Department of Health (1996); and the *Health Education Materials Store* on

a Website by Multi-Cultural Educational Services (1999).

4. *Ask the right questions and look for answers.* Ask open-ended questions that will help you understand client perspectives on staying healthy and learn their self-care practices. Teach clients to ask crucial questions when you refer them to community resources for assistance. Through open-ended interviews with 19 men living in various small, rural communities in Iowa, Sellers, Poduska, Propp, and White (1999) learned that rural Midwestern men equate health with "being able to work and meet responsibilities" (p. 326). In order to be acceptable to this population, health promotion programs must adapt to those values of independence and self-reliance, the pervasive economic competitiveness of farming and rural businesses that controls their lives, and the seasonal variation in intensity of work schedules. For example, scheduling health education programs in the winter after fall harvest and before spring planting and in conjunction with community organization meetings acknowledges that their time is valuable.

5. *Pay attention to financial issues.* Teach clients to use materials they already have on hand for health-directed behaviors such as strength building. Learn how to prepare inexpensive, nutritional foods that satisfy client cultural preferences. Teach clients how to comparison shop. Learn about community resource options for low-income clients, and act as a role model for frugal lifestyle.

6. *Find resources and form partnerships.* Partnering your health-promotion program with cultural associations in the community, private providers, public health departments, and social service agencies saves time, energy, and money while providing culturally congruent health promotion. Collaboration with indigenous outreach workers and respected local folk prac

titioners increases connectedness with clients and their lifestyles.

Practicing these principles will allow you to tailor your health promotion intervention in ways that (a) preserve your clients' cultural values, health beliefs, and health-related practices that promote and maintain their well-being; (b) accommodate health-related practices that are not harmful to their health; and (c) repattern your clients' lifestyles for new, different, and beneficial health-directed behaviors while respecting their cultural values and health beliefs (Leininger, 1997).

Role of the Health Promoter in Assuring Program Effectiveness

According to Rissel (1994), empowerment is the raison d'etre of health promotion (i.e., enabling the community to increase control over its health). Your role then as community activist in planning health promotion programs and as health promoter in conducting the program is that of facilitator. You facilitate—but do not direct—the selection of desired health outcomes, the choice of appropriate targets of change, and the design of an acceptable health promotion program. Being a role model, mentor, and teacher in the process of facilitation contributes to collective action and favorable redistribution of resources from which community empowerment evolves.

THE ELEMENTS OF A PROGRAM DESIGN

There are four elements of a program design: goals and objectives, methods, marketing plan, and budget. This section will describe the development of goals and ob-

jectives, criteria for the methods section, and characteristics of a program budget. Marketing is discussed in Chapter 6. All elements of the program design are directly related to the focus of your health-promotion program.

Program Goals and Objectives

Program goals and objectives are important because they set the direction for the program and the expectations for what it will accomplish. Objectives are essentially promises that you make to whomever is funding your program, whether a community agency you are affiliated with or a private foundation who will award you money to cover all or part your program costs. Program goals are broadly stated, long-range aims related to the selected health outcomes. As ideals, they are not achievable in the short-term life of your program nor are they measurable (U.S. Public Health Service [USPH], no date). For example, the goal for "Shedding Pounds . . . Adding Years" was to improve nutritional health and physical fitness of low-income residents in Clarendon County, thus improving their cardiovascular health and reducing the social and financial cost of chronic disease (Bilodeau et al., 1999).

In contrast to the directional nature of goals, objectives are highly specific statements that describe the means for partially achieving the goal. Well-stated objectives clearly present a result that is measurable and achievable, based on a realistic assessment of resources. The measurable quality of the objective (time frame, minimum performance standard, magnitude, and direction of change) permit evaluation of its achievement at a later, specified date (USPH, no date).

Program objectives specify the *impact* your health promotion program will have:

the expected changes or results that will be accomplished by the program during a specified funding period. In accordance with the PRECEDE-PROCEED Model, *program objectives* project changes in behavior, environmental living conditions, knowledge, attitudes, beliefs, social support, availability and accessibility of resources, policy, and skills. Program objectives are derived from the health promotion targets (selected changeable causes of health and their modifiable determinants). In writing program objectives, do not confuse impact with *process*, which is the implementation of the health-promotion activities (delivery of services) and use of human, material, and financial resources, all described in the methods section of your program design. Box 4.1 displays program objectives for "Shedding Pounds . . . Adding Years."

Methods

The methods section of the program design provides a blueprint for achieving objectives by describing the (a) setting and facilities; (b) target population, criteria for selection of participants, participant enrollment process; (c) activities timeline for implementation; (d) staff selection and training; and (e) justification for selection of methods. In designing the methods for your program, ask the following questions: Will these methods achieve our objectives within the projected time frame and resources? Are the activities and their sequence described clearly enough that a lay person who is unfamiliar with this program can understand what will occur? If challenged can we defend our choice of methods with authoritative sources? To describe methods in sufficient detail requires from 800 to 1,000 words plus the timeline for implementation of the program in the form

of a table or Gantt chart (see Figure 4.2). Approaches to health promotion and strategies for engaging your target population will be discussed under "Conducting Successful Health Promotion Programs."

Budget

The budget is a description of your program in financial terms: a line-item budget categorizing estimated costs of marketing, implementing, and evaluating the program. The budget is important because it tells those funding your program whether you know what you are doing. The budget should demonstrate that you can transform your program design into real events over time. It must be as realistic as possible because your funding source will scrutinize it. Is the budget large enough to cover all activities and resources needed? Is it "padded"? In other words, are there items included in the budget that you want but that are not directly related to the program (e.g., AV equipment, computers)? Follow this cardinal rule: "Every budget item must be accounted for somewhere in the text [of the program design]. Every expense-generating activity mentioned in the text must be reflected in the budget" (Gilpatrick, 1989, p. 157). Thus, the budget includes dollars requested from your funding source as well as financial contributions by other sources (e.g., your own organization, individuals, businesses, community agencies, or a grant), whether in real dollars or "in-kind" contributions of personnel or material resources.

The budget is comprised of three components. First, the budget summary provides a quick overview of total costs, total requested funds, and total donated funds in each major budget category for personnel and nonpersonnel costs (see Table 4.1).

Box 4.1 Program Objectives for "Shedding Pounds . . . Adding Years"

1. At the end of 3 years, the number of nutritional and physical fitness health promotion programs for low-income residents in Clarendon County will increase from 1 nutritional and no physical fitness programs by an additional 16 Exportable Wellness Packages in 12 neighborhood churches and four neighborhood organizations.

2. At the end of 6 months of participation in an Exportable Wellness Package, 90% of clients will be able to identify high-fat, high-sodium, and high-cholesterol foods from a food selection list with 80% accuracy.

3. At the end of 1 year of participation in an Exportable Wellness Package, 80% of clients will increase physical fitness, as measured by a decrease in resting heart rate.

4. At the end of 1 year of participation in an Exportable Wellness Package, 80% of clients will improve cardiovascular health, as measured by a 20% decrease in serum cholesterol level.

5. At the end of 1 year of participation in an Exportable Wellness Package, 50% of overweight clients will increase physical fitness, as measured by a 15% decrease in Body Mass Index.

6. At the end of 1 year of participation in an Exportable Wellness Package, 75% of known hypertensive clients will improve cardiovascular health, as measured by a 10 mm Hg decrease in blood pressure.

7. At the end of 1 year of participation in an Exportable Wellness Package, 70% of clients will increase self-confidence in adhering to learned behavioral modifications, as evidenced by a comparison of interviews conducted upon enrollment and at 1 year.

8. At the end of 1 year, accessibility to the Clarendon Memorial Hospital Wellness Center for low-income residents will increase from 0 to 20 low-income residents via Fitness Scholarships for 3 months of personal training and maintain 20 Fitness Scholarships for 2 subsequent years.

9. At the end of 3 months participation in a Fitness Scholarship personal training program at the Clarendon Memorial Hospital Wellness Center, 80% of Fitness Scholarship recipients will increase physical fitness as demonstrated by comparison of baseline body and target body measurements (body fat percentage, appearance measurements, and exercise performance [strength, aerobic, flexibility]) with 80% target body achievement.

10. At the end of 9 months participation in the Youth Fitness Leadership Program, 95% of middle-school and high-school students will increase their knowledge of methods to improve nutritional health and physical fitness, as evidenced by comparison of pretest and posttest scores.

11. At the end of the Master Health Advocate course, 100% of participants will increase their knowledge of methods to improve nutritional health and physical fitness, as evidenced by comparison of pretest and posttest scores.

Box 4.1 *(continued)*

12. At the end of each monthly Increased Health Awareness through Action multimedia campaign, 25% of community residents interviewed by telephone survey will be aware of the health promotion target.

Note: From *Shedding Pounds . . . Adding Years* (p. 7), by N. Bilodeau, A. Collins, and N. Hussey, 1999, Unpublished master's scholarly product. Medical University of South Carolina, Charleston. Revised with permission of the authors.

Second, the budget detail expands on the summary by listing each item and its cost calculation on a separate line, hence the name line-item budget (see Table 4.2). Finally, the budget justification is a brief narrative in which rationale is provided for items that are not self-explanatory and items which might be questioned by funders. For more information related to program budgeting, see "Planning and Writing an Annual Budget" in *Community Toolbox* (chapter 27, section 4) by Rabinowitz, Berkowitz, and Brownlee (1999).

CONDUCTING SUCCESSFUL HEALTH PROMOTION PROGRAMS

Successful implementation of your program depends on a well-planned health promotion intervention, adequate resources, strong community and organizational support, appropriate in-service training and constructive supervision of staff, and conscientious monitoring of activities and use of resources. Starting small and building on accomplishments contributes to success, as does learning by experience, adapting to circumstances, responding to staff and client needs, keeping the goal in mind, and "a sense of humor" (Green & Kreuter, 1999, p. 213). Success also depends on having selected the appropriate approach to health promotion: The approach must be congruent with the predisposing, reinforcing, and enabling factors targeted for change.

Matching the Targets of Change to Approaches to Health Promotion

According to the PRECEDE-PROCEDE Model (Green & Kreuter, 1999), there are two basic approaches to health promotion: health education and community organization. *Health education* involves planned learning experiences for the purpose of motivating, facilitating, and sustaining voluntary health-related behaviors. *Community organization* involves collective action to redistribute resources through policy change, regulatory provision, or organizational arrangements. The approach to health promotion that you choose will depend on the determinants you are targeting for modification or that you wish to strengthen. Table 4.3 displays the appropriate health promotion approaches for predisposing, reinforcing, and enabling factors (modifiable determinants).

Health Education

Motivation for behavioral or organizational change is influenced by a combination of

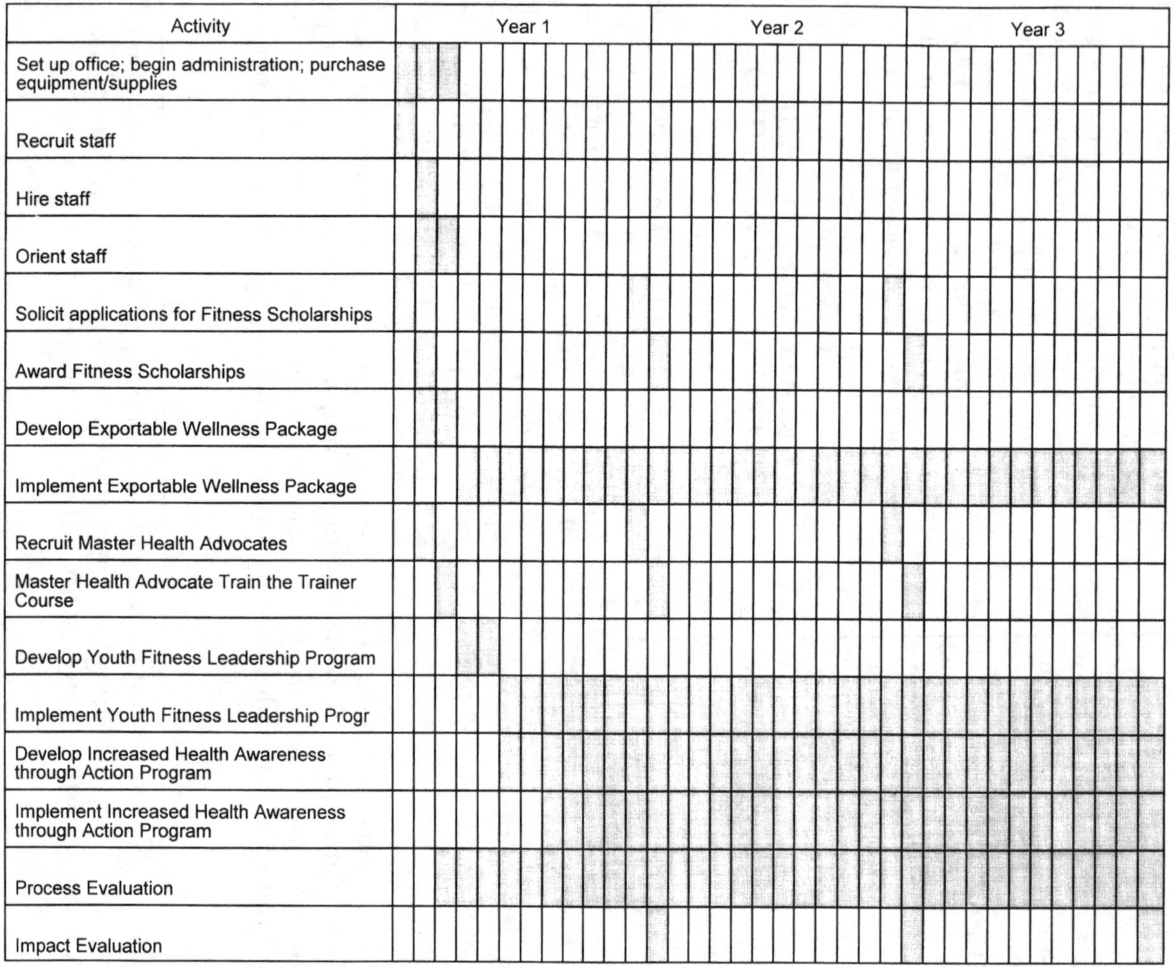

Activity	Year 1	Year 2	Year 3
Set up office: begin administration; purchase equipment/supplies			
Recruit staff			
Hire staff			
Orient staff			
Solicit applications for Fitness Scholarships			
Award Fitness Scholarships			
Develop Exportable Wellness Package			
Implement Exportable Wellness Package			
Recruit Master Health Advocates			
Master Health Advocate Train the Trainer Course			
Develop Youth Fitness Leadership Program			
Implement Youth Fitness Leadership Progr			
Develop Increased Health Awareness through Action Program			
Implement Increased Health Awareness through Action Program			
Process Evaluation			
Impact Evaluation			

FIGURE 4.2   Timeline for "Shedding Pounds . . . Adding Years."

Note: From *Shedding Pounds . . . Adding Years,* (p. 11) by N. Bilodeau, A. Collins and N. Hussey, 1999, Medical University of South Carolina, Charleston. Revised by permission of the authors.

TABLE 4.1   Three-Year Budget Summary for "Shedding Pounds . . . Adding Years"

	Requested	Donated	Total
	$283,026	**$395,308**	**$678,334**
PERSONNEL	**$194,843**	**$316,659**	**$511,502**
Salaries & wages	$116,873	$57,912	$174,785
Fringe benefits	$28,050	$13,899	$41,949
Consultant & contract services	$49,920	$244,848	$294,768
NONPERSONNEL	**$88,183**	**$78,649**	**$166,832**
Space costs	-0-	$68,400	$68,400
Rental, lease, or purchase of equipment	$11,380	-0-	$11,380
Consumable supplies (office, educational, medical)	$11,998	-0-	$11,998
Communications	$149	$10,249	$10,398
Travel	$48,360	-0-	$48,360
Other costs	$16,296	-0-	$16,296

Note: From *Shedding Pounds . . . Adding Years* (p. 15), by N. Bilodeau, A. Collins and N. Hussey, 1999. Medical University of South Carolina, Charleston. Revised with permission of the authors.

TABLE 4.2   Three-Year Budget Detail for "Shedding Pounds . . . Adding Years"

	Requested	Donated		Requested	Donated	Total
				$283,026	**$395,308**	**$678,334**
PERSONNEL				**$194,843**	**$316,659**	**$511,502**
Salaries & Wages				**$116,873**	**$57,912**	**$174,785**
Program director @ $37,440/year + cost of living/merit raise @ 4% for Years 2 and 3	$116,873					
Registered nurse Year 1 @ $15/hr × 20 hr/mo × 12 mo + Year 2 @ $15.60/hr × 30 hr/mo × 12 mo + Year 3 @ $16.25/ hr × 40 hr/mo × 12 mo (donated by Health Dept.)		$17,016				
Registered nutritionist Year 1 @ $15/hr × 40 hr/mo × 12 mo + Year 2 @ $15.60/ hr × 80 hr/mo × 12 mo + Year 3 @ $16.25/hr × 96 hr/mo × 12 mo (donated by Clemson University Cooperative Extension Service)		$40,896				
	$116,873	$57,912				
Fringe Benefits				**$28,050**	**$13,899**	**$41,949**
Program director @ 24% of salary	$28,050					
Registered nurse @ 24% of salary		$4,084				

(continued)

TABLE 4.2　*(continued)*

		Requested	Donated	Total
Registered nutritionist @ 24% of salary	$9,815			
	$28,050	$13,899		
Consultant and Contract Services		$49,920	$244,848	$294,768
Fitness instructor Year 1@ $18/hr × 40 hr/mo × 12 mo + Year 2 @ $19/hr × 80 hr/mo × 12 mo + Year 3 @ $20/hr × 96 hr/mo × 12 mo	$49,920			
Master health advocates (community volunteers):				
(5) Year 1 @ $10/hr × 40 hr/mo × 12 mo +				
(5) Year 2 @ $10.40/hr × 40 hr/mo × 12 mo +				
(10) Year 2 @ $10/hr × 40 hr/mo × 12 mo +				
(5) Year 3 @ $10.82 × 40 hr/mo × 12 mo +				
(10) Year 3 @ $10.40/hr × 40 hr/mo × 12 mo +				
(15) year 3 @ $10/hr × 40 hr/mo × 12	$244,848			
	$49,920	$244,848		

NONPERSONNEL			$88,183	$78,649	$166,832
	Requested	**Donated**			
Space Costs			-0-	$68,400	$68,400
Rent (including all utilities) @ $9.50/sq ft/mo × 200 sq ft × 36 mo		$68,400			
	-0-	$68,400			
Rental, Lease, or Purchase of Equipment			$11,380	-0-	$11,380
4 Desk chairs @ $100/ea	$400				
4 Desks @ $200/ea	$800				
2 Filing cabinets @ $125/ea	$250				
1 Telephone answering machine @ $60	$60				
3 Bookshelves @ $100/ea	$300				
4 Desk lamps @ $30/ea	$120				
1 TV/VCR @ $600	$600				
1 Desktop computer @ $2,500	$2,500				
2 Laptop computers @ $2,500/ea	$5,000				

TABLE 4.2   *(continued)*

	Requested	Donated	Total
1 Copy/printer/FAX machine @ $1,000 $1,000			
1 Portable printer @ $350 $350			
$11,380	-0-		
Consumable Supplies (Office, Educational, Medical)	$11,998	-0-	$11,998
Office supplies @ $200/year × 4 staff × 3 yr $2,400			
100 reams of copy paper/yr @ $3.50 ea × 3 yr $1,050			
5 toner refills/yr @ $40/ea × 3 yr $600			
Printing $500/yr × 3 yr $1,500			
600 Self-care books @ $7/ea $4,200			
20 boxes of nonsterile/disposable gloves @ $9.10 ea $182			
1 box cotton balls @ $10 $10			
3 Cavicide disinfectant spray (24 oz) @ $6.10 ea $18			
12 boxes alcohol wipes @ $2.30 ea $28			
10 bottles (800 ml) liquid hand soap @ $10.50 ea $105			
6 Sharps containers @ $4.50 ea $27			
2 blood pressure cuffs, adult @ $59.60 ea + $369			
2 blood pressure cuffs, large @ $65.20 ea +			
2 blood pressure cuffs, small @$59.60 ea			
6 stethoscopes @ $17.50 ea $105			
4 portable scales @ $50 ea $200			
2 tape measures @ $2 ea $4			
2 glucose/cholesterol/supplies @ $11.10/mo × 36 mo $800			
4 privacy screens @ $100 ea $400			
$11,998	-0-		
Communications	$149	$10,249	$10,398
2 telephones @ 28.95 ea/mo × 36 mo	$2,084		
Long-distance service fee @ $50/mo × 36 mo	$1,800		
1 cellular phone @ $60 + $50/mo × 36 mo $60	$1,800		

(continued)

predisposing factors. But a minimum amount of knowledge and skill (why? what? how? when? where?) is necessary before a person can adapt health-related behaviors, whether personal self-care or collective action for community wellness. Self-care skills range from personal wellness behaviors such as weight lifting to accessing health-related resources. Community wellness skills include ranking issues, negotiating, persuading, communicating with the media, networking, coalition building, fund-

TABLE 4.2   *(continued)*

		Requested	Donated	Total
1 beeper, setup fee, 1 mo service @ $89 + $7/mo × 35 mo	$89	$245		
Internet service fee @ $20/mo × 36 mo		$720		
Postage $1,200/yr × 3 yr		$3,600		
	$149	$10,249		
Travel			$48,360	-0-	$48,360
Year 1: 9 staff @ 200 mi/mo × 12 mo × $0.325/mi +				
Year 2: 19 staff @ 200 mi/mo × 12 mo × $0.325/mi +				
Year 3: 34 staff @ 200 mi/mo × 12 mo × $0.325/mi	$48,360			
	$48,360	-0-		
Other Costs			$16,296	-0-	$16,296
Liability insurance @ $1,924/yr × 3 persons	$5,772			
20 Wellness Scholarships @ $150 ea × 3 yr	$9,000			
4 software licenses @ $127 × 3 yr	$1,524			
	$16,296	-0-		

Note: From *Shedding Pounds . . . Adding Years* (pp. 16–18), by N. Bilodeau, A. Collins and N. Hussey, 1999, Medical University of South Carolina, Charleston. Revised with permission of the authors.

raising, and other social and political skills (Green & Kreuter, 1999).

No doubt you have heard that it is critical to adhere to the principles of adult learning (Knowles, 1970, 1973) in conducting health education. Norman (1999) has challenged Knowles' theory of adult learning, asserting that the principles are untested self-evident axioms and suggesting that Knowles' characteristics of adult learners can be attributed to their busy lives. Norman cautions against leaving mastery of core knowledge to chance—even self-directed adult learners need guidance in setting objectives and evaluating of their learning. In Norman's final analysis, adherence to the principles of adult learning results in a student-centered versus teacher-centered process. See Box 4.2 for principles of teaching and learning in designing educational programs for adults.

Community Organization

As an approach to health promotion, community organization engages a group or community in deliberate, collective action intended to change the distribution of community resources or the sociopolitical environment for health, enabling the community to increase control over the determinants of their health (Rissel, 1994). In the PRECEDE-PROCEED Model, this concerns increasing availability and accessibility to health-related resources and advo-

TABLE 4.3   Health Promotion Approaches by Modifiable Determinants

	Health Promotion Approaches	
Modifiable Determinants	Type of Approach	Examples
Predisposing factors: knowledge, attitudes, beliefs, values, perceptions, self-confidence	Health education: direct communication to public, clients, employees, students, etc.	Exportable Wellness Package: teaching groups or counseling individuals on positive nutrition; Increased Health Awareness through Action: multimedia campaign, "5 a Day"
Reinforcing factors: family, peers, teachers, employers, health care providers, staff, community leaders, decision makers	Health education: indirect communication through in-service, supervision, consultation, feedback	Master Health Advocate: train-the-trainer course prepares nonprofessional community volunteers as a liaison between on-site Exportable Wellness Package and professional resources for healthy lifestyles in the community
Enabling factors: health-related, political, and social action skills; availability, accessibility of resources; community, government commitment to health	Health education: skills training for clients, staff Community organization: collective social or political action to change policy, regulatory provision, and organizational arrangements	Exportable Wellness Package: teaching aerobic exercise, weight lifting, reading food labels, and measuring food portions Fitness Scholarships: Members of the coalition influenced hospital policy change for 20 low-income residents per year

Note: Compiled from *Health Promotion Planning* (3rd ed., pp. 29, 41, and 156), by L. W. Green and M. W. Kreuter, 1999, Mountain View, CA; and *Shedding Pounds . . . Adding Years* (pp. 9–10), by N. Bilodeau, A. Collins, and N. Hussey, 1999, Medical University of South Carolina, Charleston.

cating organizational policies or legislation to promote community wellness.

Media for Engaging the Target Population

Your final decision related to program design is the selection of media for engaging your target population in health promotion. No one medium is better than another, and many times a combination of different media is needed to modify distinct predisposing, reinforcing, and enabling factors. Table 4.4 lists the different types of media for engaging people in health promotion, describes their corresponding target populations, and identifies the general purpose for which each medium can be used.

Fit & Fun Carnival: Engaging the Target Population Via a Single Medium

A special event is a single medium designed to create public awareness of a problem or

Box 4.2 Teaching Tips

Principles of Teaching and Learning in Adult Education

- Facilitate student identification of learning issues and selection of learning resources
- Exploit adult learners' previous experiences as learning resources
- Adjust presentation of learning resources to the learners' level of experience
- Design problem-based learning experiences
- Facilitate application of new knowledge and skills to learners' immediate experience
- Foster shared responsibility for mutual inquiry through organizational arrangements
- Ensure recurring experiences of success
- Provide feedback about achievement of objectives at periodic intervals
- Guide student self-evaluation
- Facilitate cooperative learning skills and group process
- Arrange for a comfortable physical environment conducive to interaction with and among learners

Note: Adapted from *The Modern Practice of Adult Education: Andragogy vs. Pedagogy* (pp. 52–53), by M. Knowles, 1970, New York: Association Press.

program and usually includes incentives for attendance such as celebrity appearances and drawings for prizes. For example, a special event was used in the mythical town of Blue River, to increase the awareness among elementary school families of the benefits of physical fitness and to enable changes in exercise behavior among children and their parents. This Fit & Fun Carnival combined physical-fitness education and skills training with fun and entertainment to provide an incentive for children and their parents to participate in the 2-day health-promotion program. The well-publicized appearance of Kerri Strug, 1996 Olympic gold-medal gymnast, attracted nearly 80% of Blue River elementary school students and their families. Admission to the Fit & Fun Carnival and its activities was free, but tickets to participate had to be earned by attending physical-fitness educa-

tional events, obtaining a fitness evaluation, and participating in fitness training sessions for a variety of age-appropriate aerobic and strength exercises. Children used the tickets to ride a pony, play games, and purchase balloons and sugar-free Popsicles. Drawings were held frequently throughout the day for prizes such as Beanie Babies, Harry Potter books, Pokémon cards, and in-line skates. Adults left the carnival swinging hands with their children, and smiling children left clutching their balloons and prizes. Over the course of the Fit & Fun Carnival, a total of 1,725 people attended; 1,439 children and adults attended educational events and fitness training sessions; 463 children obtained fitness evaluations; and exercise programs were designed by personal trainers for 294 families. The special event provided an alternative approach for motivating elementary school children

TABLE 4.4   **Media for Engagement of Target Population**

	Medium	Target Population	General Purpose
Engagement Via Mass Communication			
Major mass communication	Newspaper Radio Television	Population at large	Predispose behavioral change Public awareness Notification
Minor mass communication	Newsletters Bulletins Notices	Target population defined by their membership in a group	Predispose behavioral change Public awareness Notification
Engagement Via Institutional Intervention			
Behavior-based point of intervention	Restaurant (eating) Tavern (drinking alcohol) Grocery store (buying food) Industry (work practices)	Target population defined by common behavior which occurs at the institution	Predispose behavioral change Information dissemination Enable behavior change Skill training
Center-based point of intervention	Clinic School/college/ university Fitness center Hairdresser/barber shop	Target population defined by caseload of clients receiving services from professional staff at center	Predispose behavioral change Information dissemination Enable behavior change Skill training Reinforce behavior change Providers, peers
Engagement Via Social Network			
Formal social network	Church group Community organization Fraternal organization Neighborhood association Professional association School club	Target population defined by membership in the network	Predispose behavior change Education
Informal social network	Card group Coffee klatch Dads'/moms' night out	Target population defined by participation in network	Predispose behavior change Education
Created social network	E-mail listserv Telephone tree Neighborhood watch group	Target population defined by participation in action alerts	Predispose behavior change Notification Information dissemination

(continued)

TABLE 4.4   *(continued)*

	Medium	Target Population	General Purpose
Engagement Via Special Event			
Special event characterized by guest celebrity, drawings for prizes, or entertainment in addition to health promotion	Cooking contests Health screening Health fair Immunization carnival	Population at large	Predispose behavior change Public awareness Enable behavior change Increased availability and accessibility of health resources

Note: Compiled from "Orchestrating the Points of Community Intervention," by M. A. Preston, T. Baranowski, and J. C. Higginbotham, 1988–1989, *International Quarterly of Community Health Education, 9,* 11–34.

in Blue River toward increasing exercise habits where mass communication and center-based institutional interventions had failed.

"Shedding Pounds . . . Adding Years": Engaging the Target Population Via Multiple Media

"Shedding Pounds . . . Adding Years" is a health promotion program to assist low-income residents in Clarendon County, South Carolina, sustain a healthy lifestyle. The design uses multimedia to reach a wide variety of subpopulations as well as the community at large (Bilodeau et al., 1999):

1. An *Exportable Wellness Package* will engage clients through formal social networks such as church groups and other community organizations to provide health education, health screening, counseling, and referral, tailored to meet each group's goals, reached in partnership with an indigenous master health advocate.

2. The *Fitness Scholarships* program will engage 20 low-income clients per year via a center-based institution, Clarendon Memorial Hospital, where clients will receive personal fitness training in strength building, aerobic exercise, positive nutrition, and stress management from the professional Wellness Center staff.

3. The *Youth Fitness Leadership Program* uses a center-based institution, the school system, to engage middle-school and high-school students in health education related to nutritional and physical fitness and community action for health promotion. Summer camp scholarships will provide an incentive for the community action component, which may be participation in a special event or development of a product or service promoting health in the community.

4. The *Master Health Advocate* train-the-trainer course uses a center-based institution, Clemson University Cooperative Extension Service, to provide skill-training and health education in nutrition, physical fitness, and communication to prepare 30 indigenous, nonprofessional community volunteers over 3 years to be wellness liaisons between the community and professional resources available for healthy lifestyles for the Exportable Wellness Packages.

5. *Increased Health Awareness through Action* uses major mass communication to raise public awareness related to a specific

health issue via a weekly news column and television and radio broadcasts. A speaker's bureau will engage people through formal social networks such as community service organizations and fraternal organizations to predispose people to health-directed behavior.

SUMMARY

An effective health promotion program produces changes in client knowledge, beliefs, behavior, and environmental conditions, which in turn facilitates achievement of the community's desired health outcomes. You can ensure that your health promotion program will be effective by making it part of a community partnership, by focusing on changeable behavioral and environmental causes of health and their determinants, and by making sure that it is culturally congruent. Using the PRECEDE-PROCEED Model for Health Promotion Planning and Evaluation will assist you in choosing the appropriate focus for a health promotion program. Practicing the *Six Steps Toward Cultural Competence* will ensure that the program is acceptable to your clients. The approach to health promotion that you choose will depend on the determinants you are targeting for modification or wish to strengthen. Engaging your target population may require a combination of different media to modify distinct predisposing, reinforcing, and enabling factors. Your role as a community activist in planning and conducting health promotion programs is to facilitate the community in increasing control over its health.

REFERENCES

Advisory Committee on Interpreter Standards, Working Group. (1998, September). *Profes-*sional interpreter standards, training, and skill assessment (Draft) [Online]. Available: http://www.crosshealth.com/download. htm [1999, October 29].

Bilodeau, N., Collins, A., & Hussey, N. (1999). *Shedding pounds . . . adding years: Obesity as a risk factor for chronic disease in Clarendon County, South Carolina.* Unpublished master's scholarly product, Medical University of South Carolina, College of Nursing, Charleston, SC.

Downing, B. T. (n.d.). *Guidelines for working with interpreters.* (Available from The Center for Cross-Cultural Health, Suite W227, 410 Church Street SE, Minneapolis, MN 55455)

First International Conference on Health Promotion. (1986). The Ottawa charter for health promotion. *Health Promotion, 1*(4), i–v.

Gilpatrick, E. (1989). *Grants for nonprofit organizations: A guide to funding and grant writing.* New York: Praeger.

Green, L. W., & Kreuter, M. W. (1999). *Health promotion planning: An educational and ecological approach* (3rd ed.). Mountain View, CA: Mayfield.

Institute of Health Promotion Research, University of British Columbia. (1999, October 25). *Published applications of the precede model* [Online]. Available: http://www.ihpr.ubc. ca/preapps.html

Knowles, M. (1970). *The modern practice of adult education: Andragogy vs. pedagogy.* New York: Association Press.

Knowles, M. (1973). *The adult learner: A neglected species.* Houston, TX: Gulf Publishing.

Leininger, M. M. (1997). Overview of the theory of culture care with the ethnonursing research method. *Journal of Transcultural Nursing, 8*(2), 32–52.

Leininger, M. M. (1999). What is transcultural nursing and culturally competent care? *Journal of Transcultural Nursing, 10*(1), 9.

Meleis, A. I. (1999). Culturally competent care. *Journal of Transcultural Nursing, 10*(1), 12.

Minnesota Department of Health, Refugee Health Program. (1996, October). *Translated health education resources: A listing of distributors of translated materials.* (Available from The Center for Cross-Cultural Health, Suite W227, 410 Church Street SE, Minneapolis, MN 55455)

Minnesota Public Health Association, Immigrant Health Task Force. (1996, August). *Six steps toward cultural competence: How to meet the health care needs of immigrants and refugees.* (Available from The Center for Cross-Cultural Health, Suite W227, 410 Church Street SE, Minneapolis, MN 55455)

Multi-Cultural Educational Services. (1999, September 2). *Health education materials store* [Online]. Available: http://www.mced services.com//qothe.html [1999, October 29].

Norman, G. R. (1999). The adult learner: A mythical species. *Academic Medicine, 74*(8), 886–889.

Powell-Griner, E., Anderson, J. E., & Murphy, W. (1997). State- and sex-specific prevalence of selected characteristics— Behavioral risk factor surveillance system, 1994 and 1995. *MMWR Surveillance Summaries* [Online], *46*(SS-03). Available: http://www.cdc.gov/epo/mmwr/preview/mmwrhtml/00048737.htm [1999, October 22].

Preston, M. A., Baranowski, T., & Higginbotham, J. C. (1988–1989). Orchestrating the points of community intervention. *International Quarterly of Community Health Education, 9*, 11–34.

Rabinowitz, P., Berkowitz, B., & Brownlee, T. J. (1999, June 13). Planning and writing an annual budget. In University of Kansas, *Community toolbox, Part I: Generating and managing resources for the initiative* (Chapter 27, Section 4) [Online]. Available: http://ctb.lsi.ukans.edu/tools/c27/C27s4.html [1999, November 1].

Rissel, C. (1994). Empowerment: The holy grail of health promotion? *Health Promotion International, 9*(1), 34–47.

Sellers, S. C., Poduska, M. D., Propp, L. H., & White, S. I. (1999). The health care meanings, values, and practices of Anglo-American males in the rural Midwest. *Journal of Transcultural Nursing, 10*(4), 320–330.

U.S. Public Health Service, Clinical Management Branch, Region IV. (n.d.). *Health planning, program development and evaluation.* Atlanta: Author.

United Way. (1996). *Tri-county needs assessment of Sumter, Clarendon and Lee Counties.* Unpublished manuscript.

University of Minnesota, Community Interpreter Training Program. (n.d.). *Code of ethics for interpreters.* (Available from The Center for Cross-Cultural Health, Suite W227, 410 Church Street SE, Minneapolis, MN 55455)

CHAPTER 5

Community Mobilization and Participation

Carl O. Helvie

This chapter will define selected terms that are important in community mobilization/participation, discuss process of community change and community mobilization/participation, describe the multilevel intervention model, and specify ways to gain community participation.

DEFINING COMMUNITY

A *community* can be a population within a specific time and place. A *place* can be a political subdivision, a geographical area or other boundary concepts and in practice may be a total community, a census tract, school, or industrial setting. A *time period* (interval or point in time) when coupled with statistical concepts will allow evaluation of the incidence and prevalence of diseases or health concerns and population characteristics at a point in time or changes in health factors over time in the identified place. This is the definition of community most frequently used in practice. The specific community focus should be identified (total, census tract, school, industry) before any process to improve community health begins.

A second definition of community is the demographic definition and involves viewing the community as subgroups of the population such as age, sex, social class, or race. In practice, immunization rates may be assessed in relation to age groups, or an epidemic of sexually transmitted diseases may be assessed in relation to social classes, race, and age in order to determine where priorities of service should be provided. This definition of community is often coupled with the previous definition of time and place and adds information to the assessment of the community for planning purposes.

A third way to view community is as a system that exchanges internally and externally and must continually adapt to these exchanges. Adaptation may move the community toward or away from a healthy balance. This concept of community is developed in detail by Helvie (1991, 1998).

Another important definition is community-based versus community-focused. The American Nurses Association (1995) defines community-based care as care provided outside the institution. This can be either population- or individual-focused. Examples of individual or group-focused community-based care is that provided by nurse practitioners, health maintenance organizations, and home health agencies. On the other hand, population- or community-focused care is based upon an assessment of the population and taking actions to gain participation of all people who would benefit from the services. A further discussion of this concept will be found in Helvie (1998).

DEFINING COMMUNITY MOBILIZATION

To *mobilize* is "to assemble, organize"; "to adapt or organize;" "to render mobile, put into motion, circulation, or active use" (American College Dictionary, 1953). It is believed that this concept places the credit and power to bring about change (social planning model) in the hands of the practitioner rather than the community population. There is more emphasis now on community participation (locality development model), a model that incorporates such processes as democratic procedures, voluntary cooperation, self-help, development of indigenous leadership, and education. In actual practice there is usually a combination of the two models—locality development and social planning. A further discussion of these models, and related concepts and roles appears below.

DEFINING COMMUNITY PARTICIPATION

Community participation is defined as "non-professional involvement in health-care service delivery, policy decisions, and program development" (Zimmerman, 1990) and "the social process of taking part voluntarily in formal and informal activities, programs, and/or discussions to bring about planned change or improvement in community life, services, and resources" (Bracht, 1990). This chapter focuses on ways to gain maximum community participation (citizens, organizations, professionals) that will bring about the greatest change to benefit the community. It also focuses on ways to mobilize a community to reach the most people with interventions when using the social planning model.

THE PROCESS OF COMMUNITY CHANGE

The process for introducing change into a community involves community participation at various stages. Some authors believe that community members should be involved from the assessment stage onward. Others believe that community members should be involved following data collection, but before planning, intervention, and evaluation begin. Others use community members to implement a plan developed by the practitioner (social planning model).

Assessment

Community change that moves a population to a more healthy level must be based on a thorough assessment of the problems and needs of the community. The process and resources for completing a community assessment are discussed in detail and their application with a community is presented in Helvie (1998). Some authors involve community members in this step. Usually the citizen, organization, and professional members who are selected are influential leaders in social, political, religious, and other organizations. They provide input on health problems identified by their constituency.

Planning for Community Change

After community health problems have been identified, planning to correct the problems is the next important step. This involves making a community diagnosis, setting priorities, establishing goals and objectives for the identified problems, and considering alternative ways to meet goals.

Community Diagnosis

Different approaches are used for writing community diagnoses. At the least, they should include the problem or condition and the causal factors related to the problem. The problem needs to be identified, and unless the causal factors are related it is difficult to plan a solution. For example, if the community problem is high infant mortality, causal factors should be identified to direct interventions. A causal factor for the problem of high infant mortality might be inaccessible services and resources. A diagnosis also frequently includes a statement that indicates the size or duration of the problem, such as 75% of all delivering mothers lack awareness of health promotion activities.

Community diagnosis may be specific to a particular theory. For the energy theory based upon systems, Helvie (1998) developed a specific format for community diagnosis related to that theory, which is as follows: "There is a community energy balance or deficit (identifies how well the community is dealing with the particular problem) related to (the problem or behavior and community or aggregate affected) due to (community factors that cause the

energy balance or deficit), resulting in (the effect of the balanced or deficit energies on the population)." For example, a diagnosis for an increase in measles in a school using this format would be: "An energy deficit related to a high and increasing rate of measles among children in Santos School due to (a) inadequate funding for health personnel and (b) inadequate information of immunization and prevention, resulting in a measles rate in the school of 9.2% in 1998 compared to 4.2% in 1993 and 5.0% in the state and 5.2% for the nation" (Helvie, 1998, p. 47). This diagnosis provides direction for reducing the rate of measles because the "due to" becomes the basis for the interventions and the "resulting in" can be used for evaluating the interventions. Thus, interventions would be directed toward implementing efforts to prevent the spread of the disease in the school, to teaching care of the sick child and how the disease is spread, and to making resources available for preventive and curative care. Examples of methods for teaching might include flyers sent to parents on care and prevention, spot announcements on television, and articles in the newspapers.

Priority Setting

After the diagnoses have been written, they must be prioritized because there are never enough resources, money, time, or personnel to deal with all identified problems. Several priority models have been identified. The American Public Health Association (1991) identified five factors to consider when setting priorities. These include: (a) amount of community concern; (b) community resources (time, money, manpower, equipment, supplies) available to deal with the problem; (c) solvability of the problem with current knowledge; (d) the need for special education; and (e) whether additional resources and policies are needed.

Yura and Walsh (1988) suggest a model of high, medium and low priority. Hanlon suggests a community-focused model that has elements similar to the APHA model (Pickett & Hanlon, 1990). These include: (a) the size of the problem identified (usually the larger the problem the higher the priority); (b) the severity of the disease (the more severe the problem the higher the priority and in combination, for example, a common cold may affect more but is less severe that tuberculosis which would become the priority); (c) sufficient scientific knowledge and techniques to treat and prevent increases the priority; (d) the availability of resources to carry out the program; and (e) readiness of the population for the proposed program. Pickett and Hanlon developed a formula that can be used with these factors to establish priorities of community diagnoses.

Goals and Objectives

Goals are broad guidelines and do not indicate the way to achieve the desired outcome (McKenzie & Jurs, 1993). Achieving the desired outcome is the function of the objectives that are guided by the goals. At the community level, state your goal in terms of reducing the incidence of high-risk behaviors or increasing the percentage of the population who practice a particular health activity at a particular time and place. "Reducing the level of stroke in all people in a specified census tract" would be an example of a goal for a census tract in a community where stroke levels are high because the population lacks knowledge of the importance of reducing obesity and alcohol and salt intake and is unaware of available resources.

Objectives identify the "how to" part of carrying out the goal and describe the behavior or change needed to meet the goal. Objectives have four components, which are: (a) the particular client (aggregate or community); (b) an activity to meet the goal; (c) a time frame for the accomplishment of the activity; and (d) a standard. A standard represents the proportion of the population who will accomplish the activity. An example of an objective to meet the goal of reducing strokes would be: 90% of the obese population in the identified census tract will reduce salt and alcohol intake and be provided with weight-loss information by January 1, 2001. (It is helpful for evaluation purposes to provide a specific number of the population that will be helped.)

Program Evaluation and Review Technique

When planning will be carried out over a long period of time, it is helpful to break down objectives into sub-objectives and place them on a time axis along with the planned activities related to each. The critical path in this network is the longest path in terms of time. Called a PERT chart it allows the planner to evaluate progress at each stage. For example, the objective of stroke reduction for 90% of all people in the census tract by January 1, 2001 was identified. If resources (facilities, equipment, personnel) are unavailable to carry out the activity, this will make up one set of sub-objectives with time periods for each. For example, obtaining facilities might take one year. A second set of objectives might be to advertise, hire, and train personnel, and a third would involve making the public aware of the program. Other objectives would be identified and the one that is going to take longest would be the critical path.

Alternative Actions to Meet Goals

There are many ways to reach a goal. Most of the data related to these alternatives will be found in the assessment stage when comprehensive data is collected. Some questions that might be considered before selecting the best actions for the goal of stroke reduction in a census tract include: (a) Are adequate facilities available? (b) Are the facilities conveniently located? (c) Are they in use? (d) Do people know about the services? (e) Do they value the services? (f) Can they pay for the services? and (g) Can they obtain education and treatment from private physicians or should a special program be developed? Answers to these questions will lead to further questions. For example, if facilities are available but underutilized because the community is uninformed about the services and the need for them, education could be provided on television or radio programs, in programs in the community, by meetings of key people with community groups in the identified census tract, or by telephone calls or door-to-door visits by volunteers. The best one should be selected from these and other alternatives.

Interventions

There are three major approaches to intervention in a community to improve health. These include: (a) working with the community or high risk aggregates; (b) working with other subsystems of the community on behalf of the population; and (c) working with the environment to influence the health of the population. The emphasis of all approaches is to improve the health of the population by increasing the resistance of the population or by making the environment (including disease agents) more favorable for increasing population health.

An example of interventions using the first approach would be teaching a group of obese adolescent teenagers about diet, exercise, and behavior modification to re-

duce weight and possibly prevent cardiovascular diseases, arthritis, and other weight-related chronic illnesses. An example of working with other community subsystems to improve the health of the population would be providing health information on the radio and television or writing articles for the newspaper (communication subsystem); working to produce change in health practices through the political process (political subsystem); or working to increase hours of recreational facilities to accommodate the population (recreation subsystem). Alerting environmental health personnel about rat-infested areas in a community or about neighborhood water sources that harbor mosquitos and working with them to eliminate the problem are examples of working with the environment. An additional example would be tracing the source of lead after many children in a neighborhood have been affected and arranging for eliminating the source to protect other children.

Community Participation During This Process

Community participation may take place at any point in this process and is useful during the assessment phase for identifying health concerns that are of importance to the segments of the population represented. Members of the community can also help determine the best way to validate data. For example, additional data to validate utilization of health services findings may be necessary. Community participants may help to develop questionnaires or surveys that are culturally or socially sensitive in order to gain additional information from segments of the population.

During the planning phase, community participants may assist in developing interventions that are culturally sensitive. They are also useful in identifying times and places where interventions may most effectively take place for selected segments of the population. Using community participants to present data on the intervention or as examples of those who subscribe to the intervention may be effective in gaining community acceptance. For example, if I see that my neighbor carries out a certain health behavior, I may be more likely to try it, or if my neighbor presents information on television about health behavior, I may also be more likely to try it. Thus, community participation may be effective at any step in the process of assessing, planning, and implementing community care if the focus is on bringing about community change in health behavior.

COMMUNITY PARTICIPATION OR MOBILIZATION

At times community participation may be solicited by practitioners in order to assist them in developing their skills or to empower members of the community so they become more self-sufficient in health matters in the future. This is the core of the locality-development model of community development and often the focus is on empowerment of the community.

Community Development Models

Although community mobilization and community participation have been mentioned, not all community development models involve community participation. All models involve community mobilization, however, because they have the goal of bringing about change in the community. This change may be from within (locality development) or from without (social planning).

There are three models for bringing about community change: locality development, social planning, and social action. The locality development model is also called the *community development model*. The United Nations defined community development as "a process designed to improve conditions of economic and social progress for the whole community with its active participation and the fullest possible reliance on the community's initiative." This model is based on the assumption that a local people should be involved in goal setting and in the implementation of community change. Democratic processes, voluntary cooperation, self-help, development of indigenous leadership, and education are major themes of this model development. In this approach the community members are actively involved throughout the process of assessing, planning, implementing, and evaluating. This approach both strengthens the leadership skills of the participants and increases the probability of success for the interventions or changes that are planned for the community.

The *social planning model* emphasizes a technical approach to solving social problems in a community. In this model, an expert planner (the practitioner) uses technical abilities and skills to bring about change in the community. The practitioner establishes, arranges, and delivers services to people who need them. People may be mobilized in order to reach the largest number in the community with the interventions. This model involves gaining compliance or participation of the population during the intervention phase in order to introduce the greatest community change that has been planned by the practitioner (social planning model). Concepts useful in this approach are institutionalization and diffusion theory, which will be discussed later in this chapter.

The *social action model* assumes that the disadvantaged aggregate needs to be organized in order to make demands on the larger society to increase resources or treatment more in accord with social justice or democracy. Practitioners push for change in major institutions or community practices and for a redistribution of power, resources, community decision-making, or policy changes in formal organizations. Civil rights groups such as the National Association for the Advancement of Colored People (NAACP), Congress of Racial Equality (CORE), and Southern Christian Leadership Conference (SCLC) are examples of groups who have used this approach.

SOCIAL PLANNING APPROACH

Diffusion theory and institutionalization are two important aspects for involving the community in an intervention when using the social planning approach for community change.

Diffusion Theory

Diffusion theory involves reaching the most people with community interventions. It is defined as "the process by which an innovation is communicated through certain channels over time among members of a social system" (Rogers, 1983, p. 333). Rogers defines innovation as "an idea, practice, service, or other object that is perceived as new by an individual or other unit of adoption" (p. 11). An example of an innovation adopted by individuals would be the use of seat belts, and a large increase in the use of seat belts when the innovation is introduced means the diffusion was successful. At an organizational level, a large increase in businesses and organizations including fitness programs for employees would indicate diffusion of fitness as an organizational behavioral change.

Diffusion is most effective if individuals, groups, organizations and the total community are targeted concurrently. The methods for doing this may be through the use of mass media, the political process, and organizational structures. The concept of involving individuals, groups, organizations, and the community in a multilevel intervention will be discussed later in this section.

Magnitude and Rapidity of Diffusion

Rogers (1983) identified several attributes that influence diffusion. These include the relative advantage, compatibility, complexity, "trialability," and observability of the innovation. The relative advantage of an innovation refers to its actual or perceived superiority over existing practices or ideas. Aspects of superiority include unique benefits, usefulness, economic factors, convenience, satisfaction, prestige factors, and the time involved. If an innovation is perceived as superior it is more likely to be accepted.

Trialability is the degree to which one can try an innovation on a limited basis. Trying an innovation and diffusion are more likely if it can be tried or experimented with on a limited basis. When innovations demonstrate positive results and generate positive discussions, they are more likely to be adopted and to become more diffused among the population.

The complexity of the innovation is also a factor in its adoption and diffusion. An innovation that is difficult to understand and communicate is less likely to be adopted than one that is less complex.

Other factors include reversibility, risk, cost-effectiveness, and modification (Kolbe & Iverson, 1981). Reversibility is the ease of reversing an innovation with few lasting effects. The easier it is to reverse without discomfort, the greater the likelihood that it will be adopted. Risk refers to the degree of uncertainty in adopting an innovation, and the greater the uncertainty, the less likely it will be adopted. Modification is the ability of the innovation to be updated, and the easier this is, the greater the likelihood that it will be adopted. Cost-effectiveness is the benefit of the innovation over the cost and the greater the perceived benefits the more likely it is to be adopted.

Categories of Innovation Adopters

Green, Gottlieb, and Parcel (1987) found a consistent sequential pattern of adopting innovations throughout a population. Five groups were identified: innovators, early adopters, early majority adopters, late majority adopters, and laggards. *Innovators* take risks and are anxious to try new things. They are able to deal with uncertainty and setbacks such as the loss of financial or other resources and perform a major role in introducing new things into the community.

Early adopters are respected members of the community and serve as role models. Consequently, they are the most effective opinion leaders in the community. Their adopting the innovation and communicating about it will speed adoption throughout the community. They are viewed by others as discrete users of new ideas. *Early majority adopters* are rarely leaders in the community. They are just a step ahead of the majority because they deliberate a long time before adopting the innovation.

Late majority adopters are a step behind the average citizen in adopting innovations. In their case, adoption is a result of pressure from others and economic necessity. *Lag-*

gards are the last members of the community to adopt an innovation. They are traditional and suspicious of new ideas, somewhat isolated from others, and are bound by the past.

Facilitating Innovation Adoption

There are certain things that can be done to facilitate the adoption of innovations. Green et al. (1987) identify interventions related to the five categories of innovation adopters. For example, early adopters respond to a cognitive approach whereas majority adopters respond to a motivational approach, and later adopters respond to efforts to remove environmental, economic, and behavioral barriers to adoption. Parcel, Perry, and Taylor (1989) identify social theory strategies to facilitate adoption such as modeling, incentives, guided imagery, self application of acquired skills, and social contracting.

The majority of people learn about an innovation through *modeling* (Bandura, 1986), that is by observing others use it. Factors that influence the adoption of the innovation through modeling are the characteristics of the model and the ease in understanding the outcome of using the innovation. Incentives may be used in addition to modeling and may be direct, vicarious, or self-produced. *Direct incentives* are external outcomes that result from performing the expected behavior. A *vicarious incentive* is the observation of rewards and punishments that others receive by performing a behavior. A *self-produced incentive* is one set by the individual for performing a particular behavior.

Guided imagery allows a person to practice a behavior in a simulated situation in which fear of failure is minimized. The user may receive feedback and may also observe modeling. *Self-application of acquired skills* is a strategy in which the user practices the behavior in a natural environment without a model and with responsibility for self-monitoring. *Social contracting* involves a written agreement between two or more people to demonstrate a commitment. It usually includes names of the parties involved, behaviors to be performed, goals to be achieved, how goals will be measured, incentives for successful performance, and the signatures of all parties. Additional information on diffusion can be found in Helvie (1998).

MULTILEVEL INTERVENTION MODEL

A useful model for involving the most people in a planned change in a community is the multilevel intervention model developed by Simons-Morton, Simons-Morton, Parcel, and Bunker (1988) and patterned after earlier public health models. The focus of the model is to assist individuals in the community in reducing personal risk factors for disease and concurrently to influence community organizations and local government to reduce environmental factors that contribute to the disease. Thus, interventions maximize the influence on the community population.

Two categories of factors are considered important in community interventions: personal health factors and environmental influences on personal health. Health problems may be influenced by both. Personal factors that can be changed and that are risks for certain diseases include excess weight, dietary choices, smoking, and promiscuous sexual behavior. Environmental factors influence choices about these personal behaviors and may directly influence personal health. For example, environmental influences that may influence smoking

are advertising about the glamour of smoking and the availability of cigarettes in machines. Secondary smoke in restaurants and bingo halls are examples of a direct environmental influence on health.

Personal and environmental factors occur at the individual, organizational, and governmental levels. Personal choices influence personal health behaviors whereas policies and practices of organizations affect the health of employees. Likewise, public actions and policies affect the health of the community. Thus, the intervention model is directed toward these three levels: individuals, organizations, and government. The focus is on reducing the personal risks of diseases in individuals and on influencing organizations and governments to reduce environmental risks and facilitate positive influences on personal health behaviors. Additional information on this model can be found in Helvie (1998) and in Helvie and Nichols (1998).

GAINING COMMUNITY PARTICIPATION

Citizen Participation

Citizen participation was defined earlier in this chapter. Studies show that citizen participation improves community health outcomes and long-term maintenance of programs (Bracht, 1990). Studies also show that health care is delivered more effectively by community health workers who have the confidence of the people, who understand the health needs of the community, and who can be trained in a short time to provide preventive and curative care (World Health Organization, 1978). Citizen participation has produced benefits at the national, community, interpersonal, and individual levels and has resulted in neighborhood and community improvement and feelings of personal and political efficacy (Florin & Wandersman, 1990).

Citizen Involvement in Health Care

Zimmerman (1990) identified some of the ways citizens can be involved in rural areas. These include: 1) providing emergency medical services such as caring for disabled people, screening for diseases, and helping new mothers and others to relieve shortages of personnel; and 2) improving community acceptance of programs by assisting in the tailoring of the program to the particular population. He says citizen participation ranges from the model of decision making to the model of simply delivering services with no authority for decisions.

Factors Influencing Citizen Participation

The following factors influencing citizen participation were identified by Bracht (1990): 1) concern for one's neighborhood; 2) previous leadership position experience; 3) perceived confidence in ability to recruit competent colleagues to support the project; 4) availability of resources to carry out the project; 5) faith in the sponsoring agency; 6) citizen authority that is clearly defined; 7) the citizen's ability to create, sustain, and control an organization that is effective; 8) historical perspective and broad knowledge of the community; 9) early identification and discussion of change barriers in the community; 10) volunteer roles and time commitment that are clearly stated: 11) commitment to locality ownership or partnership by the staff; 12) recognition and/or tangible benefits during the planning process that reinforce citizen participation; 13) timely use of conflict resolution, when needed.

Organization structure may also facilitate citizen participation (Bracht, 1990). Citizens may be involved in: 1) leadership boards or councils; 2) coalitions; 3) lead or official agencies; 4) grass-root organizations; 5) citizen panels; and 6) network or consortia. The author discusses each of these organizational structures and says the successful programs usually utilize parts from several of these.

Task forces comprised of citizens and professionals who report to the community advisory board may also be used. Although these focus on special assignments, members may eventually move from the task force to the community advisory board. Using citizens on task forces increases the amount of community participation and influence.

Identifying Community Members for Participation

A method for identifying community lay leaders was discussed by Michielutte and Beal (1990). Their method was a modified snowball technique in which 10 leaders were contacted and asked to identify 5 additional social, political, religious, business, or less visible leaders. This process continued until no new names were generated. From this list leaders for the study were identified.

Studies on Citizen Participation

Poland, Giblin, Waller, and Hankin (1992) evaluated the effect of using women who had received public assistance (paraprofessionals) in providing prenatal care to low income women. After six weeks of training the women assisted the prenatals with housing, food, health, transportation, and other necessities during home visits. Women were randomly assigned to prenatals or a control group. Women who were visited by the paraprofessionals kept significantly more prenatal appointments, and had infants with higher birth weights than the other group.

Ross, Loening, and Mbele (1987) evaluated the breast feeding behaviors of three groups of women supported by three types of health workers including lay workers. A fourth group received limited support and a fifth received no support. Significant differences were found between groups with the group receiving support from the lay workers being the most effective. The authors concluded that lay workers were effective in providing support during home visits.

Lacey, Turkes, Manfreidi, and Warnecke (1991) evaluated a smoking cessation program among black women in several urban public housing developments using lay health educators. Interventions consisted of televised smoking cessation classes or reminders of smoking cessation by the lay educators. The lay workers were successful in organizing the hard to reach women and in increasing their knowledge about the dangers in smoking and their interest in participating in a structured program for smoking cessation. The authors concluded that lay workers are effective in mobilizing a population to participate in health programs, but new methods should be developed to sustain the involvement of the public.

Mobilizing a community also involves gaining participation of organizations and of professionals in a community. Involvement of these segments of the population will now be discussed.

INVOLVING COMMUNITY ORGANIZATIONS

It is important to involve community organizations in community interventions because they may provide health programs or make environmental changes that coincide with the health interventions planned for the community population. They may also provide access to hard to reach populations such as low-income or minority aggregates. They may also consent to structural or cultural changes that assist in the implementation of health programs. For example, they may make environmental changes such as no smoking policies, removal of cigarette machines, the provision of exercise programs and facilities, and/or the modification of food offered in the cafeteria. This is an especially important population to reach because at least a third of our adult lives are spent at work and there are 127 million people (46% women) in the workplace in the United States (Statistical Abstracts, 1994).

Gaining Participation

Efforts to gain participation of community organization should start early in the community change process. During the assessment stage, community leaders in organizations should be identified and actively involved in assessment and planning by involvement on community boards for community changes. They may also be involved in assessing and planning for change in their own organizations by identifying worker concerns and ways to tailor community interventions to the population of workers.

Some organizations may be more willing than others to be involved. These should be targeted for early inclusion. These include those that are first to adopt new ideas and they may serve as models for others (Rogers & Shoemakers, 1971). Those organizations with a history of promoting health and making environmental changes or that have high profile in the community such as large work-sites should also be targeted.

When encouraging work-sites to participate in health programs: 1) point out the
advantages of assisting in the adoption of
the health program; and 2) identify and
remove barriers to the program. Advantages of programs from the employer point
of view include: 1) better employee morale
and productivity; 2) possible decrease in
health care costs; and 3) improved ability
to recruit and retain employees. Employer
barriers may include: 1) resistance to
change; 2) costs; and 3) concerns about
consequence of participating. Employees
may also see advantages. These include better access to care; decreased cost of care;
and environmental and social support for
changing behavior. Disadvantages for an
employee point of view include issues of
confidentiality; perceived interference of
company in personal life; and diverting of
company's attention from other important
issues (Bracht, 1990).

Organizational Interventions

Successful worksite interventions use multiple interventions directed toward employees in various stages of changing behavior
such as those who want to quit smoking,
those who have decided to quit, and those
who have quit and are afraid to backslide.
Basic interventions include motivation and
incentive; education; and environmental
change and social support. *Motivation and
incentive interventions* motivate employees to
attempt behavioral changes such as trying
new diets, starting an exercise regime or
maintaining behaviors newly started. Moti-
vations may include incentives or awards,
contests with an organization or between
organizations. Behavioral change programs such as smoking cessation, weight
loss, and exercise programs have used
these approaches.

Education provides tools for employees
to use in changing behavior. Methods that

have been effective include television or
movie presentations, pamphlets, and book-
lets. Counseling and social support used in
conjunction with these programs have been
found to increase success.

Environmental changes that restructure
the environment include smoke free environments, removing junk food and cigarette machines; and improving the food
offered in the cafeteria. The social environment may offer support for individual
behavioral changes from co-workers, supe-
riors, or family members.

Long-term behavioral changes require
ongoing educational programs and incentives that help members maintain the new
behaviors and assist other employees who
wish to make changes. Thus, there should
be periodic repeat programs for the population.

Health Interventions Reported in Organizations

Stunkard, Cohen, and Felix (1989) evaluated weight loss competition at worksites in
three studies. Team competition was more
effective than cooperation or individual
competition for men, and more effective
than individual competition for women in
the first study. Ten worksites were used in
the second study to replicate the first. Four
influencing variables were evaluated including: 1) age, sex, employment type; 2)
blue collar vs. white collar; 3) method of
assignment of team; on 4) outcomes (recruiting, attrition; weight loss; and cost-effectiveness. The authors reported that in
this study there was high recruitment, low
attrition, a large weight loss, and a favorable
cost effectiveness. The third study was a
follow up of this study and the authors reported only a limited maintenance of
weight loss over time.

Shipley, Orleans, Wilbur, Piserchia, and
McFadden (1988) evaluated a two-year

smoking cessation program at seven work-sites. Four companies offering the Live for Life program were compared with three companies that offered only annual health screening assessments. Just over 26% of the smokers quit in the Live for life program compared to just over 17% in the other companies. The authors concluded that smoking cessation programs can be effective in organizations.

GAINING PARTICIPATION AMONG PROFESSIONALS IN THE COMMUNITY

The involvement of professionals in a community health program is also important. Health professionals may assist in community wide acceptance of the program or the integration of the program into different organizations. They may also provide information on community health care practices or community health facilities and may assist in introducing structural changes into the organizations for which they work.

Health professionals may be invited to participate in boards or committees that oversee the program. Professionals should be identified during the assessment stage and should be from various health disciplines and various types of health care institutions. Health professionals can interpret health care practices in the community and in organizations, offer advice to committee members on health care, and can interpret and implement the program in their own institution.

An important aspect of some planned community changes may be to educate health professionals. Many states require continuing education of health professionals and the new program and needed skills may be offered by this method with continuing education units being given for atten-dance. A second way of involving professionals may be through presentations at professional societies.

Community participation is important to help the community members become self sufficient in health matters using a locality development approach. Likewise, mobilization of the community to bring about changes in health behavior after an assessment has been completed (social action approach) may involve citizens, organizations, and professional participation.

REFERENCES

American Public Health Association. (1991). *Healthy Communities 2000—Model Standards: Guideline for community attainment of the year 2000 national objectives.* Washington, DC: Author.

Bandura, A. (1986). *Social foundations of thought and action.* Englewood Cliffs, NJ: Prentice-Hall.

Barnhart, C. (1953). *The American College Dictionary.* New York: Harper and Row.

Bracht, N. (1990). *Health promotion at the community level.* Newbury Park, CA: Sage.

Florin, P., & Wandersman, A. (1990). An introduction to citizen participation, voluntary organizations, and community development: Insights for empowerment through research. *American Journal of Community Psychology, 18*(1), 41–54.

Green, L. W., Gottlieb, N., & Parcel, G. (1987). Diffusion theory extended and applied. In W. B. Ward (Ed.), *Advances in health education and promotion.* New York: Plenum.

Helvie, C. (1998). *Advanced practice nursing in the community.* Thousand Oaks, CA: Sage.

Helvie, C., & Nichols, B. (1998). Reconceptualization of community health nursing clinicals for undergraduate students. *Public Health Nursing, 15*(1), 60–64.

Kolbe, L. J., & Iverson, D. C. (1981). Implementing comprehensive school health education: Educational innovations and social change. *Health Education Quarterly, 8,* 57–80.

McKenzie, J., & Jurs, J. (1993). *Planning, implementing, and evaluating health promotion programs: A primer.* Philadelphia: W. B. Saunders.

Michielutte, R., & Beal, P. (1990). Identification of community leadership in the development of public health education programs. *Journal of Community Health, 17*(1), 59–68.

Parcel, G., Perry, C., & Taylor, W. (1990). Beyond demonstration: Diffusion of health promotion innovations. In N. Bracht (Ed.), *Health promotion at the community level.* Newbury Park, CA.: Sage.

Pickett, G., & Hanlon, J. (1990). *Public health administration and practice* (9th ed.). St. Louis, MO: Time Mirror/Mosby.

Rogers, E. M. (1983). *Diffusion of innovations* (3rd ed.). New York: Free Press.

Simons-Morton, D., Simons-Morton, B., Parcel, G., & Bunker, J. (1988). Influencing personal and environmental conditions for community health: A multilevel intervention model. *Family and Community Health, 11*(2), 25–35.

Stunkard, A., Cohen, R., & Felix, M. (1989). Weight loss comparisons at the worksite: How they work and how well. *Preventive Medicine, 18,* 460–474.

United Nations, International Children's Emergency Fund Health Organization Joint Committee on Health Policy. (1981). *Community involvement in decision making for primary care.* Geneva, Switzerland: Author.

World Health Organization. (1978). *Alma-Alta 1978 primary health care.* Geneva, Switzerland: Author.

Yura, H., & Walsh, M. (1988). *The nursing process* (5th ed.). Norwalk, CT: Appleton & Lange.

Zimmerman, M. (1990). Citizen participation in rural health: A promised resource. *Journal of Public Health Policy,* 323–340.

CHAPTER 6

Marketing Community Health Promotion Programs

Carolyn Chambers Clark

MARKETING DEFINED

One definition of marketing is that it includes the exchange of activities (goods, products, programs, or services) to satisfy client needs. Marketing is more than that. *Marketing* encompasses everything you do to bring your service to the community— from the name you choose to the design of your letterhead and the words you or your receptionist use to answer your phone. It includes the name you give a community workshop, the conceptual framework you work from, and how you provide services (Gerson, 1989; Gombeski, 1998; Dever, 1991).

The community will choose to work with you (or not) based on the benefits to be gained. Few people will attend a workshop or planning session out of curiosity. They will work with you because they expect a benefit. It is your job to understand what benefits they are looking for and then provide promotional materials that convinces them they will obtain what they desire. You may convene a *focus group* of community representatives or conduct a telephone survey of a random sample to find out what the needs of the targeted community are. If you choose to work with a focus group, see chapter 19 for more information.

Image marketing includes actions taken to improve the image of a program. If a community is opposed to a specific program, adverse publicity can end it. For example, in some communities, an AIDS/HIV prevention program focused on safe sex rather than abstinence can be undermined if individuals distort the message to mean that premarital or extramarital sex is being advocated (Gerson, 1989).

Although perceptions may be inaccurate, you will need to pay attention to what individuals believe because community members act on their perceptions, not on the reality of what is presented. If a program is viewed as serving only a targeted few, you may need to expand your range and serve more of the community. Promoting your program to a larger community may improve an image that has been tarnished.

When done properly, marketing will generate more participants and has the potential to create more money than it costs. Marketing successful health promotion programs involves being an available and flexible provider. You will need to study the community and find a suitable segment of it, then tailor your program to fit that niche ("3 Keys to Successful Promotions," 1996). Suppose you have planned a stress management program that meets twice a week in an adult center. You have already determined convenient times and planned beneficial content. In this case, you are in control. But suppose community participants tell you they can't meet at those times and that they already know the content? In that case, you will have to change the meeting time and content, and the participants will be in control. In either case, client satisfaction will determine whether community members wish to engage in future programs with you.

Likewise, naming programs is important. In a retirement community, "What to Do When Someone You Love Has a Heart Attack" or "Protecting Your Grandchildren with First Aid" will have more appeal than a general first-aid course (Breckon, 1997).

T-shirts, refrigerator magnets, gym bags, posters, water bottles and other products can be used to sell the program to potential clients. These products can also serve as daily reminders to clients to engage in health behaviors and can increase public awareness of your program.

Community health promotion marketing involves the following processes:

1. identifying and satisfying community needs
2. developing new programs and maintaining existing programs and services
3. targeting a specific community
4. developing a mix of strategies to influence community use of services

5. evaluating the effect of strategies on use of services

When developing a market plan, address the following processes: (a) market analysis, (b) competitive analysis, (c) target markets and entry strategies, (d) market positioning techniques, (e) marketing mix, and (f) marketing strategies and tactics (Gerson, 1989).

The following list shows what your community health promotion marketing plans should contain, and is based on information contained in Breckon (1997).

Component	Action
Targeted community	List primary and secondary audiences
Costs	Choose cost-effective ways to reach each segment of the community
Messages	Design them to appeal to your target audience, by tying them into their needs or values (use "cool" and "in control" for teens, e.g.)
Timetable	Ensure sufficient time to attain goals and provide sufficient time for testing and revising of each program with a representative audience

Market Research and Analysis

Market research and analysis helps identify whether the targeted community will be interested in your programs. *Market attractiveness* is based on whether the market is large enough to support your program and whether the program has potential to grow; the number of clients from the targeted community who are aware of and can afford the time or money to participate in your programs; the number of competitors offering similar or related services; and the ease with which you can enter and exit the market.

The demographics, sociographics, and psychographics of your client base will also give you important information. Some of the demographic categories are total population of the program area, rate of change of the population, age/sex distribution, racial/ethnic composition, socioeconomic status, housing information, and fertility patterns. Analyze each of these demographic factors when planning a community health promotion program.

Sociographics and psychographics add sociology and psychology to the demographic analysis and interpret the emotional needs, values, and lifestyles that can lead to wellness. The identification of these patterns makes it possible to predict illness lifestyles and to market wellness programs in geographical areas that could benefit (Gerson, 1989).

The next list contains specific questions to ask in order to complete market research. Answers to these questions will provide you with a useful market analysis to guide your health-promotion efforts.

1. How big is the market for this program?
2. How much will the market for this program grow in the next year or two?
3. What are the demographics (age, income, education, etc.) of the targeted community?
4. What are the emotional needs, lifestyles, and values of the targeted community?
5. What people, places, and things will influence the targeted community to participate in the program?
6. What special time, content, and other considerations must be met

in order to ensure community participation in the program?
7. How will impulse, client needs, cost, and related factors influence program usage?
8. What other factors will lead to success with this community?
9. How interested is the community in this program?
10. Is the community base stable or fluctuating?
11. Are competitors for this targeted community entering or leaving the market?

Competitive/Collaborative Analysis

As a health-promotion provider, you may be aware of other health care professionals who are also marketing to your targeted community. Duplication, overlap, and hurt feelings are only a few of the reactions that can result if you do not do a careful competitive/collaborative analysis. Use the following questions to make a competitive/collaborative analysis (Gerson, 1989).

1. Who are the current providers of programs for the client?
2. What are my strengths and weaknesses in competing for this market?
3. Is there a way to collaborate with the current providers of services?
4. What is the distinctive characteristic of my program that sets it apart from other programs?
5. What short- and long-term trends may affect program usage?
6. How can the program be positioned for the greatest degree of collaboration with competing programs?

Target Market Analysis

Before targeting a segment of the community and providing a health promotion program, you need to complete a target market analysis. Before developing a community health promotion program, find out the answers to the following questions in order to complete that analysis.

1. What is my target market?
2. Which characteristics of the community need to be included in planning a new program?
3. What plans are needed to reach the targeted community to convince them to attend my programs?
4. How can I use focus groups to generate specific messages for my target group? (See "Working with Groups," chapter 19, for more information on focus groups.)
5. What are the most effective times of the year for my program? (Losing weight may seem more desirable just before the swimming suit season or after major holidays, for instance)
6. Who are the most effective message senders and communication channels for my target group?
7. How can I present myself as an expert so people from the targeted community will listen?

(Based on information presented by Breckon [1997], Dever [1991], and Gerson [1989].)

Marketing Mix

The purpose of the marketing mix is to achieve a positive image with the targeted community. Everything in the marketing mix focuses on satisfying community needs. The marketing mix components include the Four *P*s of marketing: product or service, price, place, and promotion. These four factors act in concert for successful marketing. Use the questions that appear in the list below to analyze market mix.

The Four *P*s	Questions
Product or service	How will I determine that the community's needs have been satisfied by my health-promotion program?
Price	What is the value of the service to the community? What are the costs to have the program delivered?
Place	Where will the program be delivered?
Promotion	How can I best inform the targeted community of the existence of the program? (advertising, publicity, public relations, program promotion)

(Based on information presented by Gerson [1989], Dever [1991], Friedman and Altman [1997])

COMMUNICATION FACTOR ANALYSIS

Everything you do to market a community health promotion program involves communication. Identifying, engaging, and convincing the targeted community to collaborate with you involves communication processes. When choosing methods of program promotion, also analyze communication factors. These may greatly affect the success of your community health promotion program. Some of the barriers to success include perceptual distortions of information about the health promotion program, differences in values and attitudes between you and your target community, incorrect or improper use of words to convey specific meanings, and lack of listening on the part of the targeted community. Use Table 6.1 to decide what kind of marketing and communication media to use.

To find out if communication factors may influence your program, investigate perceptual distortions, community values, word useage, and listener skills. Below is a list of questions to ask to analyze communication factors that could influence the success of your program.

Types of Obstacles	Questions to Ask
Perceptual distortions	Have I communicated my message clearly so there is less chance that what I've said will be distorted?
Targeted community values	What values may influence how clients hear messages about my program? What attitudes may influence how clients hear messages about my program?
Proper word usage	What words or symbols should be used or avoided so the messages about my
Listener skills	program are heard? What can I do to ensure that my targeted community listens to my message?

(Based on information presented by the Office of Cancer Communications [1992].)

Decide exactly whom you want to reach. Select a segment of your target by sex, age, ethnic group, values, interests, or financial status. Be sure to pretest your message with your target audience. Some questions to ask people from your target group are:

- What do you like about the message?
- What parts of the message are difficult to understand?
- If you were hearing this message for the first time, would you act on it?
- What other message might be more effective?

Consider asking gatekeepers or community opinion leaders (political leaders or members of parent and teacher groups, activists, law enforcement) to be in your pretest target group. They can help you politically or through their programs ("Launching Effective Media Campaigns," 1988).

TABLE 6.1 Marketing Media Selection Factors

Method	Marketing Objective	Target Group
Face-to-face communication	Present a complex message Trigger or evaluate extensive behavior change; influence both long-term attitudes and behavior change; stimulate trial use or adoption of a new behavior	Low educational level
Mass media communication	Present a simple factual message Motivated to change Short-term change Create awareness or interest or interest in health and level wellness practices reinforce behavior change	High educational level

(Based on information presented by Breckon [1998] and the Office of Cancer Communications [1992].)

If you are planning a large-scale media-based intervention, you may have to spend a great deal of time marketing your program to possible sponsors because you cannot implement it by yourself. Invite a group of interested sponsors to an early organizational meeting. If you don't know whom to invite, call different organizations and businesses and speak with the director of public relations or director of advertising or sales promotion. Be sure to set an agenda for your first meeting and stick to it. Items should focus on a current, serious unmet need in the community. All invited guests should participate in brainstorming and problem-solving sessions. When you involve these community leaders in the design of your program, they will be more involved and enthused and are apt to be more active in implementing the media campaign. Later you can build coalitions by adding sponsors who will also be asked to contribute. Pretest to ensure that the language in your media messages is relevant and is understood by the targeted group (Jason & Salina, 1993).

Advertising Objective	Questions to Ask
Reaching the community	What forms of impersonal advertising might best reach the community? (newspapers, radio, television, magazines, direct mail, brochures, fliers, forms, displays and word-of-mouth)
Engaging the community	What forms of advertising are most likely to engage the community in the program? (Consider reading level, amount of funds individuals might have for health promotion, and type of media used by target community.)
Creating increased demand	What forms of advertising are apt to create an increased demand for my program? (Study ads that attract you and use the same kind of appeal in your ads.)

(Based on information presented by Gerson [1989], Breckon [1997], and Dever [1991].)

ADVERTISING YOUR PROGRAM

Advertising basics includes advertising principles, developing attention-getting ads, collaborating with an agency to develop ads, and choosing forms of media to use. Advertising includes all the ways you present your health promotion program to the targeted community. It is not always possible to determine the direct effects of advertising on community participation in your program. Despite this imprecision, it is important to fulfill two advertising objectives: publicize your program and increase the demand for your program. Use some of the questions below to determine the best forms of advertising for your community health promotion program.

Advertising Principles

When advertising a health promotion program, consider the following principles:

- Develop advertising that is based on client needs not on your own interests.
- Feature only one program per ad.
- Focus ads and circulate them only to the target population.
- Present the program as if you are the first to offer such a service.
- Establish a reputation by placing ads regularly; remember that ads must be seen and read many times before some clients will act on them.
- Be honest and open when describing the program.

• Generate local media coverage by developing a local fact sheet on your program and establishing contact with local media. Start a list of local health and medical reporters, talk-show producers and hosts, public service directors, news assignment editors, health columnists, health care reporters, and community calendar editors.

Provide background information about your program and updates when programs change. Ask public service directors to help raise awareness by airing public service announcements (PSAs) about your program. Tell all media representatives why the story is timely and interesting (newsworthy), local (relates directly to the community), and important (public needs to know this).

Always follow up by telephone after you send a news release (announcement), letter to the editor, query letter (specific story idea), or media advisory (invite media coverage of an event). Fax your news releases to the correct editor by calling first to find out. Include local statistics and quotes from specialists when you can. Develop a press kit about your program including a letter of introduction, fact sheet, source list, calendar of upcoming events, your business card, positive and informative articles or editorials, charts or graphics, brochures and fliers. Send the kits to the reporters and editors you will be contacting so they will have all the information at hand when they cover your program. Box 6.1 shows a press release for a fitness program.

Developing Attention-Getting Ads

You may have a wonderful program, but if no one knows about it clients will not participate. Use the following techniques to develop effective campaigns (Office of Cancer Communications, 1992; Di Lima & Schust, 1997; Friedman & Altman, 1997):

1. Find a slogan that is easily remembered such as Smoke-Free Forever.

2. Try your ads out on a sample of the client population you hope to reach: Ask your sample, "What are the strengths and weaknesses of this ad?"

3. Begin the headline of your ad with the word *Which*: "Which method to stop smoking do you prefer?" or "Which method of losing weight interests you?" Make sure the headline contains a grabber that will get the reader's attention.

4. Write the rest of the ad so that it ties in with the headline. Close your ad with a slogan or phrase that will stick in the reader's head: "Quality programs for 15 years."

5. Avoid making promises you can't keep. Consumers want to hear they can lose weight, get in shape, stop smoking, and control their stress levels. Tell them exactly how you will help them enhance their wellness. Be honest, sincere, and professional, and avoid quick and easy comments. Consumers are smart enough to know that it's not that easy to quit smoking, lose weight and keep it off, get along with family members, reduce stress and do all the wellness actions that result in well-being.

6. Put your program in perspective: (a) the time that is required, (b) the money or payment required, and (c) the effort expended to get the desired reward. Describe the commitment of time that will be required; for instance, "It will take an hour a day for the next 8 weeks to stop smoking, but you will be free from smoking [overeating, stress, haggling with your family] for the rest of your life. This could be the best 8-hour commitment you've ever made."

7. Highlight the benefits of committing to this program in very specific terms:

Box 6.1　Media Release for Shape-up Program

FOR IMMEDIATE RELEASE

"SHAPE UP:" A COMMUNITY HEALTH PROMOTION PROGRAM OPENS

　　"SHAPE UP," a new community fitness program that was named and chosen by residents of Stellburn, FL, begins today. Dr. Ramona Bastion, a health-promotion expert, is the facilitator for the project. Dr. Bastion surveyed the Stellburn community to find out what kinds of programs they wanted. The "Shape Up" program was developed in collaboration with the community to meet their needs. Shape Up will provide an 8-week program that will help participants set their own fitness goals and work with a Shape Up partner to meet them.

　　Dr. Bastion will present a free lecture next Tuesday to describe the program more fully and to answer questions at the Stellburn Community Center, 555 Maple Street in Stellburn. Everyone is welcome and the first 50 attendees will receive a fruit basket compliments of Stan's Fine Produce.

For more information, contact:
Dr. Ramona Bastion
(727) 322-0841
rbast@earthnet.link

END

"We've helped hundreds of people to lose weight and to feel and look better. They're living proof that our program works." Emphasize the rewards of joining the program: "Quitting smoking will help you to be healthier, happier and breathe more easily." If you're not asking consumers to make serious investments in their own wellness, rethink your strategy. A single story of how one community member turned her life around because of your program will sell consumers on your program for a long time.

　　8. Evaluate your ads periodically. Decide if you need to update them. Suppose consumers were coming to your center in the spring and summer, but aren't now that it's late fall. Call a random sampling of consumers to see what's wrong, and ask if they have any suggestions. Go with what they suggest if you can, or make a few home visits to see if it's the cold weather that is dampening their enthusiasm.

Collaborating with an Agency to Develop Ads

If you do not have the in-house capabilities to generate attention-getting ads, think about hiring an advertising agency or collaborating with another provider who does. To find the best fit with another agency, consider the following:

1. What are the advertising skills of the agency's personnel?
2. How well does the agency understand my programs so they can communicate it to the client?
3. What is the agency's past success with ads to this particular market?
4. Does the agency meet deadlines?
5. How well can the agency track the results and impact of their ads?
6. What techniques will they use to communicate with me?

7. How comfortable and satisfied am I with representatives of the agency I'll be working with?

You can communicate an important health promotion message quickly to wide and diverse audiences or to a specific population by developing public service announcements, or PSAs, for radio or television. Local TV or radio stations air PSAs during unsold blocks of advertising time or during station breaks. Contact station managers and public service directors after you've written a few PSAs.

Radio PSAs

Radio PSAs are 10, 20, or 30 seconds long. Be aware that broadcasters generally speak at the rate of 155 words per minute, so gauge your copy based on that:

    10-second PSA = 20–25 words
    15-second PSA = 30–35 words
    20-second PSA = 40–50 words
    30-second PSA = 60–75 words

When writing PSAs for radio, use the following guidelines:

1. Grab the reader's attention immediately and hold it. Your message may have to compete with the distractions of driving, work, study or reading, so it should snap with short, punchy sentences:

   - "Lose weight. It can help you feel better and ward off chronic disease such as heart disease, arthritis, chronic back problems and maybe even some cancers."
   - "Exercise. A good exercise program can relieve stress, help control your weight, and improve your heart and lungs."

2. Speak directly to the listener, using the second person *you*. The first example below switches from second to third person and is difficult to follow, while the second example stays with second person and engages the listener:

   - "Are you trying to stop smoking? Many people think they'll gain weight if they do, but they most don't."
   - "Trying to lose weight? Good for you. You probably won't gain more than a couple of pounds, if you gain any at all."

3. Write for the ear, not the eye. Use words and word combinations that reflect the way you talk. Make sure your PSAs are clear, informal and uncomplicated.

4. Use the present tense and active voice to lend immediacy to your message: "Take action." "Decide now." "Stop smoking."

5. Vary the length of your sentences, creating a pleasant flow or rhythm. Read your PSAs aloud to ensure that too many short sentences do not sound choppy or monotonous.

6. Choose your words carefully for precise meaning, color, clarity, and brevity. Avoid phrases such as "due to the fact that," "in order to," "prior to," and use "because," "to," and "before."

7. Avoid long, rambling sentences, proper names, awkward sounds, and scientific terms. Use short sentences and only essential information.

8. Since ads may be read by someone not familiar with your program, if you must mention someone's name

and it's unusual, spell the words as they are pronounced; e.g., Dr. Lined (pronounced lined) or Dr. Lined (pronounced lin ed).

9. Always mention any addresses or phone numbers at the beginning and end of your message so listeners can jot them down if they miss them the first time.

10. Avoid abbreviations, symbols, cliches, and exaggerations.

11. Use contractions to give the message a conversational tone.

12. Use titles before names such as Dr. Henniman.

13. Spell out fractions, round off numbers and use "about," "nearly," "approximately," and "more than."

Double- or triple-space your typed copy with one PSA per page, making sure not to split words at the end of lines. Include the length of the announcement and the period of time you want the ad used for; for example, "FOR USE July 10–November 11" or "IMMEDIATE TFN" (till further notice). Put the most important information in the first sentence or two in case words must be cut (Office of Cancer Communications, 1992). Box 6.2 is an example of a radio PSA.

Television PSAs

Keep the copy shorter than for radio PSAs (8, 13, 18, or 28 seconds), using 8- or 13-second spots for reminders. By keeping the copy short, you will ensure your spot will not be cut off or mistimed, and that it will fit in any station's program slot. When writing television PSAs, use all the rules for radio, but add sight and sound. Videotapes or slide/announcer copy spots are prepared, delivering action and a soundtrack. They are relatively easy to produce and are low

cost. An announcer reads the copy while 35-mm slides are shown. Treat the visual and spoken material as equal, letting each communicate a clear central message. Use the spoken message to explain and the visual message to set a tone, demonstrate, or emphasize.

These tips for developing PSAs are based on information presented by the Office of Cancer Communications (1992):

1. Repeat the main message as many times as possible.

2. Summarize or repeat the main point or message at the close.

3. Make every word count.

4. Recommend a specific action.

5. Demonstrate the problem, behavior, or skill.

6. Present the facts in a straightforward manner.

7. Use a slogan, theme, music, or sound effects to enhance recall.

8. Use only a few characters.

Box 6.2   Radio PSA

Program Material: Spot announcement

Time: 30 seconds

Log: PSA

Subject: Dieting doesn't work

Use: March 20–July 15

Dieting doesn't work. Almost everyone gains back the weight they've lost plus more. Dieting can also lead to heart, kidney, and back problems. To get all the facts, come to a free lecture given by Dr. Hilda Swenson, health promotion specialist, at the Adult Learning Center, every Tuesday from 5–6 p.m.

9. Superimpose the main point on the screen, reinforcing the main message.
10. Make the message understandable from the visual portrayal alone.
11. Use either a testimonial, demonstration, or slice-of-life format.
12. Use positive, not negative appeals.
13. Make the message and style relevant to the intended audience.
14. Pretest prior to final production.

Box 6.3 will test your creative advertising skills.

Marketing Through a Press Conference

A press conference is the perfect way to provide some dynamic new information about an important health or wellness issue and advertise your program at the same time. Make sure you have at least a week to prepare, and decide where to hold it. Send a letter to the media detailing the purpose of the conference and where and when it will be held. Describe the overall subject of the conference, objectives (if appropriate), and mention that you will answer questions.

Develop a one- or two-page fact sheet that includes descriptive information about the program and any impressive statistics you can find. Make the fact sheet available at the press conference, not before.

Box 6.3   Creative Corner

Develop an ad and a PSA for one of the following programs:

- Domestic violence
- AIDS prevention
- Smoking cessation

Have light refreshments available during the conference. When the press arrives, distribute the fact sheet along with an agenda. Be sure to limit the question-and-answer session to 15–20 minutes, then conclude the conference immediately.

Talk Show Marketing

When participating in a talk show, be sure to prepare a list of the questions you want asked of you, making sure that the last one is important. Backtiming is common, and when there are only a few minutes left the host will usually go to the final question.

Role-play your participation before going to the station. Be familiar with the answers to the questions, but in order to look spontaneous don't memorize them. Call the station in advance and ask what clothes and makeup to wear or watch talk shows and follow their example.

Arrive early at the station to become familiar with the setting and the staff. Smile and make frequent eye contact with the host so you will appear relaxed. Avoid looking down or at your notes unless you quote statistics. Breathe from your abdomen and sit up straight; bad posture is magnified on television. Bring graphics ($9'' \times 14''$ is recommended) with a wide border and good color contrast or use slides. Graphs, logos, addresses, and phone numbers can be written down and given to the studio personnel to be interjected into the interview.

Marketing on the Internet

Seek out electronic bulletin boards and make information about your program available. E-mail related organizations about your program and ask them to make the information available to their members. Consider starting a website and publishing a newsletter related to your program. Be sure to post current program information, upcoming events, learning materials, and other items of interest. Investigate the use of listservs that can permit you to distribute materials to others on the list.

DEVELOPING A MARKET PLAN

A good marketing plan includes specific goals and objectives, target groups, messages, channels, budget, tracking and evaluation, and media selection factors (Breckon, 1997).

Goals and Objectives

Be very clear about what marketing outcomes you desire and then state them in measurable terms. If your goal is to increase attendance over last year's at a weight management program, a specific objective might be to increase the number of community participation by 10%. Develop a consensus with your target community, and then go to work.

Target Groups

Be sure to define your target groups carefully prior to marketing (Gombeski, 1998). For example, if your program is meant to affect hypertension, is your target group community members who have not yet developed hypertension, those who are already being treated for hypertension, or health care practitioners who treat hypertension?

Messages

Determine the beliefs, needs, and orientation of your target group. Once assessed,

these will give you an idea of what marketing messages are needed by your target groups and in what sequence. If obstacles are anticipated, it may be necessary to dispel inaccurate beliefs first.

Many programs use three forms of media to communicate their message: television, radio, and print (newspapers and magazines). But don't underestimate the power of word-of-mouth advertising. Referrals from satisfied participants of current or past programs may be your best source of new clients.

Channels

Determine the communication channels that are used by your target group. If your target group is overweight adults, determine if they read weight loss newsletters, watch television, or listen to the radio. Maybe your marketing message can be placed as an ad in a popular weight-loss newsletter. A story on a local cable television station or during the community segment of local news may be the perfect way to capture your target group's attention.

If your budget is low, choose free or low-cost methods such as community bulletin boards, public service announcements, and fliers. You may find a printer who will donate fliers if you allow the company to put their name, address and phone number on each one.

Budget

Make sure your budget extends over a year so that it will equal the peaks and valleys of media coverage. Also include ideas for fund-raising. There is never enough money available to advertise your programs so budget wisely.

Marketing Evaluation

Monitor your marketing program. Evaluation could be as simple as asking participants, "How did you hear about our stress management program?" or "Did our cable show influence your interest in our weight management program?" Evaluating your efforts is important because it will guide future marketing. If the marketing channels you used were ineffective, they should not be repeated, or at least should be modified based on participant feedback.

A SMALL-SCALE MARKETING CASE STUDY

Janet, a health promotion specialist, asked a target group of members of her community what kind of programs they wanted. She surveyed them through a short check-off list that she had handed out at a health fair she had sponsored a few months earlier. The most popular program was one for getting in shape.

Janet had $250 to spend on promoting a new "Shape Up" community program and decided to place an ad in the local paper for a free lecture. She convinced a local produce stand to provide a small fruit basket in exchange for giving their business card to the first 50 people who came to the lecture. Janet also included a coupon for one free fruit basket in her ad to get people to come to the lecture and sign up for the program. Janet found the free public announcement section in one of the local newspapers and placed an ad in their calendar of events. A friend who was a local printer agreed to print some fliers in exchange for featuring his company name and address at the bottom of the fliers. Janet obtained a list of potential consumers who were interested in fitness from the local YWCA and mailed half of the fliers with a free packet of wildflower seeds in each. She placed the rest of the fliers on the windshields of clients at a

local hospital after obtaining permission from the administration. The flier was good for the printer's business and it saved some of Janet's publicity money, which she used to purchase T-shirts with "Shape Up" printed on the back. She also called local radio and television stations and asked them to mention the free lecture in one of their community announcements and sent them PSAs.

A LARGE SCALE MULTIMEDIA MARKETING PROJECT

The Chicago Lung Association partnered with PruCare HMO and a multimedia prevention program was born. A large-scale media project was developed and implemented without the help of state or federal funds. Voluntary associations, community groups, and for-profit agencies collaborated eagerly because of the enormous publicity their sponsorship would generate. In cooperation with Channel 5, NBC's Chicago affiliate, "Freedom from Smoking in 20 Days" was aired on the evening news. It reached approximately 500,000 viewers during the 10:00 p.m. broadcast. True Value Hardware stores participated in the program by distributing 50,000 self-help smoking cessation manuals. A group of worksite locations also provided biweekly stop-smoking support groups for the 3-week program. At the end of the 3 weeks, 41% had stopped smoking, while only 21% who had used the self-help manuals and television broadcasts had quit. At 1-year followup, smoking cessation rates were similar for both groups (Jason & Salina, 1993).

REFERENCES

Breckon, D. J. (1997). *Managing Health Promotion Programs: Leadership Skills for the 21st Century*. Gaithersburg, MD: Aspen.

Dever, G. E. A. (1991). *Marketing community health: Community health analysis.* Gaithersburg, MD: Aspen.

DiLima, S. N., & Schust, C. (1997). *Publicizing your program.* Community Health Education and Promotion Manual. Gaithersburg, MD: Aspen.

Friedman, R. J., & Altman, P. (1997). *Marketing your seminar: How to design, develop, and market health care seminars.* Sarasota, FL: Professional Resource Press.

Gerson, R. (1989). *Marketing health/fitness services.* Champaign, IL: Human Kinetics Books.

Gombeski, W. R. (1998, December). Better marketing through a principles-based model. *Health Care Leadership Review,* 6.

Jason, L., & Salina, D. (1993). Quality media connections: Another look at successful prevention interventions. *Prevention Forum, 13*(3), 1–8.

Launching effective media campaigns. (1988). *Prevention Forum, 9*(1), 1–2.

Office of Cancer Communications. (1992). *Making health communication programs work: A planner's guide.* (NIH Publication #92-1493.) U.S. Department of Health and Human Services, Public Health Service, National Institute of Health, National Cancer Institute, Washington, DC.

3 keys to successful promotions. (1996). *Health Promotion Practitioner, 5*(4), 3.

CHAPTER 7

Evaluating Community Health Programs

Sandra MacDonald

COMMUNITY SELF ASSESSMENT IN PROGRAM EVALUATION

When working with communities make sure they are involved in all phases of program evaluation, especially the assessment phase. *Community self-assessment* is the process whereby communities identify their own perception of needs and resources. A self-assessment of community strengths and resources can help communities evolve toward a higher level of wellness and promote resilience. Community strengths include such determinants of health as knowledge, coping skills, supportive environments, and education. Other determinants include biology and genetic makeup, childhood development, and health services (Minister of Supply and Services Canada, 1994; Evans, Barer, & Marmor, 1994). Resilience includes being able to avoid negative consequences when faced with adversity. Resilient communities rebound from adversity strengthened and more empowered (see chapter 1). Let a holistic wellness approach to community assessment stimulate you to think about the political, social, and cultural components of health. This in turn

can help you to help the community shape the design, implementation, and evaluation of health- and wellness-promotion programs. Involving communities during the assessment phase of program planning helps to ensure that programs address priority needs.

Ideally, community self-assessment may be initiated by representatives of the community. If that is unlikely, you can promote community self-assessment by approaching community leaders. Either way, community members can be active participants, identifying collective strengths and resources such as the number of community volunteers or existing youth programs or alcohol or drug use in young people. Effective programs are planned to respond to the perceived needs of the community. Box 7.1 outlines some areas to consider when collecting information for community self-assessment.

Stanley and Stein (1998) discussed the importance of gaining commitment for self-assessment by involving community coalitions and community members. Involving community members in the assessment phase provides an opportunity to build

---

Box 7.1 Examples of Community Self-assessment Information

(Think about what is in place **now** and what effect may occur **after** the program and use this form to evaluate change.)

Collect information on:	Now	After

Physical environment

- number of playgrounds
- water and sewage services
- environmental toxins

Social and economic environment

- self-help groups
- access to food banks

Personal health practices

- exercise
- diet
- social support
- spiritual/religious support
- stress management techniques
- environmental sensitivity

Health services

- number of healthy-baby clinics
- prevention programs

Resources in the community

- newspapers
- radio/television

Healthy child development

- immunization rates
- dental health

partnerships. Enhance community member involvement by surveying community leaders and key informants and feeding back the results to those surveyed. Box 7.2 shows examples of community self-assessment information and how it may relate to program evaluation. They can also participate by identifying priority health needs such as dietary management for older adults, violence prevention, or the need to lower rates of smoking.

Community self-assessment involves partnerships with identified communities. Choose a way to partner that supports the community in the self-assessment process and help them to identify priorities for planning, implementing, and evaluating community health promotion programs. Make sure your plan involves community members in all phases of the process from assessment to planning, development, and delivery of services (Glick, Hale, Kulbok, & Shettig, 1996). Involving the community through a self-assessment process is the first step toward identifying priority health promotion issues. When communities assess their own program needs, they feel ownership of the programs and there is an in-crease in positive outcomes (Glick et al., 1996; Kang, 1995). Community self-assessment is based on needs-assessment research and the identification of key community strengths and resilience. Use community self-assessment data to empower the community to make decisions regarding their own health.

Empowering the Community

Involving the community in identifying priorities could be considered a strategy for empowering the community. *Empowerment* can be defined as enabling communities to acquire the knowledge and skills to make informed decisions and allowing communities to make those decisions (Hitchcock, Schubert, & Thomas, 1999). This empowerment strategy could also be considered a form of social marketing. In its broadest sense, marketing includes developing a product to satisfy needs as perceived by the consumer. It also refers to the activities designed to plan, price, promote, and distribute services that will satisfy the consumer. In social marketing, programs or services

---

Box 7.2   Community Self-assessment Information

Key Informants Issues	Community Leaders Issues	Considerations for Program Evaluation
• loneliness in older adults	• social isolation	• grandparenting program reached 100% of older adults
• teen pregnancy	• teens are "bored"	• increased attendance at sponsored community teen events
• drug and alcohol abuse in adults	• Family violence R/T alcohol abuse	• AA group attendance increased

are designed to satisfy the consumer's identified need. See Box 7.3 for an example of marketing to a specific consumer need.

Social marketing refers to applying marketing techniques and concepts to social issues versus products (Lefebrve, 1992). For example, upon completion of a community self-assessment you may find that a need for a health promotion service for women at risk for cervical cancer has been identified by the consumer, the women in the community. Your next step is to offer assistance with planning, promotion, and implementation of a service that will meet that need.

Social marketing techniques include an assessment of the target group's perceived needs to identify priority issues and the feasibility of program implementation. It also involves considering the community as a consumer of services and the health program as the product. For example, a gambling addiction program may involve an educational strategy or group therapy approach depending on the identified needs of the target population. Consumer needs

are the top priority that influence the development of the program, so be sure to query the community for opinions. If you can't survey the entire community, select leaders or key informants. The main concept that can be borrowed from the social marketing approach is that health and wellness programs are developed to meet the needs of the consumer, or in this case the community. As consumers, the communities participate in the decision making about the priority health program, and thus are enabled or empowered to make decisions regarding program development.

Empowering the community involves ensuring its participation in the decision-making process. Ideally, community health professionals should work in partnership with communities. For example, a self-assessment may reveal the need to expand a family counseling program. In response to this, the health board may allocate additional financial resources to the program. The community has identified a need and recognized that a problem exists and also has been involved in the process. Thus, it

---

Box 7.3   Marketing Services for Women Experiencing Menopause

Product: Health Promotion Service	Plan	Promote	Distribute
Women's health education program	• Specific content • Educational strategies • Teaching materials • Budget	Public awareness campaign	Accessible to 100% of eligible women in the community
Self-help initiative	• Train women • Budget	Public awareness campaign	60% of eligible women participate

has been empowered to be involved in making decisions regarding programs in the community.

TYPES OF PROGRAM EVALUATION

Program evaluation is a multidimensional process that can be formative or summative. It can also occur on three levels of accountability: impact, process, and outcome. This section includes formative and summative evaluations as well as discussion of the three levels of accountability.

Formative and Summative

Formative program evaluation is conducted during the implementation phase of the program, and it addresses quality-control issues such as the physical facilities and preparedness of the health educator. It also provides evaluation of the program as you go along, so that you can make changes before you use all your resources only to find that the program was not effective. Box 7.4 provides questions that you might may ask during the formative and summative evaluation process.

Summative program evaluation is conducted at the completion of the program. It involves assessment of results such as changes in behaviors, attitudes, knowledge, or health status indicators. The health status indicators include but are not limited to such indicators as morbidity, mortality, risk behaviors, preventive practices, and sociodemographic statistics. Figure 7.1 shows daily smoking statistics for two fictitious communities that led to the development of a health-promotion program for community X to prevent or reduce smoking in women. This approach may be limited

because it overlooks other aspects such as participant satisfaction or changes in lifestyle. If you were planning a program based on the statistics presented, you would have to take further steps to achieve community involvement. This might include targeting a group of smoking females and their families to assess their need or you may want to explore with key informants whether there are nonsmoking policies in the workplace.

Communities must be viewed as complex networks with various types of leadership, cultures, beliefs, values, and strengths as well as inadequacies (Stoner, Magilvy, & Schultz, 1992). Therefore community health-program evaluation methods must be multidimensional to address the nature of the communities. A multidimensional approach to program evaluation could include using a variety of methods such as surveys, telephone interviews, key informant interviews, and focus groups. These methods are discussed in more detail in methods of evaluation later in this chapter.

Process, Impact, and Outcome

Program evaluation can also occur at one or more of three levels: process, impact, and outcome (see Box 7.5). *Process evaluation* enables the early detection of problems with the implementation of the program and provides a succinct description of the quality of the program (Green & Kretuer, 1999). Identifying problems with process can prevent failure of the program because of a lack of input into the design or content. Peer review is one form of process evaluation that seeks input from experts in the field in order to validate such areas as content and scheduling. In process evaluation, community members' reactions are assessed as well as resources such as staff,

---

Box 7.4   Formative and Summative Evaluation Questions

Formative

Is there adequate lighting?

Are there enough seats, equipment, and materials?

Is the room too cold or too hot?

Does each session have specific objectives?

Is the health professional prepared to address the topic?

Is the content of the program valid?

Is there sufficient time for community input?

Is there a relaxed, collaborative atmosphere?

Did the health professional share leadership with the community?

What other suggestions did the community have to make this process more useful
    to them?

Summative

Did the program meet the set goals and objectives?

Are the participants satisfied with the program?

Did the program achieve what it set out to achieve?

Are the health educators satisfied with the outcome?

Should the program be implemented again?

Does each session have specific objectives?

What was learned from the community that needs to change before offering this
    program again?

---

space, and budget. Process evaluation asks such questions as: Is the budget adequate to implement to program? Are facilities accessible? Has the program been reviewed by experts in the field?

Impact evaluation assesses the immediate effects of the program on participants' knowledge, attitudes, and behaviors. *Outcome evaluation* is the most difficult of the three to measure, and it entails an assessment of the indicators of health status and quality of life that were identified in the early phases of the planning process (Green & Kreuter, 1999). Outcome indicators can include epidemiological statistics such as mortality, morbidity, and disability rates; sociodemographic statistics such as smoking behavior, hunger, unemployment, and homelessness; and wellness indi-

cators such as quality of life and self-evaluation of lifestyle change. Box 7.5 illustrates several components that could be considered when conducting process, impact, and outcome evaluation of a community health promotion program.

PRECEDE-PROCEED FRAMEWORK FOR HEALTH PROGRAM EVALUATION

One way to evaluate health and wellness programs is by using a theoretical framework for planning and evaluation. One such framework is the PRECEDE-PROCEED framework developed by Green and Kreuter (1999). PRECEDE is an acronym for a process that identifies the predispos-

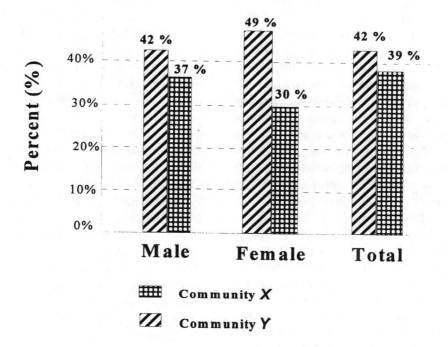

FIGURE 7.1 Daily smoking by gender, community *X* versus community *Y*.

Box 7.5 Levels of Accountability for Program Evaluation		
Process	**Impact**	**Outcomes**
Implementation	**Knowledge** **Attitudes** **Behaviors**	**Health status**
Are facilities adequate and accessible? Educator preparedness? What are attendance rates for participation?	Has knowledge improved? Have behaviors changed? Are attitudes modified?	Have risk behaviors been modified? Are preventive practices enhanced? Have sociodemographic statistics changed, e.g., homelessness?

ing, reinforcing, and enabling causes in program planning and evaluation. PROCEED is an acronym for policy, regulatory, and organizational constructs in educational and environmental development. This nine-phase sequential process can be used to identify major health issues for targeted communities and provide a database for the evaluation of programs. It represents the causal chain that is set in motion by health-promotion programs and directs attention to evaluation outcomes rather than inputs. See chapter 4 for a full description of the framework.

The epidemiological and social diagnosis of the PRECEDE-PROCEED framework lays the foundation for program evaluation. These first two phases document program evaluation indicators such as perceived health status, vital statistics, and determinants of health and are characterized by multiple information-gathering activities. These indicators then can be used to evaluate the efficiency and effectiveness of the program through outcome evaluation. It is important to target specific populations when collecting information, because their perception of need as well as their perception of evaluation indicators will vary. For example, heterosexual women who are at high risk for HIV may want family counseling rather than education. The target group's perception may be different than yours, so it is critical to involve the target population when planning and evaluating programs.

Phase 3 of the PRECEDE-PROCEED framework identifies additional health-related behavioral and environmental factors that could be linked to the outcomes of the identified health program and thus be used in program evaluation. These external factors may include preventive actions, self-care activities, household income, physical environment, access to health services, or healthy public policy. In phase 4 of the framework, the health and environmental factors are further classified as predisposing, reinforcing, or enabling factors that impact on health behavior or the environment. Predisposing factors include knowledge, attitudes, beliefs, values, and perceptions of health. Reinforcing factors are rewards or incentives from others that may encourage or discourage health-related behaviors. The enabling factors include skills, resources, and barriers that facilitate or hinder health-related behaviors. Predisposing, reinforcing, and enabling factors have an impact upon health related behaviors and the environment. These factors in turn influence the health and quality of life of the target populations and are used when evaluating programs (Green & Kreuter, 1999).

During the fifth phase, health-education components are planned, organized, implemented, and evaluated. With input from the community, health and wellness promotion strategies are chosen that are appropriate to the target population, staff are selected, and the health promotion program is launched. During phase 6, the PROCEED portion of the model is implemented. This phase guides the evaluation of the program through the three levels of accountability: process, impact, and outcome.

Resources are mobilized to evaluate the program, and time and personnel are budgeted. Developing a timeline can assist in outlining the resources required to implement the strategies and the expected time frame. Figure 7.2 outlines a possible timeline for health promotion program evaluation. Budgeting also involves consideration of personnel requirements and such items as photocopying, postage, telephone cost, and other resources as necessary.

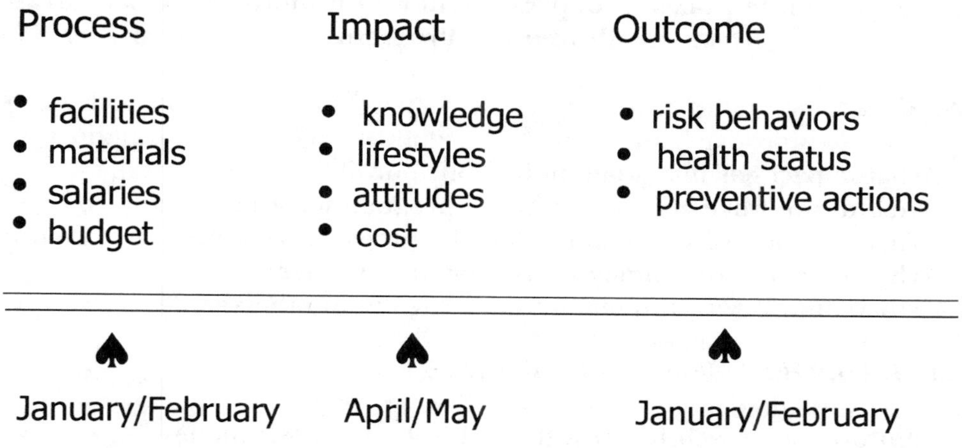

Process

- facilities
- materials
- salaries
- budget

Impact

- knowledge
- lifestyles
- attitudes
- cost

Outcome

- risk behaviors
- health status
- preventive actions

♠   ♠   ♠

January/February   April/May   January/February

FIGURE 7.2   **Possible timeline for program evaluation.**

METHODS OF EVALUATION

The methods of program evaluation discussed here include focus groups, key informant interviews, and surveys.

Focus Groups

Focus groups are small groups of key individuals who possess a unique insight into the health needs and resources of the community. Focus groups are an appropriate method for program evaluation, but the results usually cannot be generalized to apply to other groups or communities. Focus groups can consist of 8 to 12 participants who come together to discuss a common issue or concern, but they can be as small as 4 to 6 participants (Kreuger, 1988; Morgan, 1993). Generally they are a homogenous groups, but their common interest or concern may be defined by the evaluator. For example, groups may be formed based on geography or demographics or on a particular interest such as elder abuse. A moderator and co-moderator are

usually required and the session is videotaped for accurate analysis. Field notes can also be taken to ensure content validity. Focus group questions should be broad enough to encourage discussion, but limited to four or five key items (Box 7.6). Focus group questions may change depending on the flow of the discussion during the session, but the main items identified for evaluation should remain the same.

The focus group moderator can influence the nature and quality of the information collected during the session. The moderator must be involved in the group, but not dominate the discussion. The interpersonal skills of the moderator will likely influence the process of interaction and therefore it is important to be aware of the impact of the moderator's comments. Adopting a passive role and allowing the group discussion to be led primarily by the participants can facilitate the expression of sensitive information. The role of the co-moderator is to facilitate discussion. The co-moderator may also need to alert the moderator if the group is being directed

---

Box 7.6   Example Focus Group Evaluation Questions for a Cardiovascular Promotion Program

QUESTIONS

1. What impact has this program had on your life?
2. What did you like about the way the program was run?
3. What did you dislike about the way the program was run?
4. Why would you recommend this program to others?
5. Why wouldn't you recommend this program to others?

GENERAL THEMES EMERGING IN ANSWERS

1. Improved approach to stress through relaxation techniques
2. Healthier diet and exercise patterns
3. Satisfaction with educational strategies/Dissatisfied with physical facilities
4. A new outlook on life/Changed diet and exercise regime

---

or if particular items or topics are missed. The moderator and co-moderator roles are pivotal to the quality of information collected (Sim, 1998).

Key Informant Interviews

Key informant interviews are interviews with individuals who live or work in the community and who possess a special insight into its needs and resources. Interviews can be conducted by telephone or face to face and are another method of tapping into the community during program evaluation. Telephone interviews are the most frequently used method of collecting data (Burnard, 1994) and may be used to collect quantitative information (e.g., rating scale) and qualitative information (e.g., specific interviewer quotes) on the process, impact, or outcome of a program. They offer the evaluator an opportunity to discuss the health-promotion program with key informants in the community. Textual data from the interviews can be analyzed using Word

Perfect by identifying a key word such as "loneliness" and searching the document for that word, or a qualitative data analysis program such as ETHNOGRAPH or NUDIST can be used. In this way, common themes or concerns that emerge can be identified.

Below are some examples of key informants and the priority community concerns with which they would be concerned:

- Mayor: water and sewage
- Town Councillor: parks
- Police: juvenile crime
- Volunteers: parks
- Businesses: road conditions
- Contractors: road conditions
- Social Activists: access to physicians
- Social Workers: counseling
- Dentists: fluoride in water
- Physicians: elder abuse
- Lawyers: juvenile crime
- Nurses: parenting

When developing questions for the key informant interview guide, information may be used from discussions with health professionals, secondary data from such sources as health statistics, and information from program participants. The interview guide should be kept short and should address only those indicators identified for evaluation such as participant satisfaction and accessibility to the program. The development of an interview guide will help to structure and focus the content of each interview and will help the interviewer when key informants have questions about the process (Barriball, Christian, While, & Bergen, 1996). One of the drawbacks of telephone interviews is not being able to contact a person. The interviewer should keep accurate records of all calls including name, telephone number, address, time of call, length of interview, and number of attempts to reach the person. This record can then be used when reporting and analyzing results, but caution must be exercised because the results cannot be generalized to apply to other groups.

Surveys

Surveys are also an effective and popular method of evaluating community health promotion and wellness programs. The questions can be open-ended and ask for specific answers to specific questions, or close-ended and ask participants to select an answer from a range of choices (Fain, 1999). Designing good questions that are easily understood and answered can be time-consuming, and Fain suggests that they be specific and in simple language. Each question should represent one concept and be phrased in a neutral way (Box 7.7).

Surveys collect health-related information that may not be available anywhere else. They can be designed to gather infor-

mation on self-reported health status, sources of quality care, satisfaction with health services, barriers to access, and community perceptions of needs and resources. Tayler and Haley (1992) conclude that although surveys are expensive, the information collected is critical for establishing a baseline of data for development of the program and for future comparison.

Surveys can be expensive because of the costs and time associated with developing and distributing the survey and analyzing the data. When programs are being evaluated it is important to obtain a representative random sample of the participants who have used the program or obtain input from all participants. Telephone listings of program participants could be obtained during registration for the program. Contacting a random selection of that listing could provide the representative sample needed to accurately reflect their evaluation of the program. The evaluator must be aware of the limitations of each of these approaches and recognize that a combination of methods may be the best approach to any program evaluation.

COST-EFFECTIVENESS OF HEALTH PROMOTION PROGRAMS

Health care professionals have long recognized the value of health and wellness promotion programs in community practice. It can be difficult, however, to evaluate their cost effectiveness, but there are ways to do it: For example, the cost of the program could be compared to the cost of another program or to the anticipated dollar benefit for participants. It can also be difficult to prove that these programs reduce health care costs and improve the health status of targeted populations. This may be due to

---

Box 7.7   Survey Questions for Program Evaluation

Open-ended

1. Describe some reasons for attending Program X.
2. Explain your beliefs about health promotion.
3. Describe your experience with Program X.
4. What did you like about Program X?
5. What did you dislike about Program X?

Close-ended

1. Please rate your satisfaction with Program X:
   a. very satisfied
   b. somewhat satisfied
   c. unsatisfied
   d. very unsatisfied
2. Rate the teaching strategies in Program X:
   a. Excellent
   b. Very Good
   c. Good
   d. Poor

---

the difficulty of empirically measuring changes in attitudes and behaviors that may indicate improved health and well-being. It can also be difficult to establish a clear link between health promotion and changing disease rates in the future, because such changes may take as long as 20 years (Gillis, 1992).

Using a cost-benefit analysis to evaluate programs can bolster the argument that health and wellness programs are worthwhile because they will reduce health care costs by decreasing the use of health services (Gillis, 1992). Healthy people have less sick time and increased productivity in the workplace. Using a cost-benefit analysis approach can be complicated, but the basic idea is simple. Think about what the community will gain, what the costs are, and how the gains will compare with the costs (Fagin & Aiken, 1992). Costs are equal to

the actual cost of administering the health promotion program, plus the costs anticipated as a result of implementing the program, less the savings accrued because of an improved health status. See Box 7.8 for a cost-benefit example.

The cost effects or benefits could also be equal to the lives or number of years of life saved by prevention, less the lives or years of life that are lost to side effects. For example, one health promotion intervention—smoking cessation—may cost $50,000, but may save 100 years of life. Thus, the cost is only $500 per year of life saved and is therefore worth doing. Other examples include the cost associated with an HIV prevention program versus the cost of treatment of those infected with HIV; the cost associated with a healthy heart program versus the cost of treatment for cardiovascular disease, or the cost associated

---

Box 7.8   Hypothetical Cost-Benefit Analysis for a High School Parenting Program

Costs	=	Cost of administration	+	Cost of implementation	−	Savings from improved health status
		facilities (*$500*)		handouts (*$150*)		?
		secretarial (*$100*)		videos (*$250*)		
				salaries (*$5,000*)		

---

with clean air versus the costs of treatment for lung, liver, and environment-related cancers.

Cost-benefit analysis can provide critical information for evaluating community health and wellness programs. Program evaluation research should include cost-benefit analysis that substantiates an economic rationale for the allocation of resources. It may be difficult to conduct detailed cost-benefit studies that clearly link health promotion programs to changing disease rates in the future. Health and wellness are constructs not easily measured, but disease and death can be converted into monetary terms.

Be prepared to meet future community demands by sharpening specialized clinical, prevention, health promotion, and program evaluation skills (Aiken & Fagan, 1992). When assessing the cost-effectiveness of programs seek the help of a statistics consultant from a local university or medical center. With smaller programs, you may be able to analyze the resources and the budget against costs of running the program and anticipated benefits. For example, if you have been given $250 to run a parenting seminar for parents of school-aged children, you may determine that the costs of the program include photocopying ($50), secretarial support to develop educational materials ($50), coffee and tea ($50),

and transportation for parents ($50). Other resources may include reimbursement for your time and the facilities donated by a local organization. Sizing up the costs and resources, you can determine that the resources and budget are sufficient to run this program, so it could be considered a cost-effective measure. Another anticipated benefit that cannot be assigned a monetary value would be the improved parenting skills resulting from participation in the program, which could be assessed by asking the parents to self-evaluate their learning.

SUMMARY

Community health and wellness program evaluation is a multifaceted process that begins with a community self-assessment. Involving the community members in the assessment, planning and evaluation provides an opportunity to build partnerships between the community and the health care professionals working with the community. Program evaluation can be formative or summative and can focus on process, impact, and outcome. A variety of methods can be used in health and wellness program evaluation including surveys, telephone interviews and focus groups. The PRECEDE-PROCEED framework can assist you in planning and evaluating health and wellness programs for the community. One consideration in program evaluation is the cost-effectiveness, which can be difficult to conduct but is worth the effort.

REFERENCES

Burnard, P. (1994). The telephone interview as a data collection method. *Nursing Education Today, 14,* 67–72.

Barriball, K., Christian, S., White, A., & Bergen, A. (1996). The telephone survey method: A discussion paper. *Journal of Advanced Nursing, 24,* 115–121.

Beddome, G., Clarke, H., & Whyte, N. (1993). Vision for the future of public health nursing: A case for primary health care. *Public Health Nursing, 10*(1), 13–18.

Evans, R., Barer, M., & Marmor, T. (1994). *Why are some people healthy and others not?* Hawthorne, NY: Aldine de Gruyter.

Fagan, C., & Aiken, L. (1992). *Charting nursing's future.* New York: J. B. Lippincott.

Fain, J. (1999). *Reading, understanding and applying nursing research.* F. A. Davies.

Gillis, A. (1992). Allocation of health care resources: The case for health promotion. *Nursing Forum, 27*(4), 21–16.

Glick, D., Hale, P., Kulbok, P., & Shettig, J. (1996). Community development theory: Planning a community nursing center. *Journal of Nursing Administration, 26*(7/8), 44–50.

Green, L., & Kreuter, M. (1999). *Health promotion planning: An educational and environmental approach.* Toronto, Ontario, Canada: Mayfield.

Hitchcock, J., Shubert, P., & Thomas, S. (1999). *Community health nursing: Caring in action.* Toronto, Ontario, Canada: Delmar.

Kang, R. (1995). Building community capacity for health promotion. *Public Health Nursing, 12*(5), 312–318.

Kreuger, R. (1988). *Focus groups: A practical guide for applied research.* London: Sage.

Lefebrve, C. (1992). Social marketing and health promotion. In R. Bunton & G. MacDonald (Eds.), *Health promotion; Disciplines and diversity* (pp. 153–181). London: Routledge.

Minister of Supply and Services. (1994). *Strategies for population health: Investing in the health of Canadians.* Ottawa, Ontario, Canada: Publications Health Canada.

Morgan, D. (1993). *Successful focus groups.* California: Sage.

Pike, S., & Banoub-Baddour, S. (1991). A nursing intervention: The design and implementation of a cardiovascular health education program. *Canadian Journal of Cardiovascular Nursing, 2*(3), 3–8.

Sim, J. (1998). Collecting and analyzing qualitative data: Issues raised by focus groups. *Journal of Advanced Nursing, 28*(92), 345–352.

Taylor, B., & Haley, D. (1990). The use of household surveys in community-oriented primary care health needs assessment. *Family Medicine, 28*(96), 415–421.

Stanley, S., & Stein, D. (1998). Health Watch 2000: Community health assessment in South Central Ohio. *Journal of Community Health Nursing, 15*(94), 225–236.

Stoner, M., Magilvy, T., & Schultz, P. (1992). Community analysis in community health nursing practice: The GENESIS model. *Public Health Nursing, 9*(4), 223–227.

CHAPTER 8

Health Promotion in Rural Settings

Julia W. Aucoin and Sheilda G. Rodgers

This chapter will explore the cultural characteristics of the rural population, describe the elements of promoting health in rural settings, discuss access to service issues for the rural population, differentiate between health beliefs in the rural culture and other settings, and discuss strategies to promote the health of rural dwellers.

RURAL VERSUS METROPOLITAN LIVING

Rural implies an escape from the hustle and bustle of the city, being out in the country, or living off the land. For many rural dwellers this is a choice, yet for many more it is a legacy passed down through generations. Population density most often defines a rural setting. The federal government applies the term in order to describe locales for funding opportunities; sociologists apply the term to describe communities. The definition of *rural* can range from a community of less than 100,000 people to densities of 6 or fewer persons per square mile (American Nurses Association, 1996).

Recently recommended refinements to the term metropolis may yield megapolis, macropolis, and micropolis to reflect the blending of city and suburban boundaries into larger communities (Mayhew, 1997). In terms of health care, *metropolitan* living implies access to services in close proximity, although there may be restrictions on access due to transportation, affordability, and managed care penetration.

As of the 1990 census, approximately 27% of the 250 million people in the United States were living in rural areas, and 73% were classified as urban (U.S. Department of Commerce, 1991). In the last decade there were population shifts in and out of the rural and metropolitan domains, with projected slower growth in rural settings. At present, the findings of the 2000 census are being evaluated, with the intent of assigning a location to individuals' residences in order to appropriate funding accurately.

Many urban dwellers do not know their neighbors and may not have family in close proximity, but rural dwellers demonstrate a reliance upon friends and families for many of their needs, including health care.

Additionally, the excitement of an urban setting overwhelms the tranquility of a rural setting for many health care practitioners who are seeking a location for their practice. Family and financial needs may take precedence over the desire to serve a particular population when a practitioner is choosing a home. The characteristics of the rural dweller and the personal preferences of health care providers create the need to provide care using different strategies in the rural setting than in the urban setting.

ACCESS TO CARE

Today's managed care environment has transformed how people access health care. The introduction of the primary care provider as the gatekeeper has forced people to choose a practitioner and seek assistance from that individual for all their health care needs until such time as they are referred to a specialist. The Health Maintenance Organization Act of 1973 offered hope that health care costs could be managed and that health would be the primary focus of care. However, the system has remained illness-oriented with little emphasis on health promotion activities and affordability.

The merger and acquisition arena has created large health care systems that are intended to provide seamless care to clients, but that in reality create a bureaucratic maze that is difficult for the average person to navigate, especially when they don't feel well. Furthermore, it has become increasingly difficult for a solo practitioner to hang out a shingle and take on the financial and liability risks that are assumed in the health care industry.

Urban settings feature large medical centers that contain many primary care practices. In order to entice more clients to a particular managed care plan, a variety of services are offered at many locations convenient to home and work. However, urban settings may have inner city congestion problems with difficult parking and busy streets that make travel to the practitioners' offices inconvenient and time-consuming. The complexity of the health care system may make it undesirable to even attempt to seek assistance, as knowing who to call for which problem can be confusing.

Until recently, only traditional services were covered by managed care plans. A recent trend indicates that offering a discount on complementary therapies and health promotion activities has become popular with consumers. However, health promotion activities are not as available or as utilized as envisioned by the HMO Act of 1973. The proliferation of health clubs can be viewed as a wave passing through cities with varying effect, following a cycle like made and broken New Year's resolutions.

Rural dwellers have little access to an HMO for their insurance coverage or health care delivery unless they work for a large employer who can subscribe to such a plan. Frequently the rural dweller must rely on self-insurance as they are often self-employed. The local physician or nurse practitioner may work on a cash or barter basis for services rendered, but when specialty or emergency care is needed the rural dweller may have to travel up to hundreds of miles for service. Many of the largest medical centers have made a reputation for themselves as the best health care provider within a vast region and influence their rural colleagues to refer clients who must then travel long distances for their care.

The advent of telehealth practice has enhanced the rural practitioner's ability to provide services at long distances. Computers, modems, and satellites make possible the transmission and interpretation of diagnostic studies, team consultations, and daily monitoring of patient status. This enables the rural patient to stay closer to home and obtain health care of similar quality to those who have better access.

INTERRELATIONSHIPS

Any attempt to implement health promotion activities in rural settings must identify key informants who will be able to assist you in establishing programs of interest. The type of informant will vary from one area to another but would almost always include prominent clergy and local government leaders. Local stores that service a majority of residents such as a general supply or hardware store can be helpful especially in terms of disseminating information. If at all possible you should refrain from giving the impression of knowing what's best for the community without prior assessment. Contact with existing community groups and, most important, with the family and friends network can assist you in identifying community leaders who may be able to provide valuable information. It is crucial that you not alienate individual subgroups, subcultures, or the people in general. Becoming a part of and being accepted by the rural community first is essential to success in this setting.

Within the context of health promotion in rural settings, you will be required to examine the interrelatedness among the people of interest. Bushy (1994) suggests that in providing care you should consider the rural dwellers' social support system. Family members, including an extended family, may positively influence one's willingness to engage in or even entertain activities to regain and maintain health. You will need to assess the structure of the family and friends network system to determine

their perceived roles in health promotion activities. In many rural communities there are casual systems in place to help residents meet their health needs, and oftentimes these systems rely on the strong sense of family and friends. This interrelatedness constitutes the community in which the persons requiring health promotion activities exist; therefore, any behavior modification of the individual or the community to improve health will be molded by the values of this network.

The family should be viewed as an extension of the person of focus and his or her environment. Health promotion activities will need to consider the presence or absence of family as an influencing variable in health activities. In rural areas, family can include a wide variety of relatives not just immediate kin. The interrelatedness of these people and their strong sense of kinship make them ideal as health care providers. Rural families, including extended members, tend to have an emotional dependency on one another. Therefore, your plan for health promotion should include how family support systems and informal health delivery systems can be incorporated. Failure to do so may alienate the community you are trying to serve and the residents may suffer negative health outcomes.

When family relationships are strained or missing you will need to seek out friends and acquaintances to assume the role of health care provider, or enabler, or to encourage participation in health promotion activities. Characteristic of many rural areas, people often live close to one another and work with the same people for many years. Over the course of time a strong sense of friendship and commitment evolve and the network becomes far-reaching. For many the "friends network" may be as strong as the "blood kin network." Commitment to one's friends is serious and the responsibility to assist in times of hardship or need is common place. When you tap into this resource as a means of achieving health promotion goals, remember that several members of the friends network may be willing participants in your effort.

When examining health care practices in rural areas you should identify the community's and the individual's existing social network early on in your efforts. With recent reports of shortages of health care providers in rural areas, friends should be included as a possible resource for implementation of health promotion activities. It may be necessary for you to visit people at nontraditional sites to elicit participation in health promotion. Social gathering places for rural dwellers may include gas stations, popular breakfast stops, and general stores. Visiting in these places creates a trusting relationship and a sense that you are comfortable in their normal environments, a much-needed first step to make inroads into the community's health. For example, in one small rural community a local service station was the regular meeting place for many retired mill workers to gather for coffee in the early morning hours. These men met each morning to observe other people going to work and stopping for gas. This site would be an ideal place to begin discovering the community's needs and implementing small-scale activities such as distribution of literature and blood-pressure screening.

Reliance on friends and family creates a strong network of assistance. Providing transportation and picking up prescriptions are two health care activities that often become a shared responsibility of the social support system. You should build on this network to increase services and participation in activities that focus on health promotion. Friends who take the responsibility of assisting another in being healthier may

be encouraged to do the same for themselves.

In areas rich with health care workers, professional support is thought to be required for success in health promotion activities (Serembus, 1998). This support is usually not available to you in rural settings, so relying on friends and family for reinforcement and motivation will be necessary. Serembus (1998) suggests that support from family and friends is consistently associated with success in adherence to certain types of health behaviors. Through effective collaboration with friends and families you can be instrumental in meeting the challenges of health promotion in rural settings.

CULTURAL COMPETENCE

In any attempt to institute health promotion activities in rural areas you must be aware of the culture in which you are to function. Cultural competence involves creating an atmosphere of mutual respect and open communication. The combination of economic, educational, and cultural differences between you and rural dwellers creates a challenge in health promotion endeavors. You should not attempt to interact with rural residents with a priori beliefs about their culture. Categorizing, stereotyping, and generalizing will denigrate the rich culture of many and should be avoided. Rather, you should identify a means by which to amass cultural data. It will be difficult to know every aspect of the diverse cultures of the rural area, but a holistic assessment approach would identify cultural influences on health. Tools exist that systematically appraise individuals and groups within a community; use these for a richer, more meaningful database. Two examples are the "Cultural Assessment Interview Guide" (DeLaune & Ladner, 1998) and the "Data Base for the Culturally Diverse Client" (Leininger, 1978). The cultural diversity in most rural areas will make this effort challenging, but the rewards of positive health outcomes warrants the effort.

Individuals should not be expected to give up their cultural practices to fit in with the existing system of health care delivery; health care providers must be socialized to be culturally competent caregivers. Kavanagh and Kennedy (1992) posit that culturally congruent approaches to care and effective communication and interventions require consideration of the clients' perspective and understanding. You will need to do a cultural self-assessment, but you may also need specific training or course work in dealing with culturally diverse populations, including rural people.

Culturally sensitive programs should be the goal of those seeking to implement health promotion programs. Care should be taken so that efforts are not perceived as an attempt to change the culture. Any perception that you lack sensitivity to rural people's needs inhibits effective utilization of services available. With few health professionals to turn to for help, it is crucial that you develop health care professionals who are culturally competent and who are committed to the special needs and concerns of the rural dweller. You need to be socialized to the health practices, beliefs, religious structures, and social networks of the community. The degree to which you impart a feeling of acceptance, support, and encouragement will help to determine the rural resident's ability to engage in appropriate interactions for health promotion.

As you plan projects for rural areas, keep in mind the possible utilization of rural areas as sites for clinical experiences for students. Registered nurses completing bachelor's degrees could bring a wealth of knowledge and experience to the setting, adding to the number of available health care professionals. Student exposure to rural environments increases the likelihood that they will seek out future employment there, but it also provides them with the opportunity to add to their repertoire of skills in dealing with diverse groups. See the case study in Box 8.1 for a typical scenario resulting from poor planning.

Language is an integral part of any culture or geographical locale. Pay attention to the language patterns of the groups in the rural community. Accept existing dialects as a vital part of the culture and never give the impression that the dialect is incorrect or bad. You should use theories of communication to enhance verbal exchanges between you and culturally different rural dwellers. Consulting the individual or members of the group to explain or clarify terms will prevent your making incorrect assumptions. Avoid the use of jargon, technical terms, and slang and keep information simple. An interpreter may be required when working in rural areas with large numbers of non-English speaking groups. Your effort to communicate effectively conveys to the people that your interest in their health is genuine. Whether you are in eastern South Carolina or Cajun south Louisiana, learning to listen to a dialect allows you to experience the richness of the peoples' lives.

According to Kavanagh and Kennedy (1992), mutual communication has as its goal the maintenance or restoration of the integrity of individuals or groups. When communicating in rural settings the approach must project trust and genuineness so that people will be receptive to the health care activity you are presenting. Artificial barriers created by the poor use of language and inadequate communication will be difficult to overcome later, if not impossible.

Box 8.1   Case Study: Cultural Competence with Rural Diversity

A small town is the focus of a health promotion activity to prevent heart disease, which has been sponsored by a grant. You are ready to implement the activities that will involve exercise and nutrition education. Sample diets have been constructed and a video has been purchased to demonstrate exercise. The video is in English only and depicts no people of color. On the evening of implementation, you note that of the 20 attendees, 6 are Hispanic with limited English-speaking ability, 5 are African American, and the other 11 are European-American.

Study questions

1. What cultural issues may negatively impact the program's effectiveness for the audience?
2. What steps were necessary to ensure that the program is culturally competent/sensitive?
3. What aspects of culture would enhance the health promotion programs?
4. How can the nurse handle the current situation and prevent negative outcomes?
5. What are the possible outcomes of this situation and how can the nurse address each of them?

HEALTH BELIEFS

Different health beliefs exist for the different subgroups of the rural setting: ethnic, geographic, religious, and economic. A person's health belief dictate what type of behaviors will be employed to maintain or regain health. Health can only be defined within the context of the person experiencing it and what is considered health for one rural dweller may not be for another. Value systems and environments will define what is believed about health. For example, many rural dwellers may consider themselves healthy if they are able to work, carry on normal duties, or engage in desired activities, despite the presence of disabilities and chronic illnesses.

As a middle-class health care professional you cannot impose on that definition by creating false meanings of health that are not attainable for the individual. This will create barriers, frustrations, and misunderstandings that could cause your health promotion to fail before it begins. Many rural dwellers may only seek health care for the treatment of illnesses rather than for promoting health. Through interaction with health care workers they trust, they may be persuaded to try health promotion, particularly if you are able to demonstrate that it can prevent diseases that result in loss of work and decreased ability to enjoy life as they define it. The successful approach is to determine the most prevalent health beliefs or practices and incorporate them into whatever plan is being developed.

Sortet and Banks (1997) suggest that rural people may be suspicious of health professionals and may rely on folk remedies, healers, or family members when they become ill. The use of home remedies and folk medicine is widespread in rural areas and is an outgrowth of an era when organized health care was nonexistent. Affordability, accessibility, and prior practices are variables that impact on a person's belief about health requirements. Home remedies are passed down through the years from one family member to another and are tried before seeking health care from the more formal system of health care delivery. People who use folk remedies believe in their effectiveness and you should respect any person's use of them. Failure to do so reflects an attitude of cultural insensitivity.

Home remedies and practices are part of the *folklore* passed to each new generation. Some that are still in practice in rural central North Carolina include pressing keys at the upper middle back for a nose bleed; a paste of oatmeal for itchy skin; garlic around the neck for general health; and a paste of snuff or chewing tobacco for bee and wasp stings. Drinking vinegar for high blood pressure and eating garlic to clear constipation are still common practices as well. One older man reported that reading certain passages in the Bible will stop nosebleeds.

While it is difficult to substantiate the outcomes of these home remedies, it is equally difficult to refute them. The perceived benefit to those practicing them is unquestionable. Many rural dwellers continue to use home treatments before seeking a professional practitioner for a variety of reasons, not the least of which are cost and availability.

Several home remedies in use in rural settings are in fact cost-effective and can be used in many settings.

1. Use clean white washcloths or handkerchiefs rather than expensive gauze for wound care.
2. Make your own saline by dissolving 1 teaspoon of table salt in 2 cups warm water.
3. Sit in bathroom with door closed, using steam from hot water in shower to decongest.
4. Use a strip of cloth to make a sling rather than purchase one.
5. Use bags of frozen peas or corn to make ice packs for injuries or arthritis.
6. Use hot wet washcloths wrapped in plastic or a bag as a heating pad for aches and pains.

STRATEGIES FOR HEALTH PROMOTION

Setting priorities is important in every aspect of community health. In order to gain support and acceptance, it is necessary to focus on small and immediate success. In beginning an alliance in a new rural community, you would want to identify one area that can be improved upon with little effort and maximum visibility. For example, take advantage of the social nature of church groups and promote exercise by starting a walking program that enables churchwomen to walk while they are doing another activity they enjoy—talking among themselves. Other residents will see these community leaders enjoying themselves and will model their own behavior after these women. As the walkers get out more, they will begin to feel better, have more energy, and be able to continue the good works of the church with more vibrancy.

Another opportunity exists in partnering with industry. In a rural farm community where many accidents may have occurred while using heavy equipment, you could invite the factory representative to show the operators how to use the equipment properly. This could potentially improve efficiency, and therefore possibly the economy, but it can also show the farmers how to prevent loss of limb or life. Demonstrating the proper use to children will also prevent needless mutilating injuries. The factory representative has a responsibility to teach the farmers how to operate the equipment at no charge and may reap increased sales as a result. Constant review on equipment operation is a standard in industrial settings, and implementing this standard in the rural setting will prevent lost time and lost lives.

Using the existing resources within a community is the most important strategy that can be employed in a rural setting. The Rural Clinic and Community Health Promotion Project was designed to assist communities served by National Health Service Corps Clinics to develop or expand health promotion activities in seven of its rural Oklahoma communities (Bender & Hart, 1987). A needs assessment was completed after support was established by town leaders, clinic personnel, and residents. It was found that little health promotion activity was currently underway and that the greatest needs were in accident prevention, exercise and fitness, environmental sensitivity, nutrition, self-care, personal responsibility, alcohol abuse, drug abuse, smoking cessation, and stress management. A threefold strategy was designed:

1. An information campaign was planned to increase awareness and to motivate community residents to attend the community meeting. It included fliers, newspaper articles, church presentations, and walking around town spreading the word.

2. Community meetings provided a forum for clinic personnel to sell health promotion and conduct health risk appraisals. Scheduling avoided conflicts with important activities such as prayer meetings and other local events.

3. A directory of health-promotion resources was a valuable part of the project. An up-to-date listing of available services helped increase awareness and promote referrals to appropriate settings. Several non-health-care experts were noted in the directory. For example, the police department may be the best resource for accident prevention and security.

Each of the seven towns found that it possessed the ability to provide for health promotion; it just needed to be packaged in such a way that made residents more aware and more comfortable participating in activities.

Hjelm (1995) suggests that improving the availability of more educated nursing staff in established facilities can be an asset. Because staff development and continuing education may be limited for nurses in a rural setting, it can be helpful to recruit a nurse with a master's degree to supplement the cultural knowledge of the nurses with the scientific knowledge of the clinical nurse specialist (CNS). However, this can be an expensive venture. Hjelm offers that two or more small rural hospitals can share the cost of employing a CNS to bridge the gap between patient needs and delivery of care. This CNS could become an internal consultant to the nursing staff and patients with the intent of improving patient outcomes through coordination of multidisciplinary teams.

Along the same lines, implementing a rural nursing course within the baccalaureate curriculum can also serve the needs of the community. Rural Canada suffers from the same sparsity of practitioners that the rural United States experiences. Using a partnership model, Baird-Crooks, Graham, and Bushy (1998) report that undergraduate nursing programs and rural Alberta communities have worked together to improve residents' access to health promotion. A course including theory and clinical content has been operational for several years, using case-study strategies in conjunction with a clinical practicum. Students have reported a new awareness of life in rural communities and the ability to apply a broader and more holistic approach to their total nursing care. Many students have been inspired to seek employment in rural settings. As a result of this course, faculty have developed two resources on rural nursing, a "Book of Readings" and "Readings for the Road," which are now in demand by schools and agencies. Offering students the opportunity to experience rural nursing can improve the health of a community by bringing potential practitioners to the community before they make their employment decisions.

The American Nurses Association's Rural/Frontier Health Care Task Force has proposed several recommendations to facilitate necessary changes in the health care system that can positively affect health promotion in rural settings (ANA, 1996). These changes include working at the national and state levels to promote and support the public health infrastructure so that care is continually provided at the county level regardless of the number of private practitioners available. The ANA should continue efforts on national and state levels to eliminate legislative and reimbursement barriers that restrict rural clients' access to health care and other social services by collaborating with consumer organizations and community employers. Cultural competency should be an expectation of nurses in all settings.

Healthy People 2010 represents the newest health care objectives that are established as guidelines for our practice in any setting (U.S. Department of Health and Human Services, 2000). A new feature this year is the establishment of 10 leading indicators

of the health status of this nation. As you might surmise, it is expected that tobacco, alcohol and drug use should decline, while nutrition and personal responsibility should increase. These objectives are useful in setting goals with the community, writing grant applications, and planning programs. The specific goal of eliminating disparity in health care applies to rural settings. According to the authors of *Healthy People 2010,* 25% of Americans live in rural areas; that is, places with fewer that 2,500 residents. Injury-related death rates are 40% higher in rural populations than in urban populations, and heart disease, cancer, and diabetes rates exceed those in urban areas. People living in rural areas are less likely to use preventive screening services, exercise regularly, or wear seat belts. In 1996, 20% of the rural population was uninsured compared with 16% of the urban population. Timely access to emergency services and the availability of specialty care are other issues for this population group.

SUMMARY

The rural setting is inherently different from the urban setting because of the nature of the people that live there. The increased reliance upon family and friends makes these communities unique and makes it difficult for a health care practitioner to make a difference. Utilizing the resources within the community, building upon the strengths of the residents, and establishing small, meaningful goals are strategies for success. Funding continues to be an area of concern, as does acknowledgment that the rural residents are slow to adapt to the current health care delivery system. As cultural competency becomes better emphasized, it's the health care system that will need to adapt, accepting the practice of folk remedies and recognizing that health care is not a priority—often survival is the best we can expect.

ORGANIZATIONS

Federal Office of Rural Health Policy
Health Resources and Services Administration
5600 Fishers Lane, Room 9-05
Rockville, MD 20857
(301) 443-0835
www.nalusda.gov/orhp

National Rural Health Association
One West Armour Boulevard Suite 301
Kansas City, MO 64111
(816) 756-3140
www.nrharural.org

Rural Health WebRing
www.rural-health.org.au
The Rural Health WebRing is a collection of sites that focus on rural health issues. These include health agencies.

National Rural Health Resource Center
www.ruralcenter.org/nrhrc
A non-profit providing publications, technical assistance, and educational seminars in managed care and network and community development.

National Farm Medicine Center
www.marshmed.org/nfmc/
Offers up-to-date information about rural and agricultural health issues, other rural health links, and center research and education activities.

Rural Policy Research Institute
www.rupri.org/
Examine texts that discuss the impact of public policy on rural populations. Explores such topics as health and communications.

REFERENCES

American Nurses Association. (1996). *Rural/frontier nursing.* Washington, DC: American Nurses Publishing.

Baird-Crooks, K., Graham, B., & Bushy, A. (1998). Implementing a rural nursing course. *Nurse Educator, 23*(6), 33–37.

Bender, C., & Hart, J. P. (1987). A model for health promotion for the rural elderly. *The Gerontologist, 27*(2), 139–142.

Bushy, A. (1994). When your client lives in a rural area. *Issues in Mental Health Nursing, 15,* 253–266.

DeLaune, S., & Ladner, P. (1998). *Fundamentals of nursing: Standards and practice.* Albany, NY: Delmar Publishers.

Hjelm, J. S. (1995). The rural health care setting: Is there a need for a CNS? *Clinical Nurse Specialist, 9*(2), 212–115.

Kavanagh, K. H., & Kennedy, P. H. (1992). *Promoting cultural diversity.* Newbury Park, CA: Sage.

Leininger, M. (1978). *Transcultural nursing.* New York: Wiley.

Mayhew, S. (1997). *A Dictionary of Geography.* Oxford: Oxford University Press.

Serembus, J. F. (1998). The healthy heart: Health promotion and maintenance. *Holistic Nursing Practice, 12*(2), 44–51.

Sortet, J. P., & Banks, S. R. (1997). Health beliefs of rural Appalachian women and the practice of breast self-examination. *Cancer Nursing, 20*(4), 231–235.

U.S. Department of Commerce, Bureau of the Census. (1991). *Census of population 1990: Preliminary counts.* Washington, DC: U.S. Government Printing Office.

U.S. Department of Health and Human Services. (January 2000). *Healthy People 2010* (Conference Edition, in two volumes). Washington, DC: U.S. Government Printing Office. *www.health.gov/healthypeople*

CHAPTER 9

Health Promotion on the Internet

Judy L. Sheehan

THE EVOLVING ROLE OF THE INTERNET IN SELF CARE

The explosion of interest on the Internet and the World Wide Web has provided a valuable resource for consumers and professionals alike as it offers exceptional opportunities for information collection, dissemination and exchange (Leiner, Cerf, Clark, Kahn, Kleinrock, Lynch, Postel, Roberts, & Wolff, 1998). The vast amount of material available at the touch of the keyboard has changed the flow of information.

Over time we have come to understand that information alone does not lead to knowledge or power. In fact, too much information or faulty information can be potentially harmful and immobilizing. It is probable that too much information can result in *information overload*, which can be defined as the inability to ascertain the relevancy of information due to an overabundance data. It results in a diminished ability to make decisions based on the information obtained and has been described by Weil and Rosen (1997) as a primary social stressor. It is possible to have unlimited access to information and still have a knowledge deficit. In order for information to be valuable it must be accurate, timely, relevant, and have significance (Graves & Corcoran, 1989).

It is clear that the infiltration of the Internet into everyday society is increasing the opportunity for consumers to obtain information. Information-seeking, a task critical to self care, is easily accomplished on the Internet and is especially effective when a health provider works as a coach with the consumer. This evolving role requires a coaching rather than directive expert approach. Such an approach includes working from the sidelines with the consumer to assess need, plan an information search, evaluate the results, and determine together the appropriate meaning of the information. The coach facilitates information-processing and interpretation and thus empowers the consumer to use the computer as a tool much like a blood-pressure cuff or an at-home diabetes screening kit. Health providers are well suited to assist consumers in processing information, developing knowledge and facilitating decision making. We can anticipate the increased involvement of consumers in health-related Internet sites as they become increasingly popular and continue to grow rapidly. The participation of health care providers in this process is essential if a true client-provider health partnership is to occur. The ability to obtain information, communicate with others, make purchases, and engage in social interactions from the comfort of one's home has the potential to solve some of the perennial access problems often faced by clients. Technological innovations such as voice recognition, computer vocalizations, user-friendly mouse design, and touch screens provide greater opportunity for users with physical limitations. Individuals experiencing health care access problems—a family member monitoring the wanderings of a parent with Alzheimer's disease, a mother with young children and minimal child-care opportunities, a young man in the rehabilitation center—can participate freely in health-related activity on-line. Clients can obtain health information, communicate with providers, purchase products, join support groups, or otherwise extend into the world more easily. Economic constraints do exist for some people, and computers continue to be expensive and target the literate and well-educated. Still, there has been movement to create programs to expand availability. Internet access is available at many if not most public libraries and at some community centers, which diminishes disparities caused by economic conditions. Computers can be found at senior meal sites, libraries, and coffee shops (cyber cafés), as well as in homes. A survey conducted in 1999 by Seniorlink found that 40% of surveyed seniors (defined as individuals older than 50) had computers in their homes. Clients can—and do—attend seminars, receive answers about specific symptoms, order books, magnets, crystals, vitamins, or pharmaceutical supplies all on-line.

STRATEGIES FOR PROMOTING HEALTH ON THE INTERNET

Developing strategies for promoting health on the Internet via your own Web site requires setting goals. What is your intended purpose? What population do you want to target? What are your goals? How will you evaluate success? Do you want the Internet to act as a primary practice setting or will you use it to market other activity that takes place at a specified location? Will you use the Internet as a support for other areas of practice—communication with clients, follow-up to consultation, or selling of products and materials? The answers to these questions are critical to the planning of an Internet strategy. Because the Internet is changing at a rapid pace, it is important to stay current regarding technological trends—many of your clients are. If you have not yet done so, surf the Web frequently to review new sites and opportunities for practice applications. Join technology groups or collectives (such as holisticinstitute.com) to access consultation and computer services. Read magazines targeted at small-business owners and telecommuters to learn about advances in hardware and software. Incorporate computer seminars in your ongoing continuing education plan in order to keep up to date. Include technology-based practice in your professional business plan and address target population, Web site development, chat rooms, bulletin boards, on-line conferencing, and distance consultation. Perform a technological assessment when you are conducting a client assessment and working with a client to create a treatment plan.

When determining the target population consider the nature of the Internet, its geographic openness allows interaction with individuals that is unrestricted by location. Services designed with a world view

Box 9.1   Technological Assessment

Name: Date:

Address:

1. Do you use a computer at work?   yes   no

2. Do you use a computer at home?   yes   no

3. How many hours a day do you use a computer
   - ❐   less than one hour
   - ❐   1 to 3 hours
   - ❐   3 or more

4. Do you have an email address?   yes   no
   - ❐   If yes, what is your email address? _____

5. Select the best description of your computer usage patterns:

I am uncomfortable	computer	Internet
I am somewhat comfortable	computer	Internet
I am very comfortable	computer	Internet
I enjoy	computer	Internet
I would like to learn more	computer	Internet

6. Do you experience any of the following when using a computer (circle all that apply):
   headache
   wrist, back, or arm pain
   eye irritation
   dizziness
   confusion
   disorientation
   nausea
   irritability
   other:

Please include any additional information you think might be important regarding your experience with computers and the Internet.

in mind can be distributed globally with few problems. Keep this in mind when discussing measurement (metric system) and prices (American dollars) and identify country in the address information or survey data forms. Most computers have translator capabilities and language is not a problem. Do not assume technological ignorance based on age, race, education, or gender. Remember this when designing programs and think about the population you wish to reach. The Internet can be incorporated into a wide variety of health promotion areas: stress reduction including the use of assessment tools and access to biofeedback equipment, nutrition and diet, follow-up after direct provider contact especially when complementary techniques are being used, and the provision of supplemental information either individually or in a group support environment. Box 9.2 contains health promotion activities suitable for the Internet.

Developing a Web Site

Web sites can be designed using prepackaged programs that are user-friendly and usually sufficient for most health care providers. Prepackaged Web-design programs save time since you do not have to learn how to program HTML (the programming language of the Web) but are limited in flexibility. Examples of such programs include Top Page, Adobe PageMill, Microsoft FrontPage, and Netscape Composer. A consultant can be hired to design a Web site or you can develop one yourself. Some collaboratives offer design services as part of the membership package and are worth exploring (holisticinstitute.com).

The first step in designing a Web site is to define your goals. What information do you wish to include? The site will represent you or your organization on the Web and first impressions count. The home page, the first page seen by someone browsing the Internet, provides initial contact with the consumer. This must be motivating and engaging. Graphics and pictures are often used to add interest to the content. Keep the upload time in mind when designing a site with graphics, and make the site easy to navigate. Colors vary on different computer monitors, and sticking with clear primary colors to accent a white background provides a clean and professional look. If

---

Box 9.2   Sample Areas for Health Promotion Activity on the Internet

1. Consultation and follow-up for any face-to-face interaction
2. Identification of complementary techniques with related information
3. Provision of useful information
4. Evaluation of information related to condition or treatment
5. Assessment tools—stress, health status, etc.
6. Dietary and nutritional assessment
7. Self-help and support groups for any condition
8. Provision of health information and resources for the homebound client
9. Behavior modification, any area, evaluation of self-reporting tools, or consultation
10. On-line conferencing on any topic, with the Internet used for follow-up

you wish to add a background color, consider blue, gray, or red tones instead of brown, green, and yellows, which tend to change tone easily.

Link to additional pages or related sites provide a value-added service to visitors to your site. If you are using a Web site to expand practice opportunities you want to encourage visitors to return frequently. Enticing users to revisit your site offers a number of benefits. It increases the potential pool of clients, creates opportunities for additional revenue, and increases name recognition. If the dissemination of information is a primary concern, the greater the number of visitors the greater the dissemination of information. Health promotion E-zines, or electronic magazines, can be readily developed and distributed as health promotion tools and can be attached to content sites easily. Once a Web site is launched, anyone can visit it. The site should then be registered with various search engines (such as Yahoo) to bring visitors to the site.

Regardless of its intended use it is safe to assume that the home page is open to view by the public. Private areas such as chat rooms or on-line conferences may be added as separate pages and accessed via password. (The process and criteria for obtaining a password varies from site to site and is established by the developer.) Including chat rooms for a monitored or facilitated discussion on various topics is another strategy for health promotion. The professional acts as monitor and clarifies or verifies information, makes referrals to sources, or otherwise intervenes as an information broker and participant in the chat. One example of such a monitored chat room is webmd.com. Include a bulletin board in a Web site plan in order to ensure feedback and delayed communication with clients. A survey page added to the Web site allows an ongoing collection of opinion and feedback. This is especially useful for TQM (total quality management) activities and trend analysis. Health professionals can also visit online community bulletin boards and promote health events, provide information, or referrals or otherwise contribute information to boards separate from the Web site. Monitoring other Web sites and bulletin boards is recommended as a mechanism for identifying need and monitoring public opinion.

On-line Conferencing

Hosting an on-line conference is a means of holding an educational conference or providing an interactive learning experience on the computer. A health provider can develop such a conference in a number of ways, a presentation can be developed using a program such as PowerPoint, Astound, or Macromedia for example. This presentation may or may not include an interactive component. The program is compiled and prepared for distribution on the Web. It is uploaded by the Webmaster and sits on the Web site until activated by a user either by password or by triggering a button on the assigned page. If the program is taking place in real time with interactive conferencing, the facilitator or conference leader runs the program from his or her computer station. Participants log on and interact with each other from individual computers at various locations. An interactive box appears on all screens, and participants and leaders questions and comments appear on everyone's screen at the same time. The conference may include visuals when whiteboards or video cameras are used by the instructor. Video cameras can be mounted on the top of computers for visual imaging, and voice can also be added, although delays often can occur when uploading. Depending on the type of presentation, real-time interaction may not be necessary. A presentation can be developed by the instructor that includes decision making by the participant. This may be in the form of decision trees or multiple-choice answers. The response moves the participant to another section of the presentation and in this way allows the learner to set his or her own pace. This is especially useful for information that is repetitive and requires consistent presentation. Orientation or safety information, teaching a client and family how to operate home health equipment, or providing a decision-making model for diet control are all examples of applications for this type of presentation. In some instances, depending on the program used, feedback or scoring can be downloaded by the instructor at a later time and the instructor can then provide additional information or feedback to the user.

Distance Consultation

Providing consultation on-line is an effective and efficient mechanism for using the Internet as a means of providing information to individuals or groups. This is especially useful for peer group supervision and specialty consultation where geographic boundaries create access problems. Practitioners in remote areas of the country or in isolated practices can benefit from the contact with more experienced providers and peers. Reducing the need for costly travel encourages more frequent contact and is economically realistic. Computer contact combined with telephone contact creates a more personal exchange but is not necessary in all instances. The ability for doctors to obtain diagnostic consultation from colleagues all over the world is changing the way medicine is practiced. EKGs,

X-rays and visual images exchanged over the Internet have created the backbone of the current medical practice known as telemedicine. *Telemedicine* is the process of providing medical consultation to patients or other physicians over the Internet. In some remote locations, technicians provide the face-to-face contact with clients, performing medical testing (e.g., blood pressure, X-ray) and sending this information out over the Net to physicians at other locations. The information is reviewed, diagnosis made, and treatment established. Issues of licensing, accountability, confidentiality and ownership of information continue to be discussed and addressed as telemedicine evolves. It is time for health providers to participate in telemedicine and utilize it for health promotion. Sites such as holisticinstitute.com or other such collaborative sites offer opportunities to establish holistic practice sites.

GUIDELINES FOR USING THE INTERNET

The evolution of the Internet pose new opportunities, many of them good but all with inherent potential for problems. Issues such as confidentiality, fraud and abuse, user health and safety, licensing and accountability along with such issues as computer-generated stress and social isolation are of concern for frequent users of the Internet. As the role of geographic boundaries in professional practice changes, state regulated licenses, practice standards, and protocols will need to be reviewed. The privacy of both the provider and the consumer must be protected, and standardized guidelines are one mechanism that can make the Internet a positive factor in a person's life. Health on the Net Foundation, an international organization, has articulated a code of conduct for medical and health Web sites. Eight principles address authority, the role of information, confidentiality, attribution, justification, authorship, and honesty in advertising (Health on the Net, 1997). Agreement regarding these principles and the development of a process for self-regulation are critical in order to establish the credibility of Internet-transmitted information.

Technological Assessment

Technological assessment is a necessary standard operating procedure for all clients in this day and age. It is important not only as a health-promotion tool, but research has shown that computer-based activity increases the levels of epinepherine in the bloodstream and can create a chronic stress response in some people (Arnetz & Berg, 1993). Excessive computer use can disrupt relationships and alter cognitive functioning (Weil & Rosen, 1997). It is important to identify the role a computer plays in a client's life and whether any problems may be related to computer use patterns. It is through the assessment of a client's technological activities that plans can be made to develop a role as an information coach or that identification of health-threatening behaviors can be identified. A thorough assessment will provide data that can be used for treatment planning and strategy development. Box 9.3 presents a case study of how one woman used the Internet for health-promotion activities. The integration of technology into a client's treatment plan may not appeal to everyone, and certainly it requires the health provider to ensure that his or her technological skills are up-to-date and competent.

Safety

The health and safety of Internet users is a major concern. The Internet is an open

system much like a city or town and requires that safety policies and procedures be followed consistently. This is especially important for children and their parents. Encourage the placement of household computers in common areas where parents can observe and monitor Internet activity. Never agree to meet an Internet friend at a private location, never give out personal information to strangers, and encourage clients to follow these safety guidelines. Promptly report any lewd or unsolicited pornographic activity to the Internet access provider.

Health

It is advised that a regular computer user schedule 15-minute rest periods every hour away from electronic devices and intersperse sedentary activity with physical activity on a regular basis. The same strategies used for reducing the effects of chronic stress are recommended for reducing the physical effects of working with computers (Sheehan, 1999). Opportunities abound to access instructions for bomb-making, cults, and pornography among others. Obsession, whether with work or with surfing the Web, can disrupt relationships and interfere with daily functioning. Evidence of psychological or emotional symptoms such as paranoia, depression, or obsession warrants investigation. Appropriate referral may be necessary if behavioral symptoms are exacerbated by computer use or Internet contacts.

Confidentiality

Confidentiality is an ongoing issue as hackers continually challenge the computer industry to find new ways to protect personal information. One simple strategy for protecting the confidentiality of client identities during on-line consultation or

Box 9.3   A Case Study

Mary Smith is a 45-year-old woman who has four small children between the ages of 18 months (twins) and 5 years. Mary's husband owns his own business and she stays home with the children, taking occasional jobs as a freelance writer. A 14-year-old girl comes to help Mary 3 days a week after school. The winter brought many colds into the house as the oldest child began first grade this year and the next oldest started kindergarten. Mary does not get out much and is concerned about her weight and an intermittent sense of isolation. She uses herbs and vitamins often and is interested in providing nutritious meals for the family. Mary finds time to go to the local YMCA with the children. While there she begins an exercise program and is introduced to a health-promotion coach (new role). The health coach maintains a Web site and Mary is given the Website address and encouraged to "come on line."

The health coach begins an online program with Mary, combined with occasional face-to-face meetings at the YMCA activity center. Mary participates in the following ways:

Using E-mail

- she updates the health coach on any problems she may be having finding time to get to the exercise room. The coach suggests at-home exercises when time is limited due to children's illness or weather.
- she submits a daily nutrition diary and the coach makes recommendations and refers her to various links for vegetarian recipes specific to her likes and dislikes.
- she passes along schedule changes, questions, etc.

The health coach has also begun an on-line facilitated chat about nutrition and exercise. Mary participates with four other at-home mothers and has begun to establish a support group. In addition, the health coach has recommended the following links:

http://ahha.org
http://www.integrativemedicine.org/library/education.html
http://nccam.nih.gov/nccam/clearinghouse/

These are credible sites that provide information about holistic health and would provide a location to verify other information acquired from the Internet. The coach has also suggested that Mary enjoy some of the more recreational sites such as craft sites (*MarthaStewart.com*); an on-line mothers' resource site (*http://www.cyberrmom.com*); cooking sites (*epicurious.com*) or (*sierrahome.com*); and keep up with current events (*MSNBC.com*).

supervision is the practice of assigning code names or numbers to each client. The last name can be abbreviated using the last initial, or a hard copy of the coding sheet can be distributed by mail or fax prior to the conference. More sophisticated and expensive encryption processes must be in place for the transfer of medical or visual records such as X-rays. Credit cards and banking information are usually handled using sophisticated encryption software programs that are readily available or that can be obtained by contracting with an outside company. The industry's rapid response to hacker threats is critical to the continuing development of Internet applications and growth; without an assurance of privacy the Internet will fail. Personal information collected about visitors to a Web site or a conference comes under confidentiality guidelines. Privacy issues continue to be a grave concern especially around health sites. Web sites are encouraged to declare and maintain privacy policies as standard operating procedure and should be boycotted when they do not.

Fraud and Abuse

Providing credit card numbers over the Internet continues to involve some risk. This risk decreases when common sense purchasing rules are followed:

1. Verify vendor name, address, and telephone number as well as E-mail address.
2. Purchase by credit card whenever possible.
3. Review credentials and credibility or references before buying.
4. Review credit card bills and bank statements for duplicate or unauthorized billing and report any discrep-

ancies to the company or bank immediately.

In addition to credit-card fraud, charlatans and snake-oil salesmen have the capability to operate on the Web. Some clients may be especially vulnerable due to disease states, despair, or belief systems. Warn clients to be skeptical about promises that are too good to be true and assist in on-line searches to verify information or evaluate vendors. Stay well-read and develop an awareness of news stories about the Web and any new fraudulent practices. Check on licenses and state regulations, verify businesses with the attorney general's office, and otherwise check on references.

Teaching Discernment

Teaching clients how to discern the value of a Web site can be tricky. Discernment is subjective by nature and individuals may have different standards. Teach clients to review the credentials of the author, the site, the date of the material, and any backup references or bibliography. Encourage clients to look beyond graphics and style and to examine the content carefully. Determine the reason for the existence of the site. Is it a commerce, government, organizational, or network site? Substantiate any facts by reviewing additional Web sites and encourage the client to ask questions as needed. Printing out material and organizing it in a binder or folder helps keep track of information obtained and makes it more usable over time. Provide clients with a list of reliable links to use as necessary or maintain a list of good links on your Web site for access by your clients like rnnetwork.org does.

THE FUTURE

The evolving role of the Internet will stimulate new roles for every person participating in the health care arena. Questions will continue to be debated: Who will own the information transferred across cyberspace? Will insurance reimburse for medication that is purchased on-line? How will a client know who is providing the information? The answers to these questions will continue to change in response to new developments in technology, regulation, and education. In the beginning, direct care providers were protected from technology. Today, computers are at the bedside, in schools, kitchens, senior centers, and nursing homes. Health providers cannot ignore or reject the role technology will continue to play, and they must become active in the discussions, the planning, and the entire cyber experience.

REFERENCES

Arnetz, B., & Berg, M. (1993). Techno-stress; Psycho-physiological consequences of poor man-machine interface. In Michael J. Smith & Gabriel Salandy (Eds.), *Human Computer Interaction: Applications and Case Studies*. Amsterdam: Elseview, 891–896.

Biomed. (1999). *Cybermed*. Berkeley, CA: Biomed General Corporation.

Eager, B. (1994). *Using the internet*. Indianapolis, IN: Que Corporation.

Graves, J. R., & Corcoran, S. (1989). The study of nursing informatics. *Image: Journal of Nursing Scholarship, 21*(4).

Hart, J. A., & Reed, R. R. (1992). *The Building of the Internet*, Telecommunications Policy (Nov. 1992), 666–689.

Internet Society. (2000) Reston, VA.

Jones, S. (1997). *Virtual culture: Identity and communication in cybersociety*. Sage Publishers.

Leiner, B. M., Cerf, V. G., Clark, D. D, Kahn, R. E., Kleinrock, L., Lynch, D. C., Postel, J., Roberts, L. G., & Wolff, S. (1998). *A brief history of the internet* [On-line] Available: http://www.isoc.org/internet-history/brief.htm.

Little, R. P. (1999). *Web design for health care professionals*. Berkeley, CA: Biomed General Corporation.

Miller, R. L. (1994). 10 good reasons for multimedia training. *Multimedia Today, 2*(4), 34.

Sheehan, J. (1999). *Managing and coping with computer generated stress*. Rehoboth, MA: Two Hawk Productions.

Smith, A. (1997). *Criteria for evaluation of Internet information resources* [On-line]. Available: http://www.vuw.ac.nz/~agsmith/evaln/index.htm

Symmetrics. (1999). *What are data, information and knowledge?* [On-line]. Available: http://www.symmetrics/What_are_DIK.htm.

Weil, M., & Rosen, L. (1997). *TechnoStress: Coping with Technology @Work @Home @Play*. New York: Wiley & Sons.

PART III

Strategies for Wellness

CHAPTER 10

Nutrition and Weight Management

Carolyn Chambers Clark

SUGGESTED DIETARY GOALS

The United States Select Committee on Nutrition adopted seven dietary goals in 1977. They have been used in *Healthy People 2010* as a basis for action. Use them to counsel clients about wellness-promoting foods.

Goal 1. To avoid overweight, consume only as much energy (calories) as expended. Decrease energy intake and increase exercise if overweight. One in three Americans is overweight. The Dietary Goals recommends reducing foods high in fat, refined and processed foods, sugars, and alcohol, and increasing high-fiber foods such as fruits, vegetables, whole grains, and legumes.

Goal 2. Increase consumption of fresh fruits and vegetables and whole grains to 48% of food intake. Complex carbohydrates are satisfying and protect against cardiovascular disease, constipation, cancer, and overweight (Thun, 1992; Ames et al., 1994). To consume 55%–60% of total calories as carbohydrate, meat becomes a condiment, as in Oriental cooking and rice, pasta, potatoes and other starches the main dish. Guide-

lines for increasing complex carbohydrates and fiber in the diet:

- Choose whole and fresh foods over processed and refined ones; if fresh local foods are not available, choose fresh-frozen ones, avoiding heavy sauces.
- Choose whole wheat products over white, refined flour. The average white flour retains only 76% of the original wheat grain. When refined to white flour, 10–100% of the trace minerals, vitamins, and fiber are lost; only a small minority is replaced in "enriched" products.
- Select whole grain products for breakfast; leftovers from brown rice, bulgar, kasha, or whole grain noodles can be used as cereal. If no leftovers are available, choose hot cereals (avoiding "instant" or "quick cooking" varieties, which imply greater processing) over cold, ready-to-eat cereals made from refined grain products.
- Become creative in increasing complex carbohydrate meals, e.g., chili without beef, salads, soups, sandwich

spreads from one or more types of beans and other vegetables, pocket bread sandwiches, vegetable and pasta or rice casseroles.

Goal 3.   Reduce consumption of refined and processed sugars to 10% of daily intake. Refined sugars add empty calories that increase weight, rob the body's stores of vitamins and minerals during metabolism, and replace nutritious foods or lead to weight gain. Guidelines for reducing sugar in meal planning are:

- Read labels and avoid foods containing sucrose, raw sugar, glucose, brown sugar, turbinado honey, dextrose, fructose, corn syrup, corn sweetener, and natural sweetener; the closer the sugar is to the beginning of the list of ingredients, the greater the amount of sugar present.
- Substitute fruit juices, nonfat milk, unsweetened tea, mineral water with a slice of lemon, vegetable juice, and water for sugared, fruit-flavored drinks and soft drinks. Although commercial diet soft drinks are low in sugar, they may be high in additives, dyes, phosphates (calcium-robbing), and caffeine.
- Choose fresh fruits or fruits canned in unsweetened juice.
- Choose ready-to-eat cereals with sugar listed as the fourth or lower item on the ingredients list; sweeten cereal with fruit.
- Begin reducing sugar in recipes gradually; use a juice concentrate instead of sugar in recipes.

Goal 4.   Reduce fat consumption to 30% of daily intake.

*Goal 5.   Reduce intake of saturated fat to 10%, and take in 10% of calories in polyunsat-*urated fats and another 10% in monounsaturated fats.

Goal 6.   Reduce cholesterol consumption to 300 grams/day. Saturated fats and cholesterol are strongly associated with increased risk of cardiovascular disease, hypertension, obesity, atherosclerosis, and other degenerative diseases. Polyunsaturated fat is associated with increased risk of cancer. Some guidelines for meeting goals related to dietary fat include:

- Reduce intake of high fat foods: french fries, hamburgers, whole milk, whole milk cheeses, ice cream, bacon, prepared salad dressings, cream, nondairy creamers, hydrogenated oils (available on the grocery shelf and in many prepared foods; read ingredients list on all foods purchased), and whipped cream substitutes.
- Obtain needed essential fatty acids from vegetable oils that are relatively nonprocessed (virgin olive oil; dark, unprocessed oils), unprocessed nuts and seeds, fish, and unprocessed whole grains.
- Reduce dietary cholesterol by lowering intake of eggs, liver, and organ meats, red meats, animal fats (lard and chicken fat or skin), and high-fat dairy products.
- Use low- or nonfat yogurt or cottage cheese as a garnish for baked potatoes.
- Prepare salad dressing from yogurt, nonfat cottage cheese, garlic, onion, spices, vinegar, and lemon juice.
- Select broiled or baked meat, fowl, and fish; remove fat and skin prior to eating.
- Avoid foods implying that fat is used in the preparation, including descriptions such as: refried, creamed, cream sauce, au gratin, parmesan, escalloped, au lait, a la mode, marinated,

prime, pot pie, au fromage, stewed, basted, casserole, hollandaise, or crispy.

- Choose foods that are steamed, in broth, in its own juice, poached, roasted, or in tomato or marinara sauce; these imply low-fat preparation.
- Read nutrition information panels prior to purchasing processed foods. Avoid purchasing foods containing: animal fat, egg and egg yolk solids, butter, bacon fat, lard, palm oil, shortening, vegetable fat, hydrogenated or partially hydrogenated oils, whole milk solids, cream and cream sauces, coconut oil, coconut, milk chocolate.
- Elevate meat, fowl, or fish when roasting or broiling; do not baste with drippings; use wine, fruit juice, or broth instead.
- Roast at a low temperature (325–350° F) to enhance flavor and fat removal. High temperatures seal fats into the meat.
- Chill meat or fowl drippings and remove fat prior to preparing sauces or gravies.
- Sauté vegetables in defatted chicken stock.

Goal 7. *Limit intake of table salt to 5 grams/ day.* Use the following guidelines to reduce sodium:

- Read food and medication labels to identify and eliminate foods processed with salt or containing sodium additives, including baking soda, monosodium glutamate (MSG), cough medicines, laxatives, aspirin, sedatives, sodium phosphate, sodium alginate, sodium nitrate, etc.
- Reduce consumption of food processed in brine—olives, sauerkraut, pickles—or soak in water prior to eating.

- Avoid commercial snacks including potato and corn chips, salted peanuts, pretzels, and crackers.
- Avoid salted or smoked meats, sandwich meats, bacon, hot dogs, corned or chipped beef, sausage, and salt pork.
- Reduce or eliminate salted condiments: catsup, mustard, Worcestershire sauce, bouillon cubes, soy sauce, barbeque sauce.
- Limit processed and high salt cheeses; choose the low salt varieties.

Be aware that there still is no solid evidence that lowering salt (NaCl) intake will prevent or control high blood pressure. If it does, only 30 to 40% of adults are salt-sensitive (Muntzell & Drücke, 1992).

VITAMINS AND MINERALS

The Case for and against Vitamin and Mineral Supplementation

There are arguments for and against the need for vitamin and mineral supplementation. The American Dietetic Association National Center for Nutrition and Dietetics and the President's Council on Physical Fitness and Sports now recommend using the Food Guide Pyramid including 6–11 daily servings of bread, cereal, rice, and/or pasta; 3–5 daily servings of vegetables; 2–4 daily servings of fruit; 2–3 daily servings of milk, yogurt and/or cheese; 2–3 daily servings of meat, poultry, fish, dry beans, eggs, and/ or nuts; and sparing use of fats, oils, and/ or sweets (1995).

Loomis (1992) compared fatalities due to vitamin supplements versus prescription and nonprescription, legal drugs to illustrate the safety of vitamin use. For example, in 1990, there was one fatality due to niacin abuse and none for any other vitamin, compared to 487 fatalities due to pharmaceutical drugs. His statistics from 1983–1990 show that vitamins are 2,500 times safer than prescription and nonprescription pharmaceuticals. Some of the reasons cited in favor of proper vitamin supplementation are due to changes in the available food sources.

Justification for Supplementation

- Some soils are depleted and produce crops that are nutritionally inferior.
- Toxic insecticides leave harmful residues on food and kill important soil microorganisms and earthworms.
- The increasing use of chemicals in the processing of food has depleted them nutritionally.
- Increasing numbers of people eat vitamin-free sugar as 25% of their daily food intake.
- Chemical additives replace other essential food elements and may also be toxic.
- Numerous life experiences require additional vitamin and mineral stores to reduce stress, including: any difficulty with the digestive tract (diarrhea, colitis, liver or gall bladder disorders); pregnancy; breastfeeding; increased physical activity; infections; the use of antibiotics, aspirin, estrogen, steroids, sulfa drugs, or anticoagulants; inhaling polluted air; drinking polluted water; prolonged emotional stress; smoking or being in a smoke-filled room; fractures; alcohol intake.
- A change in lifestyle in America to a more hectic pace has decreased effective meal planning and led to more "fast-food" meals.

For these reasons, even if it were possible to eat a wide variety of foods, vitamin and mineral supplementation may be necessary. As early as 1943 the Food and Drug Administration (FDA) recognized that food processing was destroying important nutrients. Regulations were passed requiring "enrichment" of processed foods; at the time, the FDA noted that enriched foods were second best to unprocessed ones.

The argument against vitamin and mineral supplementation is that if everyone eats a wide variety of foods, all essential nutrients are available. This argument may be most relevant for the ambulatory, well-informed consumer who is able and willing to eat the wide variety of foods necessary.

Additional information that may be useful as a reference source for practitioner and client appears in the following tables: Wellness-Enhancing Foods (Table 10.1), Vitamin Functions, Deficiency Symptoms, and Food Sources (Table 10.2), RDAs and Reasons for Supplementation (Table 10.3), and Reference to Minerals (Table 10.4).

NUTRIENTS FOR PREVENTION: A REVIEW OF THE RESEARCH

This section provides a review of the nutrition literature. Use this information with clients in whatever way is helpful to them.

HIV/AIDS

Patrick (2000) reviewed the literature on HIV/AIDS and nutrition and found compelling evidence that micronutrient deficiencies (zinc, magnesium, vitamins A, E and specific B vitamins) can profoundly affect immunity and are widely found in HIV/AIDS, even in individuals who do not yet have symptoms. These findings clearly illustrate the need for nutritional supplementation with this condition.

TABLE 10.1   Wellness-Enhancing Foods

Eat these often	Vitamins provided	Minerals provided	Other advantages
Raw spinach*	A_1, B_2, B_6, C, folic acid, E, K	calcium, magnesium, potassium, copper, iodine, manganese	provides fiber and complex carbohydrate
Wheat germ (toasted)	B_1, B_2, B_3, B_{12}, inositol, choline, E	magnesium, potassium, chromium	high protein
Brewer's** yeast	B_1, B_2, B_3, B_6, B_{12}, pantothenic acid, biotin, inositol, choline, E, folic acid	selenium, chromium, copper, zinc, magnesium, calcium, potassium	can be sprinkled on foods or in drinks
Kale	A, B_2, C	calcium, magnesium, copper, iodine, manganese	provides fiber and complex carbohydrate; neutralizes free radicals and is associated with lowering cancer risk
Cantaloupe	A, folic acid, inositol, C	manganese	provides fiber and is a good dessert substitute for "sweets," neutralizes free radicals and lowers cancer risk
Sunflower seeds	B_1, B_2, B_3, B_6, pantothenic acid	manganese	easy to carry for a quick snack, provides fiber to lower risk of colon cancer and diverticulitis
Onions	C, inositol		reduces cancer risk, lowers cholesterol
Mustard Greens	C, inositol, B_5		lowers cancer risk
Sweet potatoes/yams/ pumpkins	E, inositol, A		high fiber, lowers cancer risk
Garlic	A		natural antibiotic action, reduces cholesterol, reduces cancer risk
Parsley	Most nutrient-dense food known		protects against cancer risk
Rosemary			inhibits carcinogens or co-carcinogens

(continued)

TABLE 10.1 *(continued)*

Eat these often	Vitamins provided	Minerals provided	Other advantages
Brown rice	B_1, B_6, inositol	magnesium, iodine	inexpensive, good source of protein when combined with beans, eggs, or milk products
Broccoli	A, folic acid, pantothenic acid, C, E	calcium, magnesium, potassium, copper, iodine, manganese	provides fiber and complex carbohydrate; neutralizes free radicals and protects against cancer risk and diverticulitis
Chicken (no skin)	B_2, B_3, B_6, folic acid	copper, chromium	low fat; very usable protein
Whole grains	B_1, B_2, B_{12}, choline, biotin, inositol, E	calcium, magnesium, iron, selenium, manganese, chromium	provides fiber, lowers colon cancer risk, natural laxative, protects against diverticulitis
Cauliflower	pantothenic acid, C, E, K	manganese	provides fiber, lowers cancer and diverticulitis risk, complex carbohydrate
Peas	B_2, inositol, K	magnesium, manganese	low calorie, complex carbohydrate, provides fiber, lowers cancer and diverticulitis risk
Lima Beans	folic acid, biotin, inositol, B_2	manganese	complex carbohydrate, provides fiber to lower cancer and diverticulitis risk
Grapefruit (and citrus fruit)	inositol, C, P	magnesium, manganese	lower calorie, complex carbohydrate, corrects acid imbalance; white material beneath the peel contains flavonoids and pectin to reduce pain, lower cholesterol, heal bruises
Soybeans (and other dried beans)	B_1, B_2, B_3, choline, K	manganese	inexpensive source of protein, provides fiber, associated with low cancer rate

TABLE 10.1 *(continued)*

Eat these often	Vitamins provided	Minerals provided	Other advantages
Asparagus	B_1, folic acid, C, E	manganese	low calorie, complex carbohydrates, provides fiber to lower cancer and diverticulitis risk
Cabbage	B_6, C, E, K	potassium	low calorie, complex carbohydrate, provides fiber, lowers cancer and diverticulitis risk
Carrots	A, K	potassium, manganese	low calorie, complex carbohydrate; provides fiber, associated with low cancer rate
Fish (especially salmon, mackerel, and sardines)	B_3, B_6, B_{12}, biotin, choline, co-enzyme Q10	calcium, zinc, copper, selenium	low fat, highly usable protein, reduces cancer risk, protects heart
Yogurt (lowfat; plain)	D	calcium	high protein, low fat, provides helpful bacteria
Sprouts	A, B_2, B_3, folic acid, pyridoxine, pantothenic acid, E, K	calcium, iron, phosphorus, potassium	low calorie, inexpensive, high protein, provides fiber, lowers risk of diverticulitis

*Spinach contains oxalic acid that can decrease the amount of available calcium, so be sure to eat enough calcium from other sources to make up for this.
**Not recommended for people who have yeast infections.

Source: Extracted from Simone, C. B., M. D. *Cancer and Nutrition: A Ten-Point Plan to Reduce Your Risk of Getting Cancer.* Garden City Park: Avery Publishing Group, 1992.

Alzheimer's Disease

Grundman (2000) reviewed the literature on vitamin E and Alzheimer's disease. Many lines of evidence suggest that oxidative stress is implicated in the development of Alzheimer's disease. Beta-amyloid, found in the brains of individuals with Alzheimer's disease, is toxic due to free radicals. Grundman reported on a placebo-controlled clinical trial of vitamin E in individuals with moderately advanced Alzheimer's disease showing that vitamin E may slow functional deterioration that leads to nursing home placement.

CANCER: FOOD AND SUPPLEMENTS

Food and Supplements

Animal Fat

Giovannuci and colleagues (1993) found dietary fat to be a risk factor for prostate

TABLE 10.2   Vitamin Functions, Deficiency Symptoms, and Food Sources

Vitamin	Functions	Deficiency symptoms or signs	Sources
A and its precursor, beta-carotene	helps fight infection, maintains cell wall strength, and prevents viruses from penetrating and reproducing; blocks production of cancerous tumors	night blindness, itching and burning of eyes, redness of eyelids, drying of mucous membranes, colds or respiratory troubles, dry rough skin, pimples or acne, susceptibility to eye infections, difficulty urinating or performing sexually	carrots, broccoli, kale, turnip greens, watercress, beets, dandelion greens, spinach, eggs, milk fat, papayas, parsley, red peppers, fish liver oils, sweet potatoes, pumpkin, yellow squash, apricots, cantaloupes, organ meats*
B_1 (thiamine)	promotes appetite and good digestion, plays an important role in oxidation, blood and protein metabolism, and growth	tiredness with inability to sleep, swelling legs, loss of appetite, lack of enthusiasm, forgetting things regularly, aching or tender calf muscles, rapid heartbeat, overreacting to normal stress, constipation, feeling of going crazy	sunflower seeds, brewer's yeast, beef kidney,* whole wheat flour, rolled oats, green peas, soybeans, beef heart, lima beans, crabmeat, brown rice, asparagus, raisins, desiccated liver, wheat germ
B_2 (riboflavin)	contributes to protein and carbohydrate metabolism, tissue repair and formation, growth in infants, proper nitrogen balance in adults, light adaptation	feeling trembly, dizzy, or sluggish, burning feet, chapping lips, tiring easily, being overly nervous, having bloodshot eyes	beef, liver, kidney, or heart,* ham, chicken, hazelnuts, peanuts, hickory nuts, soybeans, soy flour, wheat germ and whole wheat products, spinach, kale, peas, lima beans, brewer's yeast, sunflower seeds, eggs
B_3 (niacin)	dilates blood vessels, aids in carbohydrate metabolism and the use of vitamins B_1 and B_2	having cold feet or body numbness, having a swollen bright red tongue or gums, feeling overly anxious, weak, or tired, having memory loss, developing prickly heat rash	wheat germ, wheat bran, brewer's yeast, salmon, prunes, lentils, chicken, peanuts, sunflower seeds, tuna, turkey, rabbit

TABLE 10.2 *(continued)*

Vitamin	Functions	Deficiency symptoms or signs	Sources
B_6 (pyridoxine)	activates enzymes, aids in metabolism of fats, carbohydrates, potassium, iron, protein, and formation of hormones, nucleic acids, and antibodies, hemoglobin, and lecithin, dissolves cholesterol and regulates water imbalance, may be useful in fighting off cancer, one form of anemia, and tooth decay	feeling tense, irritable, or nervous, not being able to concentrate or sleep, having tics, tremors, twitches, bad breath, seborrheic dermatitis or eczema, bloating, puffiness, soreness, or cramping in menstruating or menopausal women	brewer's yeast, sunflower seeds, toasted wheat germ, brown rice, soybeans, white beans, liver, chicken, mackerel, salmon, tuna, bananas, walnuts, peanuts, sweet potatoes, cooked cabbage
B_{12}	maintains normal red blood cell formation and nervous system, aids in RNA and DNA manufacture, conversion of folic acid to folinic acid, carbohydrate, fat, and protein metabolism, fertility, and growth and resistance to germs	feeling apathetic, moody, forgetful, suspicious, soreness in arms or legs or having difficulty walking or talking, jerking of arms or legs	organ meats,* raw beef, clams, oysters, sardines, crab, crayfish, mackerel, trout, herring, eggs, some cheeses, nutritional yeast, sea vegetables (kombu, dulse, kelp, wakame), fermented soyfoods (tempeh, natto, and miso)
Folic acid	vital to blood formation, cell growth, synthesis of RNA or DNA, resistance to infections and to proper mental functioning	looking pale and wan, feeling "pooped," brownish spots on face and hands, panting with slight exertion	asparagus, desiccated or fresh liver,* fresh dark green uncooked vegetables, wheat bran, turnips, potatoes, orange juice, black-eyed peas, lima beans, watermelon, oysters, cantaloupe
Pantothenic acid	protects against environmental stress and infection, works with pyridoxine and folic acid to create antibodies, assists in production of body energy, protects against side effects of some antibiotics, aids in expelling trapped intestinal gas	balky bowels, chronic gas or distension, feeling fatigued or not hungry, constant respiratory infections, strange itching or burning sensations	soy flour, sunflower seeds, dark buckwheat, sesame seeds, brewer's yeast, peanuts, lobster, wheat bran, broccoli, mushrooms, eggs, oysters, sweet potatoes, cauliflower, organ meats*

(continued)

TABLE 10.2   *(continued)*

Vitamin	Functions	Deficiency symptoms or signs	Sources
Biotin	aids in metabolism of carbohydrates, proteins, and fats, assists in growth, maintenance of skin, hair, nerves, sebaceous glands, bone marrow, and sex glands	poor appetite, sore mouth and lips, dermatitis, nausea and vomiting, depression, pallor, muscle pains, pains around the heart, tickling sensation in hands and feet	nutritional yeast, liver,* eggs, mushrooms, lima beans, yogurt, and a variety of nuts, fish, and grains
Inositol	not clear, but seems to be useful in controlling cholesterol level, hair, growth, fat metabolism	not known	wheat germ, oranges, grapefruit, watermelon, peas, cantaloupes, whole grain breads and cereals, molasses, nuts, brewer's yeast, bulgar wheat, lima beans, oysters, peaches, lettuce, brown rice
Choline	essential to nerve fluid, liver functioning, keeping blood pressure down, increasing body resistance to infection	not known, possibly poor thinking ability	egg yolks, soybeans, liver,* brewer's yeast, fish, peanuts, wheat germ, lecithin
C (ascorbic acid)	contributes to health of blood vessels, gums, teeth, and bones, essential to assimilation of iron, aids body in fighting off infection and cancer-producing substances and in normalizing blood cholesterol level, detoxifies some of the poisons due to smoking, aids in healing process, essential to collagen (body "glue"), slows down aging, and protects against stress, works synergistically with vitamin E	frequent bruises, poor healing, bleeding gums when toothbrushing, frequent infections, feeling run down, having an aching back due to disc lesions	green peppers, honeydew melon, cooked broccoli or brussels sprouts or kale, cantaloupes, strawberries, papaya, cooked cauliflower, oranges, watercress, raspberries, parsley, raw cabbage, grapefruit, blackberries, lemons, onions, sprouts, spinach, tomatoes, rose hip tea or powder

TABLE 10.2 *(continued)*

Vitamin	Functions	Deficiency symptoms or signs	Sources
D	vital for maintaining health and growth of bones, for using calcium, and for metabolic functions affecting eyes, heart, and nervous system, should be taken with calcium	weakness and generalized bone aches, localized back pain on arising or bending over, pain in areas where spinal vertebrae may have collapsed, brittle bones that break easily, pain in mid- to lower back	fish, liver oil, vitamin D-enriched milk, eggs, salmon, tuna
E	seems to be useful in any condition where there is actual or threatened clotting, decrease in blood supply, increased oxygen need, externally when there are burns, or sores to heal, or to protect against exposure to radiation, body needs zinc to maintain proper levels of vitamin E	not known	nutritional yeast, wheat germ, peanuts, outer leaf of cabbage, leafy portions of broccoli and cauliflower, raw spinach, asparagus, whole grain rice or wheat or oats, cold pressed wheat germ cottonseed, or safflower oil, cornmeal, eggs, sweet potatoes
K	essential to blood clotting	some types of bleeding without clotting	spinach, cabbage, cauliflower, tomatoes, pork liver,* lean meat, peas, carrots, soybeans, potatoes, wheat germ, egg yolks

Note: Any chemicals ingested by animals concentrate in their organs and especially their livers; if you decide to eat organ meats to ensure adequate intake of vitamins, you might consider extra amounts of the vitamins that detoxify your body, such as vitamin C and pantothenic acid.

cancer. Red meat represented the food group with the strongest positive association with advanced cancer. Fat from dairy products, with the exception of butter, and fish were unrelated to risk. High intake of foods from animal sources (meat, eggs, cheese) was slightly, but not statistically, related to elevated risk for endometrial cancer. The only significant dose-response relation observed was for processed fish and meat (Zheng et al., 1995b).

Risch and associates (1994) found that eating 10 g per day of saturated fat may raise a woman's risk of ovarian cancer by 20%. They compared the eating habits of 450 women age 35 to 79 years with newly diagnosed ovarian cancer to those of 540 demographically similar healthy women in Ontario, Canada. Participants were surveyed about their number of pregnancies, history of oral contraceptive use, and diet. For every 10 g of saturated fat consumed daily, the risk of ovarian cancer rose 20%. Women who lowered their saturated fat consumption by 10 g per day experienced a 20% drop in risk. Nonsaturated fat had

TABLE 10.3   Recommended Amounts of Vitamin For Adults; Reasons Supplementation May Be Needed

Vitamin	RDA	Alternative Recommendations**	Reasons supplementation may be needed
A* or beta-carotene	Adults: 5,000 I.U. daily Nursing mothers: 4,000 I.U. daily Pregnant women: 6,000	10,000 I.U. daily; children require less, based on their weight Pregnant women require more	Americans are eating 30 pounds less fresh fruit and 20 pounds less vegetables per capita per year than in 1950; cooking dramatically decreases the value of the vitamin; widespread use of fertilizers and pesticides interferes with body's ability to convert carotene into vitamin A; high-protein diets require more vitamin A to process; cold temperatures, air pollution require additional amounts of the vitamin.
B_1 (thiamine)	1.2–1.5 mg daily	50 mg	Cereal and rice producers remove thiamine when germ and outer coating are removed; large quantities are lost in cooking water; people who eat little or no organ meats, fresh vegetables, oatmeal, potatoes, and beans may receive little thiamine, as do people who have diarrhea, who eat excess sugars or carbohydrates, drink coffee or alcohol, take antibiotics, or smoke, and those exposed to stress or aging processes.
B_2 (riboflavin)	1.3–1.7 mg daily	50 mg	Supplements are needed by people who eat snack foods, processed desserts, or commercial baked goods; the vitamin is destroyed by cooking or when antibiotics or oral contraceptives are taken; it is destroyed when milk bottles or meat containers are left exposed to light.
B_3	18–20 mg daily	100 mg daily	Heavy intake of highly refined and/or carbohydrate foods requires more B_3 to metabolize; it is lost during cooking; its metabolism is interfered with when taking oral antibiotics; illness and taking alcoholic beverages decreases its absorption.
B_6 (pyridoxine)	Male adults: 2 mg daily Nursing and pregnant women: 1.6 mg daily	50 mg daily	Losses of B_6 are due to refining, cooking, processing, storing, and to eating a high-protein diet; there is an increased need when taking steroids (such as cortisone and estrogen), oral contraceptives, or when pregnant or menstruating.

TABLE 10.3 *(continued)*

Vitamin	RDA	Alternative Recommendations**	Reasons supplementation may be needed
B_{12}	2 micrograms (mcg) daily	300 mcg daily	When eating only vegetarian meals.
Folic acid	400 mcg daily		Needed during pregnancy for an adequate development of fetal nerve cells, when taking oral contraceptives, when growing or aging, when faced with trauma, infection, or chronic daily stress, or when drinking alcoholic beverages; works best when combined with Vitamin B_{12}.
Pantothenic acid (PABA)	4–7 mg daily	25 mg daily	Needed to supplement processed food; greater need when subjected to infection, environmental stress, x-rays, surgery, or antibiotics; helps protect against sunburn.
Biotin	No RDA	30 mcg daily	Needed when eating raw eggs or taking antibiotics or sulfa drugs or when eating beef (cattle are routinely given antibiotics and hormones).
Choline	No RDA	100 mg daily	Infants need it if not breast fed (cow's milk does not contain this vitamin but breast milk does).
Inositol		100 mg daily	Caffeine may rob the body of this nutrient.
C	30–45 mg daily	1000–3000 mg daily	Needed to slow down aging processes, increase healing of infection, disease, or injury; decrease effects of toxic chemicals in the environment; if taking aspirin, more of this vitamin is needed; when smoking or drinking, more is required; soaking vegetables and fresh fruits in water or exposing fruit or juices to air destroys this vitamin.
D*	200–400 I.U. daily		Calcium is not absorbed without sufficient vitamin D; needed at times of insufficient sun exposure in winter, when soot and air pollution filter out sun rays, when spending long hours in offices or indoors; when taking steroids, or when smoking.

(continued)

TABLE 10.3 *(continued)*

Vitamin	RDA	Alternative Recommendations**	Reasons supplementation may be needed
E	12–15 I.U. daily	600 I.U. daily	When outer leaves of vegetables are not eaten; when vegetables are placed in vigorously boiling water to cook (rather than bringing the water to a boil); when eating processed foods, exposed to smog, drinking chlorinated water, undertaking strenuous exercise, when exposed to air purifiers, static electricity, sun, x-rays; by those who take oxygen as a therapeutic measure, have had a heart attack or burn.
K	65–80 mcg	100 mcg of alfalfa	People who are elderly, women with prolonged menstruation, people with liver disease, diarrhea, colitis or who take antibiotics or anticoagulants (blood-thinners).

Note: Vitamins A and D are the only two vitamins that can be toxic if taken in excess; extra amounts of other vitamins are excreted by the body. If you note symptoms overdosage in vitamins A or D, discontinue taking it until symptoms disappear, then take a smaller dose. Symptoms of vitamin A overdosage: bone or joint pain that comes and goes, fatigue, insomnia, loss of hair, dryness and fissuring of the lips, loss of appetite, peeling and flaking skin, dizziness. Symptoms of Vitamin D overdosage: nausea, weight loss, loss of appetite, head pain, calcification of bones, and in children a reduction in growth rate. RDAs are based on information provided in *Vitamins and Minerals* by Ellen Moyer, Peoples Medical Society, Allentown, PA, 1993.

**Balch & Balch (1990). *Prescription for Nutritional Healing.* Garden City Park, NY: Avery Publishing Company. The authors suggest working with a health care professional to settle on the appropriate supplements and doses. Individual needs are unique and ever-changing. RDAs were formulated for borderline health, not maximum wellness. Even Balch & Balch agree that nutrition (including supplements) must be combined with exercise and a positive attitude to obtain the best results. Suggested doses are based on the Balchs' extensive study of the literature.

no effect on ovarian cancer risk. Women who added 10 g of vegetable fiber to their diet lowered their risk of ovarian cancer by 37%. Full-term pregnancy lowered risk by 20%, and each year of oral contraceptive use lowered it another 5% to 10%.

Potter (1996) found that meat consumption was associated with increased risk for colorectal cancer but was not fully explained by its fat content. Yo (1997) reported a case-control study finding an increased risk of stomach cancer for people who frequently consumed broiled meats and fish.

Peters and others (1994) found a persistent significant association for childhood leukemia and children's intake of hot dogs and fathers' intake of hot dogs with no evidence that fruit intake provided protection. Their results are consistent with experimental animal research and the hypothesis that human N-nitrosos compound intake is associated with leukemia risk.

Citrus Pectin/Citrus Oils

Pienta and colleagues (1995) examined the ability of citrus pectin to inhibit spontaneous metastasis of prostate cancer cells in rats. Compared with 16 control rats that had lung metastases on day 30 of the study, 7 of 14 rats in the 0.1% and 9 of 16 rats in

TABLE 10.4   Reference to Minerals, Recommended Amounts, Functions, Sources, and Factors Leading to Insufficient Intake

Mineral	Functions	Best Sources	Factors leading to insufficient intake
Calcium RDA: 800 mg/day 1.5 g for menopausal women Alternate recommendation*: 1,500 mg/day	Keeps body framework rigid and teeth strong; creates tranquility in nervous system and calms nervousness; necessary for transmission of nerve impulses and for muscle contraction, clotting, some enzymes, "glue" (collagen) that holds body together and cells in place, and to regulate transport of substances in and out of cells	milk, cheese, eggs, green leafy vegetables, fish, butter, tomatoes, whole wheat bread, yogurt, canned sardines, molasses, almonds, soy milk, buttermilk, tofu (Because 1500 mg may be difficult to achieve by eating, supplementation may be necessary, especially for menopausal women. Calcium citrate is the most absorbable, safe form.)	dieting to restrict calories or cholesterol; eating snack foods; drinking soft drinks; having a high protein intake
Chromium RDA: 50–200 mg Alternative recommendation*: 150 mcg	Helps to keep blood sugar levels in check	brewer's yeast, wheat germ, calf's liver, and animal proteins except fish	refinement of cereal and grain products removes chromium; the elderly and those who are pregnant or protein-calorie malnourished are at risk for deficiency
Copper RDA: 1.5–3 mgm		almonds, avocadoes, barley, beans, dandelion greens, lentils	body levels are reduced by high intake of zinc or vitamin C (and vice versa)
Iodine RDA: 150 mcg		sea vegetables, kelp	depleted soil
Iron RDA: 15 mg to age 50 then 10 mg/day Alternative recommendation*: 18 mg/day	Works with copper to produce hemoglobin, an essential substance that carries oxygen to and from the body	organ meats, red meats, kidney beans, molasses, egg yolk, whole-grain breads and cereals	infants remaining on milk for long periods of time or those who are born of women who have low stores of iron; women who are menstruating, pregnant, breastfeeding or postmenopausal
Iodine/Kelp RDA: 130–150 mcg/day Alternative recommendation*: 225 mcg/day	Necessary for normal functioning of thyroid gland; may protect against breast cancer	seafood, brown rice, beans, bananas, green leafy vegetables, kelp	living in areas where soil is low in this mineral (Great Lakes and Rocky Mountain regions)

(continued)

TABLE 10.4 *(continued)*

Mineral	Functions	Best Sources	Factors leading to insufficient intake
Magnesium RDA: 250–350 mg/day Alternative recommendations*: 750 mg/day	Works with calcium to ensure good muscle movement and a strong heart beat; seems to prevent blood vessel and heart disease	whole grain breads and cereals, fresh peas, brown rice, soy flour, wheat germ, nuts, swiss chard, figs, green leafy vegetables, citrus fruits, dolomite	having diarrhea, vomiting, taking diuretics, drinking soft water, eating processed foods
Manganese RDA: 2.5–5 mg/day Alternative recommendation*: 2.5–5 mg/day needed	Important to fat metabolism, bone formation, brain function, reproduction, and may protect against cancer of the pancreas	nuts, seeds, whole grains, fruits and vegetables, dry beans and peas, oatmeal	high levels of calcium and phosphorus diminish absorption of manganese
Phosphorus RDA: 800 mg/day	Helps form nucleic acids; a component of cell membranes; aids in metabolism and storage and release of energy; a component of B vitamin coenzymes	liver, yogurt, milk, brown rice, wheat germ, sunflower seeds, brewer's yeast, meat, seafood, nuts, eggs, peas, beans, lentils	people with kidney disease; taking high doses of antacids
Potassium RDA: 1600–2000 mg Alternative recommendation*: 99 mg/day	Works in concert with sodium to move materials through cell walls (osmosis) and maintains acid-base balance; helps muscles contract, heart to beat regularly, nerves to carry impulses properly, and food to be turned into energy	shredded raw cabbage, bananas, turkey, apples, fresh apricots, cooked broccoli, baked potato, wheat germ, spinach, dried fruit, fresh fruits and fruits and vegetables of all kinds	using convenience foods and highly processed foods; profuse sweating; taking certain diuretics (water pills) to lose fluid; taking cardiovascular drugs, steroids, laxatives, enemas; eating licorice candy; breastfeeding, having depression or ulcerative colitis
Selenium RDA: 50–70 mcg/day Alternative recommendation*: 200 mcg/day	Protects against heart disease and cancer; detoxifies the body from effects of pollutants and radiation; important for healthy skin and hair and for production of sperm cells	high protein foods such as meats, seafoods; whole-grain breads and cereals; brewer's yeast; asparagus, garlic, mushrooms	eating beef fed on corn or eating grains grown in selenium-poor soil (northeast, Florida, parts of Washington and Oregon, parts of the Midwest); exposure to industrial pollutants

TABLE 10.4 *(continued)*

Mineral	Functions	Best Sources	Factors leading to insufficient intake
Sodium RDA: needed amount not established	Maintains osmotic pressure in the fluid outside the cells	celery, carrots, beets, cucumbers, string beans, asparagus, turnips, strawberries, oatmeal, cheese, eggs, coconut, black figs	some kidney and adrenal diseases; diarrhea; vomiting
Sulfur RDA: needed amount not established	Part of the structure of amino acids, such as keratin, the protein of the hair; component of thiamine and biotin (vitamins); required for many oxidation-reduction reactions and coenzymes; contained in blood and other tissues: detoxifying agent; part of material found in skin, bones, tendons, and cartilage	cabbage, peas, beans, cauliflower, brussels sprouts, eggs, horseradish, shrimp, chestnuts, mustard greens, onions, asparagus	no information available
Zinc RDA: 10–15 mg/day Alternative recommendation*: 30 mg/day	Necessary for adequate breathing and digestion; important to taste, hearing, smell, appetite, normal growth and sexual functioning and reproduction, wound healing, healthy hair, good complexion; decreases lead toxicity	oysters, herring, liver, eggs, nuts, wheat germ and red meats	exposure to lead in gasoline, paints, joints in food cans, lead dust, drinking water that comes through lead pipes; eating canned tomatoes in quantity; foods containing phytate (beans, whole grains, and peanut butter) or calcium interfere with zinc absorption; being a vegetarian; regularly eating imitation meats, fast foods, white bread, fried potatoes, and rich desserts; drinking alcohol; being pregnant; having a cold infection, kidney disease, heart problems, cancer, or taking birth control pill.

Note: Extracted from Balch & Balch (1990). *Prescription for Nutritional Healing.* Garden City Park, NY: Avery Publishing Company, pp. 11–12.

the 1.0% modified citrus pectin group had statistically significant reductions in lung metastases. Studies showing the ability of modified citrus pectin to inhibit human prostate metastasis are needed. Citrus fruit oils and d-limonene, the major constituent of citrus fruit oils, have cancer inhibitory effects (Ren & Lien, 1997).

Coenzyme Q10

Low blood levels of CoQ10 have been found in American and Swedish women diagnosed with breast cancer, and clinical success with small populations has been reported (Ren & Lien, 1997).

DHEA and Cancer Prevention

Epidemiologic studies have shown subnormal plasma levels of DHEA and DHEAS in people with breast cancer, as compared to controls; additionally, DHEA has been shown in animal studies to be broadly cancer chemopreventive.

Essential Oils of Vegetables

Celery seed oil, parsley leaf oil, dillweed oil, and caraway oil are essential oils present in *Umbelliferae* plants. All have shown promise in cancer chemoprevention (Ren & Lien, 1997).

Olive Oil

Increased olive oil consumption (more than once a day vs. once a day) was associated with significantly reduced breast cancer risk, whereas margarine consumption was associated with a significant risk increase, in a large study of Greek women (Trichopoulou et al., 1995). This study duplicates findings of the protective effect of olive oil in a study of American women (Martin-Moreno et al., 1994).

Protective Plant Foods and Supplements

Epidemiologic evidence indicates that diets high in fruits and vegetables are associated with a reduced risk of several cancers, including cancers of the stomach and esophagus. One explanation is that vegetables, especially green ones, contain chlorophyll, a green plant pigment, which limits carcinogen bioavailability by interfering with cytochrome P450-mediated activation of chemical carcinogens.

Blot and colleagues (1993) found that lower mortality, especially due to lower stomach cancer rates, occurred among those receiving supplementation with beta-carotene, vitamin E, and selenium.

Using data from the Iowa Women's Health Study, Zheng and colleagues (1995a) reported intakes of carotene and vitamins C and E were related to lower risks of both gastric and oral/pharyngeal/esophageal cancers. Retinol was associated with a lower risk of gastric cancer only. Zheng and associates (1995b) suggested that intake of energy from plant foods (vegetables, fruits, etc.) may be inversely associated with endometrial cancer risk. In another study, frequent consumption of vegetables, fruits, and grains was associated with increased polyp prevalence (Witte et al., 1996). After adjusting for potentially anticarcinogenic constituents of foods, high carotenoid vegetables, cruciferous vegetables, garlic, and tofu (or soybeans) remained inversely associated with polyps (Zheng et al., 1995b).

Potter (1996) reviewed the epidemiologic evidence on the relation between nutrition and colorectal cancer. Vegetables were associated with lower risk, unless they were pickled (Yo, 1997), as were folate and calcium.

Freudenheim and colleagues (1996) found only intake of vegetables had a strong inverse relationship to premeno-pausal breast cancer risk, while in the Iowa Women's Health Study, Kushi and colleagues (1996) found that vitamins A, C, and E may play a protective role in preventing and reversing postmenopausal breast cancer.

Gerster (1997) found an inverse relationship between lycopene (found almost exclusively in tomatoes and tomato products) and cancers of prostate, pancreas, and, to a certain extent, stomach.

Key and associates (1997) found statistically significant associations between vitamin B6, garlic, baked beans, and garden peas and prostate cancer. Giovannucci and colleagues (1995) found that four foods were inversely associated with risk of prostate cancer: tomatoes, tomato sauce, tomato juice, and pizza. All contain lycopene. Franceschi and colleagues (1994) found that tomatoes provided a significant protection against all digestive tract cancers.

Whole grains and legumes have anticarcinogenic properties in animal and human cells and have been associated with reduced cancer risk in epidemiological studies (Kurzer, Lampe, Martini, & Adlercreutz, 1995; Ziegler, 1994).

Yong and associates (1997) examined the relationship between the dietary intake of vitamins E, C, and A (estimated by a 24-hour recall) and lung cancer incidence in a study of 3,968 men and 6,100 women age 25 to 74. A strong protective effect was observed. While smoking is the most important risk behavior to reduce, a daily consumption of a variety of vegetables and fruits provided the best dietary protection against cancer of the lung.

Helicobacter pylori (HP) infection is involved in the development of stomach cancer. Antitumor stomach defense is weakened by the decrease in the stomach of ascorbic acid (vitamin C), carotene, and

tocopherol (vitamin E) resulting from HP-infection.

The incidence of stomach cancer is lower in individuals and populations with *Allium* vegetable intakes, particularly garlic.

Sivam and colleagues (1997) investigated garlic's antimicrobial activity against *H. pylori,* the bacterium implicated in the etiology of stomach cancer. The researchers suggest the use of garlic as a low-cost intervention, with few side effects, in populations at high risk for stomach cancer, particularly where antibiotic resistance and the risk of reinfection are high. Riggs, DeHaven, and Lamm (1997) also found evidence that garlic may provide a new and effective form of therapy for transitional cell carcinoma of the bladder. Pinto and colleagues (1997) found that garlic may modulate tumor growth in human prostate carcinoma cells in culture.

The milk thistle family of plants (including artichokes) may provide protection against skin cancer (Katiyar et al., 1997). Unlike sunblock, the therapeutic effects work just as well when applied after sun exposure. A compound called silymarin or milk thistle acts as an antioxidant and prevents swelling associated with free radical damage. Although only tested on mice, when used before and after exposure to UV rays, the tumor rate was 25% in treated mice and 100% in unprotected ones. It is not clear if eating artichokes or taking silymarin supplements will reduce skin cancer risks, but clinical testing is warranted.

Vitamin E and beta-carotene inhibited progression of preneoplatic foci to colon cancer, while wheat bran and folic acid had a weak cancer-preventive potential at a late stage of carcinogenesis (Alabaster, Tang, & Shivapurkar, 1997).

Trichopoulou and colleagues (1995), at the Athens School of Public Health, found evidence that vegetables and fruits are inversely and significantly associated with breast cancer risk. Another study found that flaxseed contains omega-3 fatty acids, which may inhibit cancer growth and metastasis, especially in mammary tumorigenesis (Serraine & Thompson, 1992).

Dietary supplements that have a reported positive effect on cancer (Boik, 1996) are DMSO (may perform as a free radical scavenger), bovine and shark cartilage (may be useful as antiangiogenic agents in treating solid tumors, stimulating the immune system, or inhibiting collagenase), multienzyme formulas and bromelain (may stimulate the immune system, enhance globulin degradation, and inhibit inflammation and platelet aggregation), and urea (may affect the fibrin matrix of tumors and inhibit angiogenesis).

Vitamin D, a nutrient made by the skin when exposed to sunlight, may be an important breast cancer protective (Ren & Lien, 1997). Southern women get more exposure to year-round sunlight. In laboratory studies, vitamin D–related compounds inhibited cancer cell growth (Rozen, Yang, Huynh, & Pollak, 1997). John (1997) found that exposure to sunlight significantly reduced the risk of breast cancer. Besides exposure to sunlight, which is a risk factor for skin cancer, vitamin D is available in fish oil, fatty fish, egg yolks, and liver. Fortified foods, including milk and some breads and cereals, also contain vitamin D.

Polyunsaturated Fatty Acids

Polyunsaturated fatty acids of the omega-6 class (found in corn and safflower oils) can act as precursors for the growth of mammary tumors, but polyunsaturated fatty acids of the omega-3 class (found in fish oil) can inhibit these effects. Bagga and colleagues (1997) found that by feeding women with breast cancer a low-fat diet and a fish oil supplement, they could alter breast tissue, significantly reducing the total omega-6 polyunsaturated fatty acids in their plasma.

Processed Foods and Sugar

Moerman (1993) examined 111 case studies of biliary tract cancer and compared them to 480 controls for dietary factors. She found a more than double risk for biliary tract cancer associated with the intake of sugars independent of any other energy source. The researcher suggested that sugars may be a risk due to their relationship with blood lipids and gallstone formation.

Slattery and associates (1997a) also found a connection between dietary sugars, especially a diet high in simple carbohydrates relative to complex carbohydrates and increased risk of colon cancer. Wu, Yu, and Mack (1997) found a risk of small intestinal adenocarcinoma in men and women associated with adding sugar regularly in coffee or tea and daily intake of nondiet carbonated soft drinks.

Franceschi and colleagues (1995) conducted a study involving 2,569 women with incident breast cancer (median age: 55 years) and 2,588 control women hospitalized with nonacute neoplastic diseases. The researchers found significant trends increasing breast cancer risk with increasing intake of the following foods, many of which are highly processed and/or contain sugar: bread and cereal dishes, pork and processed meats, sugar, and candies. High intake of milk, poultry, fish, raw vegetables, potatoes, coffee, and tea exerted a protection against the development of breast cancer.

Retinol and Squamous Cell Skin Cancers

Moon and others (1997) reported the results of two chemoprevention randomized clinical trials to evaluate retinoids in the prevention of skin cancers. People with high risk (at least four prior skin cancers) received either 25,000 IU retinol, 5 to 10 mg isotretinoin, or placebo daily for 3 years. Daily retinol was effective in preventing squamous cell cancers in people with moderate risk, but the retinols had no significant benefit for the high risk group.

Sesame Oil

Frequent consumption of semame oil was found to decrease risk of stomach cancer in a case-control study (Yo, 1997).

Soybeans and Peanuts

Seeds of many plants belonging to the legume family, especially soybeans and peanuts, are rich sources of protease inhibitors associated with a decrease in prostate, colon, breast, oral, pharyngeal, pancreas, and stomach cancers (Ren & Lien, 1997). A great deal of evidence suggests that compounds present in soybeans can prevent cancer in many different organ systems (Knight & Eden, 1996; Stoll, 1997). There is also evidence suggesting that diets containing large amounts of soybean products (tofu, tempeh, soy milk, etc.) are associated with overall low cancer mortality rates, particularly for colon, breast, endometrial, and prostate cancer (Goodman et al., 1997; Wu et al., 1996; Zava et al., 1997).

Other Protective Food Substances

Chinese medicines showing the most promise, based on clinical studies, include indirubin, rhein, emodin, psoralen, matrine, and oxymatrine (Boik, 1996). Turmeric, a spice, is a major phenolic antioxidant and has been used as a naturally occurring medicine for the treatment of inflammatory diseases. The spice also has strong anticarci-

nogenic effects in several tissues, including skin, stomach, colon, small intestine, breast, and tongue (Ren & Lien, 1997).

LeMarchand, Murphy, Hankin, Wilkens, and Kolonel (2000) investigated the relationship between intake of flavonoids and lung cancer risk, examining the food intake of 582 patients with incident lung cancer and 582 age-, sex-, and ethnicity-matched controls. They found that onions, apples, and white grapefruit had statistically significant inverse associations with lung cancer.

Deneo-Pellegrini, Stafani, Boffetta, Ronco, and Mendilaharsu (1999) examined the relationship between dietary intake and the risk of rectal cancer in 216 newly diagnosed and microscopically verified cases of adenocarcinoma and 433 controls hospitalized for diseases not related to long-term changes in diet. Controls were matched to cases on age, sex, residence, and urban versus rural status. Dietary iron was associated with significant increases in risk in men, women and in both sexes together.

Garland, Garland, and Gorham (1999) noted that the geographic distribution of colon cancer is similar to the historical geographic distribution of rickets. Colon cancer mortality and breast cancer death rates in white women rise with distance from the equator where the sun does not provide sufficient vitamin D. The authors conclude that most cases of colon cancer can be prevented with regular intake of calcium (1800 mg/day) and 800 IU/day (20 micrograms) of vitamin D_3. Vitamin D can be obtained from vitamin D-fortified milk or fatty fish.

Botterweck, van den Brandt, and Goldbohm (2000) studied the association between intake of vitamins, carotenoids, dietary fiber, and vitamin supplements use and the incidence of stomach cancer in 120,852 men and women ages 55–69. Intake of folate, vitamin E, alpha-carotene, lutein, lycopene, and dietary fiber were not associated with gastric carcinoma. Individuals who used supplements containing vitamin A had a lower risk of stomach cancers than those who did not.

Mammographic breast density is a significant risk factor for breast cancer. Vachon, Kushi, Cerhan, Kuni, and Sellers (2000) studied the association of diet and mammographic breast density in 1,508 women in a historical cohort study of breast cancer families in Minnesota. For premenopausal women, breast density was positively associated with intakes of polyunsaturated fat, polyunsaturated:saturated fat and vitamins C and E and was inversely correlated with saturated fat and total dairy intake. For postmenopausal women, taking supplemental vitamin B_{12} and vitamin C was associated positively with breast density as was white wine; red wine showed an inverse association with breast density.

Trevisanto and Kim (2000) reviewed the effects of tea on health. It is the richest source of antioxidants called flavonoids and contains other beneficial compounds such as vitamins and fluoride. A growing body of evidence suggests that moderate consumption of tea may protect against several forms of cancer, cardiovascular diseases, the formation of kidney stones, bacterial infections, and dental cavities.

ARTHRITIS: FOOD AND SUPPLEMENTS

Hansen and colleagues (1996) used a food diary with a prospective, single-blind study of 6 months' duration with 109 active rheumatoid arthritis participants, who were randomly assigned to either treatment with or without a specialized diet. The ones who followed the special diet (adjusted energy intake, fish meal, and antioxidants) demonstrated a significant improvements in morning stiffness, number of swollen joints, pain status, and reduced cost of medicine.

A significant improvement can also occur with a vegetarian regime (Kjeldsen-Kragh, Haugen, Borchgrevink, & Forre, 1994). Other studies have indicated that the inflammatory process can be reduced by switching to a vegetarian diet because it significantly alters the intake of fatty acids (Haugen and colleagues, 1994).

The effect of fish oils was evaluated in a multicenter, randomized, double-blind study with fifty-one participants who were allocated 12 weeks of treatment with either six *n*-3 polyunsaturated fatty acid (PUFA) capsules (3.6 g) or six capsules with a fat composition averaging the Danish diet. Small but significant improvements in morning stiffness, joint tenderness, and C-reactive protein were observed. A study of women (Shapiro et al., 1996) examined the relationship between ingestion of fish and arthritis. Consumption of broiled or baked fish, but not of other methods of preparing fish, was associated with a decreased risk of rheumatoid arthritis in the 324 incident rheumatoid arthritis cases (as opposed to the controls). Their results support the hypothesis that omega-3 fatty acids may help prevent rheumatoid arthritis.

Flynn, Irvin, and Krause (1994) examined the effect of cobalamin-folate supplements in 26 participants diagnosed for an average of 5.7 years with idiopathic osteoarthritis of the hands who had been medicated with prescribed nonsteroidal and anti-inflammatory drugs (NSAID). After a 10-day washout period from use of all anti-arthritis drugs, vitamins, and minerals, participants were randomly assigned to 6,400 mcg folate or 6,400 mcg folate plus 20 mcg cobalamin (vitamin B_{12}) or lactose placebo each for 2 months within self-selected diets. Grip values were higher and pain lower with combined vitamin B_{12}–folate ingestion than with other "vitamin" supplements and were equivalent to NSAID use. There were many side effects with NSAID, whereas there were no side effects with the vitamin combination and the cost was lower.

Kremer and Bigaouette (1996) found that people diagnosed with rheumatoid arthritis tended to ingest too much total fat and too little polyunsaturated fat, and their diets are deficient in zinc, magnesium, pyridoxine, copper, and folate. They suggested that routine dietary supplementation with multivitamins and trace elements is appropriate for this population.

Leventhal and colleagues (1994a) used a randomized, double-blind, placebo-controlled, 24-week trial. Thirty-seven individuals attending a rheumatology clinic of a university hospital were randomly assigned to treatment with 1.4 g/d gammalinolenic acid in borage seed oil or cottonseed oil (placebo). Treatment resulted in clinically important reductions in the number of tender and swollen joints compared to the control group. Leventhal, Boyce, and Zurier (1994b) used blackcurrant seed oil (BCSO) in a randomized, double-blind, placebo-controlled, 24-week trial. The oil is rich in gammalinolenic acid as well as alphalinolenic acid. Both are known to suppress inflammation and joint tissue injury in animal models. The treatment group in this study showed a significant reduction in disease activity.

Selenium may be an essential factor in many of the biochemical pathways associated with rheumatoid arthritis because it is involved in the production of prostaglangins and leukotrienes, which regulate the inflammation process. In one study, symptoms improved in 40% of participants after selenium supplementation.

Evidence suggests that pathophysiologic processes in bone are important in the development of osteoarthritis of the knee. Low intake and low serum levels of vitamin D may compromise usual protective re-sponses and predispose individuals to progression of the condition (McAlindon et al., 1996). People taking middling to high doses of vitamin C (in food or supplements) had a threefold reduction in risk for osteoarthritis and knee pain. A reduction in the risk of progression also occurred possibly due to beta-carotene and vitamin E, but only in men (McAlindon, 1997).

ASTHMA

Asthma is an allergic overreaction to airborne particulates, such as pollen and dust, in which a flood of antibodies can lead to lung inflammation, airway restriction, and a life-threatening shortness of breath. Most authorities recognize an emotional component of asthma and allergies, often associated with stress.

Adult-onset asthma has been linked to estrogen use. In an analysis of more than 23,000 postmenopausal women participating in the ongoing Nurses' Health Study (Troisi, Speizer, et al., 1995), past or current users of hormone replacement therapy had a 60% higher risk of being afflicted with asthma than women who had never taken estrogen. The risk for women who had been on the hormone therapy for 10 years or more was double that of nonusers.

Dietary Approaches

In a complementary approach to asthma, the diet consists primarily of fresh fruits and vegetables, nuts and seeds, oatmeal, brown rice, and whole grains. Processed foods are avoided because they often contain allergy-producing preservatives such as BHA and BHT. Dairy products are avoided because they generate additional mucus.

Vitamin E may have a modest protective effect for asthma (Troisi, Willett, et al.,

1995). Indian diets tend to include more vegetables, less meat, and fewer additives and processed and packaged foods than the typical Western diet and may reduce the risk of asthma and allergic disease (Carey, Locke, & Cookson, 1996).

Salt has been implicated as an asthma aggravator, at least in men. In one study (Carey, Locke, & Cookson, 1993), 22 men with mild to moderate asthma were placed on a low-sodium diet (80 mmol a day). Half received a tablet containing 200 mmol of sodium (the amount many Americans ingest daily), and the other half were given a placebo. Those on the low-sodium regime were found to use bronchodilators less often, were able to exhale more air, and had fewer symptoms, such as wheezing. Another study found that selenium supplementation increases glutathione peroxidase activity, thus improving cellular oxidative defense, which might counteract the inflammation and disordered respiration associated with asthma (Hasselmark et al., 1993).

Vitamin C

Preliminary results by E. Neil Schachter, M.D., of Yale University, provide evidence that 500 mg of vitamin C reduced bronchospasm in 12 participants with exercise-induced asthma.

BLADDER PROBLEMS

Almost 40 million American women develop cystitis each year. The two main types of cystitis are bacterial and interstitial. Symptoms can be triggered by environmental and food allergies and by general infections in the body.

Cranberry Juice

A study by Fleet (1994) indicated that bacterial infections (bacteriuria) and associated influx of white blood cells into the urine (pyuria) can be reduced by nearly 50% in elderly women who drank 300 ml of cranberry juice cocktail each day over the course of 6 months. Avorn and colleagues (1994) replicated these findings with a sample of 153 elderly women volunteers.

Fiber Protects

Le Marchand and colleagues (1997) conducted a population-based case-control study among different ethnic groups in Hawaii using personal interviews with 698 males and 494 females diagnosed during 1987–1991 with adenocarcinoma of the colon or rectum as compared to 1,192 population controls matched by age, sex, and ethnicity. They found a protective association in both sexes with fiber intake from vegetable sources (but not from fruits, except bananas, and cereals). Intakes of carotenoids, light green and yellow-orange vegetables, broccoli, corn, carrots, garlic, and legumes (including soy products) reduced risk, even after adjustment for vegetable fiber. The data supported a protective role of fiber from vegetables against colorectal cancer independent of its water solubility property and the effects of other phytochemicals.

HEART AND BLOOD VESSEL CONDITIONS

Kendler (1997) reviewed the literature on the use of nutrition with heart conditions. Favorable effects have been reported with the use of unsaturated fatty acids, vegetarian and semivegetarian food regimes, dietary fiber, plant sterols, vitamins (niacin, H C, B$_6$, B$_{12}$, folate). minerals (potassium, calcium, magnesium, selenium), other supplements (coenzyme Q10, L-carnitine, taurine, and botanical agents (garlic, hawthorn, gugulipid). Nutritional substances associated with undesirable heart and blood vessel effects include transfatty acids, homocysteine, carbohydrate intolerance, and excessive sodium and iron intake.

Coffee and Its Negative Effects

Nygard and colleagues (1997) reported an association between coffee consumption and the concentration of total homocysteine in plasma, a risk factor for cardiovascular disease and for adverse pregnancy outcome. Guttormsen and associates (1996) also found a relationship between lower plasma folate and cobalamin levels, as well as lower intake of vitamin supplements, coffee consumption, and smoking. Folic acid, a B vitamin found in leafy green vegetables and other produce, could provide a deterrent.

Magnesium Protects

Magnesium deficiency increases the risk of cardiovascular damage, including hypertension, cerebrovascular and coronary constriction and occlusion, arrhythmias, and sudden cardiac death. High intakes of fat and/or calcium can intensify magnesium inadequacy, especially under conditions of stress (Seelig, 1994).

Magnesium intake may be important in preventing heart attack. Singh and colleagues (1996) studied the relationship between dietary and serum levels of magnesium in a case-control study of primary and secondary care for acute myocardial infarction. They found that for individuals with ventricular arrhythmias,

magnesium intake was relatively low compared to the control group.

Brodsky and colleagues (1994) conducted a double-blind, placebo-controlled study of magnesium supplementation and its effect on atrial fibrillation. After 24 hours, the group receiving magnesium had an average heart rate of approximately 80, whereas the group receiving only digoxin had an average heart rate of 105. The results provide evidence that magnesium either greatly improves the efficacy of digoxin or exerts significant effects on its own.

Murray (1994) pointed out the benefits of magnesium over drugs. Magnesium has no side effects and is more effective. Also, over a 24-hour period, 6 g of esmolol (costing $400) or 300 mg of diltiazem (costing $200) are used for an individual with new-onset atrial fibrillation. These prices are much higher than the cost of 10 g of magnesium sulfate ($1) or 2 mg of digoxin ($2), or their combination.

Protective Effect of Fish and Fish Oil

The risk of death from coronary disease is lower among people who eat fish. However, frequent consumers of fish do not appear to have lower coronary risks than those who eat it once or twice per week (National Institutes of Health, 1995).

Studies have consistently demonstrated that fish oils may prevent cardiac arrhythmias (Kang & Leaf, 1996) and lower total cholesterol, triglycerides, and lipoprotein levels (Pauletto et al., 1996).

Garlic and Fish Oil

Adler and Holub (1997) found the coadministration of garlic with fish oil was well tolerated by people with moderately high cholesterol levels and had a beneficial effect on serum lipid and lipoprotein concentrations by lowering total cholesterol and triglycerol concentrations as well as the ratios of total cholesterol to HDL-C and LDL-C to HDL-C.

Morcos (1997) had similar results with a fish oil and garlic combination.

Folic Acid and Vitamin B₆

A number of studies have shown the protective effect of folic acid (Chasan-Taber et al., 1996; Tucker, Selhub, Wilson, & Rosenberg, 1996) on the heart. Eating more green leafy vegetables (brussels sprouts, spinach, lettuce) and fruits (apples, oranges, etc.) or including folic acid supplements could protect against heart attacks and strokes. Other researchers (Dalery et al., 1995) found that low folic acid and vitamin B_6 blood levels were associated with high homocysteine levels (a heart risk factor). Vitamin B_6 is plentiful in whole grains, legumes (e.g., peanuts and dry beans), and fish.

Coenzyme Q10 (CoQ10)

CoQ10 supplementation has been used successfully to enhance heart action, stabilize blood pressure, reduce shortness of breath and palpitations, and lessen heart muscle thickness (Lampertico, 1993: Mortensen, 1993). As the safety of prescription cholesterol-lowering medications is increasingly questioned, natural, nutritious alternatives are being used to prevent clogged arteries and lower the risk of heart attack.

Citrus Pectin Lowers Cholesterol

Studies of more than 200 individuals have shown that the equivalent of the pectin in two whole grapefruit can lower the LDL (bad) cholesterol between 25% and 30% in just 4 weeks (Cerda, 1996).

Nuts Protect the Heart

Nuts have shown to be heart protective in several studies. In one, walnuts decreased serum levels of total cholesterol and favorably modified the lipoprotein profile in healthy men (Sabate et al., 1993). In another, researchers examined the eating habits of 25,000 Seventh Day Adventists, looking for a relationship between 65 different foods and good health. People who ate nuts five or more times per week were half as likely to suffer a heart attack or die of heart disease than those who rarely or never ate nuts. The benefit held constant despite age, weight, or activity level.

Another study found that women who ate nuts more than two times per week reduced their heart disease risk by 60% (Fraser, Lindsted, & Beeson, 1995). Even though nuts contain a high percentage of fat, volunteers who ate 3.5 oz of almonds per day (590 calories) did not gain a pound. Nuts also contain mono- and polyunsaturated fats, fiber, and vitamin E, all of which protect the heart. Walnuts also contain omega-3 fatty acids (found in fish oils) and the amino acid arginine, which inhibits blood clotting and protects arteries.

Oats and Buckwheat Are Helpful

Oats and buckwheat intake has been associated with lower body mass index, lowering blood pressure and total cholesterol, and increasing the ratio of HDL (good) cholesterol to total cholesterol (He et al., 1995).

L-Arginine May Increase Exercise Capacity

Ceremuzynski, Chamiec, and Herbaczynski-Cedre (1997) studied the effect of supplemental oral L-arginine on exercise capacity in individuals with stable angina pectoris (heart pain). A randomized, double-blind, placebo-controlled study showed that 6 g per day for 3 days of L-arginine increased exercise capacity (tested on a Marquette case 12 treadmill according to the modified Bruce protocol).

Importance of Reducing Saturated Fat and Sugar

The best way to lower triglycerides, now linked with the risk of heart attack (Stampfer et al., 1997), is to cut down on saturated (animal-source) fats, candies, and fruit juice (rich in simple sugars). Vitamin E offered the strongest protection against heart attack and angina in a study conducted by Meyer (1994).

Vitamin E Decreases Risk of Death

Vitamin E supplementation lowered the risk of death from ischemic heart disease in a 5-year study that tracked 2,226 men, 45 to 76 years old. The study controlled for high blood pressure, high cholesterol, and heart disease risk factors.

A study by Martin, Foxall, Blumberg, and Meydani (1997) may explain why vitamin E is helpful in decreasing heart disease risk factors. They found that vitamin E has an inhibitory effect on LDL-induced production of adhesion molecules and adhesion of monocytes to human aortic endothelial cells, one of the early events in the development of atherogenesis.

The Cholesterol Lowering Atherosclerosis Study (CLAS) found less carotid wall thickness for a group of 29 subjects who took 250 IU per day of supplementary vitamin E versus 22 who took 100 IU or less per day (Azen et al., 1996).

Vitamin C Protects

Vitamin C may exert a protective function by lowering atherogenic risk (Hallfrish et al., 1994).

Combined Antioxidants Lower Risk

Losonczy, Harris, and Haulik (1996) examined vitamins E and C supplement use and found the two vitamins were associated with a lower risk of total mortality and coronary mortality.

Stephens and colleagues (1996) used a double-blind, placebo-controlled, randomized trial of vitamin E in individuals with coronary disease in the Cambridge Heart Antioxidant Study. Of 1,035 individuals, 546 were assigned capsules containing 800 IU vitamin E daily. The rest were given 400 IU daily. Both treatment groups showed a significantly reduced risk of nonfatal heart attacks, and the effects were apparent even after 1 year of treatment.

Singh, Niaz, Rastogi, and Rastogi (1996) combined antioxidant vitamins A, C, E, and beta-carotene in the treatment group and compared the results with the control group. They found that the vitamin combination protected against cardiac necrosis and oxidative stress and suggested it could be beneficial in preventing complications and cardiac event rate.

Kushi and colleagues (1996) studied the role of vitamins A, E, and C from food sources in women ($S = 34,486$ postmenopausal women). The researchers concluded that the intake of vitamin E from food sources could lower the risk of death from heart disease in women.

Selenium Lowers Risk

Low levels of selenium are associated with a significantly higher risk for developing ischemic heart disease (J. Stratment & Lardy, 1992), and selenium and other antioxidant supplementation (at least for men) improves the cardiac risk profile and reduces the risk of cardiovascular disease (Salonen et al., 1991; Suadicani, Hein, & Gyntelberg, 1992).

Temple, Luzier, and Kazierad (2000) reviewed the role of homocysteine as a risk factor in atherosclerosis. They completed a MEDLINE search from 1966 through January 1999 and found that studies demonstrated a positive correlation between hyperhomocysteinemia and atherosclerosis and that using folic acid (650 micrograms/day) reduced homocysteine concentrations to within normal therapeutic range after 2 weeks. Vermeulen (2000) found that folic acid plus vitamin B_6 lowered homocysteine levels in healthy siblings of patients with premature atherothrombotic disease. Bunout (2000) also found that folic acid reduced homocysteine levels in patients diagnosed by angiogram with coronary artery disease. The researchers combined the vitamin with other antioxidants in a multivitamin preparation containing 150 IU of vitamin E, 150 mg vitamin C, 12.5 mg of beta-carotene and .4 mcg of vitamin B_{12}.

DIABETES

Food and Supplements

According to Barnard and colleagues (1994), diabetes can be controlled without insulin or any medication by following a low-fat, low-cholesterol, high-complex-carbohydrate, high-fiber diet combined with daily aerobic exercise. In the study, 652 men and women, all diagnosed with type II diabetes, attended the Pritikin Longevity Center's 26-day live-in program. Seventy-six percent of the participants reduced their blood glucose levels to the normal range within 3 weeks. The second part of the study involved 197 people who were taking oral hypoglycemic agents. Seventy percent were able to discontinue their medication, and their glucose levels decreased to the normal range within 3 weeks.

The third group in the study consisted of 212 participants taking insulin injections. After 26 days, 39% were able to discontinue insulin injections. Additionally, participants in all three groups reduced their cholesterol levels by more than 20% over the 26 days.

Garg and colleagues (1988) compared a high-carbohydrate diet with a monounsaturated fat diet (MUFD) for people with non-insulin-independent diabetes (NIIDM). The MUFD lunch included a main dish of chicken breast sautéed in olive oil with seasonings and a small serving of rice, lettuce salad with olive oil and lemon juice dressing, bread, peaches, and iced tea.

The most pronounced difference in results between the two diets was the effect on total triglycerides (25% lower on the MUFD). The MUFD also excelled in raising good cholesterol (HDL) 13% and in lowering blood sugar levels and daily insulin requirements for most participants. The results suggest that partial replacement of complex carbohydrates with a diet higher in fat is beneficial and more palatable.

Salmeron and colleagues (1997) found that people, especially women, who eat high-glycemic-index foods like white bread, white rice, and potatoes and do not also include whole or less refined grains are at risk for non-insulin-dependent diabetes mellitus. The researchers' findings support the hypothesis that there is an increased risk of NIDDM associated with a high glycemic load and low cereal-fiber content diet.

Bitter Melon

Two ounces of bitter melon juice from the bitter melon (balscem pear), long used in folk medicine as a remedy for diabetes, has been shown in clinical trials to improve glucose tolerance (Srivastava et al., 1993; Welihinda et al., 1982).

Chromium

Anderson and colleagues (1997) reported on the effect of chromium picolinate taken two times per day. The data provided evidence that supplemental chromium had significant beneficial effects on glucose, insulin, and cholesterol variables in men and women with type II diabetes.

Fenugreek

Fenugreek seeds show significant antidiabetic effects in clinical and experimental studies (Sharma, Raghuram, & Rao, 1990). These results suggest that fenugreek seeds or defatted fenugreek powder should be considered as part of the diet for those with diabetes.

Onions and Garlic

Onions and garlic have demonstrated the ability to help lower blood sugar levels. Experimental and clinical evidence supports the theory that allyl propyl disulphide lowers glucose levels by competing with insulin for insulin-inactivating sites in the liver. The results are similar in both raw and boiled onion extracts (Augusti, 1996; Sharma, 1977; Sheela & Augusti, 1992). The cardiovascular effects (lowering blood pressure and cholesterol) provide further support for the liberal use of onions and garlic by people with diabetes (Murray, 1994).

Vitamins A, C, and E

People with diabetes face an increased risk of atherosclerosis, or hardening of the arteries, which can be curbed with high doses of vitamin E (1,200 IU/day) (Fuller and colleagues, 1996). The supplemented group (including people with both type I and type II diabetes) had significant reductions in LDL oxidation. Participant dietary

surveys revealed that the more vitamin A reported, the more effective insulin was in controlling blood sugar (Facchini, 1996). This suggests that vitamin A may help control blood sugar. Ting and colleagues (1996) found that vitamin C improves vascular reactivity in NIDDM.

HEADACHES

Food and Supplements

Detection and removal of allergic/intolerant foods can reduce headache symptoms. The most common allergens are milk, wheat, chocolate, food additives (MSG by itself or in foods like bouillon cubes, some canned foods/soups, and soy sauces), artificial sweeteners, tomatoes, and fish (Murray, 1994). Chocolate, aged cheese (e.g., cheddar or blue), beer, scotch, champagne, red wine, and aspartame can precipitate a headache because they contain compounds known as vasoactive amines, which cause blood vessels to expand. Too much caffeine (coffee, tea, colas) can also cause a rebound headache as blood vessels dilate (Murray, 1994).

Magnesium may be a useful supplement to prevent and treat headaches. One of the key functions of magnesium is to maintain the tone of blood vessels. Low magnesium levels have been implicated in chronic daily headaches (Gallai et al., 1994; Ramadan et al., 1989; Swanson, 1988). Low brain tissue magnesium concentrations have been found in people with migraines, indicating a need for supplementation.

Aloisi, Marrelli, and Porto (1997) treated children suffering from migraine with and without aura in a headache-free period. A 20-day treatment with oral magnesium picolate normalized the magnesium balance in 90% of the children and lowered migraine attacks.

Magnesium deficiency has also been linked to mitral (heart) valve prolapse, which in turn is linked to migraines because it leads to a change in blood platelets, causing them to release vasoactive substances. Eighty-five percent of people with mitral valve prolapse have a chronic magnesium deficiency that can be improved with supplementation (Galland, Baker, & McLellan, 1986).

McCarty (1996) theorized that magnesium taurate and fish oil could prove useful in preventing headaches. Clinical investigations and known drug activity suggest that taurine and magnesium could dampen hyperexcitation, counteract vasospasm, increase tolerance to focal hypoxia, stabilize platelets, and lessen sympathetic outflow. Fish oil, too, has promising qualities, especially platelet stabilization and antivasospastic action.

HIGH BLOOD PRESSURE

Food and Supplements

Intake of vitamin C and carotene were found to be inversely related to blood pressure (Stamler et al., 1994). In a systematic review of epidemiological studies of vitamin C and blood pressure, Ness and colleagues (1997) found a consistent cross-sectional association between higher vitamin C intake or status and lower blood pressure.

Calcium supplementation has been shown to have a protective effect on blood pressure to inner-city children (Gillman et al., 1994), men (Gillman, Cupples, & Gagnon, 1994), and pregnant women (Bucher et al., 1996). Potassium, too, has been shown to lower blood pressure, even in people with normal blood pressure. Whelton and colleagues (1997) combined results from nearly three dozen experiments involving more than 2,000 participants to show that taking potassium supplements can help reduce blood pressure. Potassium was found to be even more helpful for people with severe high blood pressure, with high salt intake, and slight more helpful for African-Americans who are particularly susceptible to hypertension. Potassium-rich foods may also be helpful: bananas, cantaloupes, orange juice, baked potatoes, and low-fat yogurt.

Appel and associates (1997) studied the relationship between diet and blood pressure. They found that a healthy diet high in fruits, vegetables, and low-fat milk can help lower blood pressure.

He and colleagues (1995) found that a higher intake of total protein (39 g) was associated with a lower systolic and diastolic blood pressure. High fiber intake (19 g) was significantly associated with both a lower diastolic and systolic pressure.

Epidemiologic studies from divergent geographic locations have consistently shown an inverse correlation between potassium intake and hypertension. Potassium depletion is associated with an increase in blood pressure (Krishna, 1994).

Smith, Klotman, and Svetkey (1992) found that potassium chloride can lower blood pressure in older people with hypertension.

Fotherby and Potter (1997) also used a randomized cross-over study using a potassium supplement versus placebo and checked its effect on blood pressure in eight hypertensive people. They found a significant fall in mean 24-hour systolic blood pressure between 4 months of potassium supplementation and placebo treatment. They concluded that a modest increase in dietary potassium intake could have significant effect on lowering blood pressure in the large proportion of older adults with hypertension.

HIP FRACTURES

Dirschel, Henderson, and Oakley (1995) examined 97 older adults with acute fractures of the proximal femur. Mean daily calcium intake was well below the recommended levels, and calcium intake less than 500 mg per day was associated with lower lumbar spine bone mineral density scores. The researchers suggested that calcium supplementation may play a role in decreasing the incidence of hip fracture.

Meunier (1996) reported a 3-year controlled prospective study of daily supplementation of 1.2 g of calcium and 800 IU of vitamin D3 for 3,270 older women living in nursing homes. The treatment reduced hip fractures and other nonvertebral fractures by 23%.

Bonjour, Schurch, and Rizzoli (1996) found that a deficiency in vitamin K may also contribute to bone fragility. In their study, reduced protein intake was also associated with lower femoral neck bone mineral density and poor physical performance. The clinical outcome after hip fracture was significantly improved by daily oral nutritional supplements normalizing the protein intake. The supplementation also resulted in a reduction in complication rate and length of hospital stay.

Meyer and colleagues (1996) used a matched case-control study in Oslo to assess risk factors for hip fracture in older adults. The researchers found increased risk of hip fracture in the lean, those who had reported weight loss because of poor appetite, and people who had low food intake. No relationship was found between calcium intake and hip fracture, but higher risk was suggested in people with low vitamin D intake, low physical activity, low hand grip strength, smoking, low level of education, and frequent admissions to the hospital prior to the study.

Meyer, Pedersen, Loken, and Tverdal (1997) used dietary data from a prospective study to relate factors influencing calcium balance to the incidence of hip fracture. There was an elevated risk of fracture for women with a high intake of protein from nondairy animal sources in the presence of low calcium intake. Women who drank nine or more cups of coffee per day also had an increased risk of fracture.

JUVENILE DELINQUENCY AND VIOLENCE

Schoenthaler and Bier (2000) reviewed two controlled trials comparing the behavior of offenders who received either placebos or vitamin-mineral supplements designed to provide the micronutrient equivalent of a well-balanced diet. Institutionalized offenders aged 13 to 17 years produced about 40% less violent and other antisocial behavior when taking the vitamin-mineral supplements. Scholenthaler and Bier designed a stratified randomized, double-blind placebo controlled trial for schoolchildren aged 6 to 12 years in two working class, primarily Hispanic elementary schools in Phoenix, Arizona. Daily vitamin-mineral supplementation at 50% of the U.S. recommended daily allowance (RDA) for 4 months versus placebo was investigated. The children who took the supplements showed lower rates of antisocial behavior in threats and fighting, vandalism, being disrespectful, disorderly conduct, defiance, obscenities, refusal to work or serve, endangering others, and nonspecified offenses.

LUNG PROBLEMS

Food and Supplements

Landon and Young (1993) discussed the interaction of magnesium and calcium.

The possibility exists that magnesium deficiency contributes to lung complications. Serum magnesium levels are used to detect deficiencies, but cells can be deficient despite normal serum values. The researchers suggested that people being treated for lung conditions should be monitored routinely for magnesium deficiency.

Britton and colleagues (1994) studied a random sample of 2,633 adults age 18 to 70 in the United Kingdom. Britton and colleagues concluded that low magnesium intake may be involved in the etiology of asthma and chronic obstructive airway disease.

Sempertegui and colleagues (1996) assessed the effect of zinc sulfate supplementation on respiratory tract disease, immunity, and growth in malnourished children at a day care center in Ecuador. On a random basis, 25 received zinc supplementation and 25 did not. The incidence of fever, cough, and upper respiratory tract secretions was lower in the supplemented group than in the nonsupplemented group at day 60.

Dow and colleagues (1996) investigated whether dietary antioxidant intake in older adults was related to lung function in 178 men and women age 70 to 96. For every extra milligram increase in vitamin E in the daily diet, forced expiratory volume increased by an estimated 42 ml and forced vital capacity by an estimated 54 ml. The results suggest that vitamin E may influence lung function in older adults.

Fawzi and associates (1994) examined the relationship between dietary vitamin A intake and cough, diarrhea, and mortality in children. The researchers found that vitamin A intake was especially protective for children who were wasted or stunted or who had cough or diarrhea symptoms. Rahman and colleagues (1996) found that a large proportion of infants remained vitamin A deficient even after large doses of vitamin

A supplementation because of frequent respiratory infections, particularly those accompanied by fever.

Humphrey and colleagues (1996) conducted a placebo-controlled trial among 2,067 Indonesian neonates who received either 50,000 IU of orally administered vitamin A or a placebo on the first day of life. Infants were followed for 1 year. The researchers concluded that giving neonates vitamin A could reduce the prevalence of severe respiratory infection.

Peters, Goetzsche, Grobbelaar, and Noakes (1993) studied the effect of daily supplementation with 600 mg of vitamin C on the incidence of upper respiratory tract (URT) infections after participation in competitive ultramarathon races. Vitamin C was shown to enhance resistance to URT infections in ultramarathon runners and may reduce the severity of infections in those who are sedentary.

MACULAR DEGENERATION

Macular degeneration or the slow deterioration of the center of the retina destroys some or all vision in 1 in 20 people in the United States age 70 or older, an estimated 10 million Americans. A diet rich in saturated fat and cholesterol and low in lycopene (tomato products primarily) may increase the risk of macular degeneration by 80% (Mares-Perlman, 1995), whereas a diet rich in vegetables containing carotenoids (especially spinach and collard greens) may decrease the risk of macular degeneration by 43%. Sweet potatoes, cabbage, cauliflower, brussels sprouts, and squash also may be beneficial, whereas supplements of vitamins A, C, E and retinol (a form of vitamin A) do not decrease the risk (Seddon et al., 1994).

In a multicenter study at eight medical centers, Richer (1996) found that a specific

14-antioxidant capsule (20,000 units of beta-carotene, 200 units of vitamin E, 750 mg of vitamin C, plus zinc, selenium, and other nutrients) twice daily stabilized patients' vision. The researcher concluded that eating green leafy vegetables provides an adequate supply of antioxidants, but high-dose supplements may be needed to stabilize advanced macular degeneration.

West and colleagues (1994) found alpha-tocopherol (vitamin E), vitamin C and beta-carotene exerted a protective effect for age-related macular degeneration.

Mares-Perlman and associates (1996) found a weekly protective effect for zinc in the development of some forms of early age-related maculopathy. Ishihara, Yuzawa, and Tamakoshi (1997) compared serum levels of vitamins A, C, and E and carotenoid, zinc, and selenium in 35 people with age-related macular degeneration with the levels of 66 controls. Serum zinc and vitamin E levels were significantly lower in the condition group, as compared to the control group. The researchers concluded that subnormal levels of zinc and vitamin E may be associated with development of age-related macular degeneration.

Snodderly (1995) examined the epidemiologic data on other risk factors for macular degeneration. The researcher found that individuals with low plasma concentrations of carotenoids and antioxidant vitamins and those who smoked cigarettes were at increased risk for age-related macular degeneration.

MEMORY PROBLEMS

Antioxidants

Swiss researchers (Perrig et al., 1997) concluded that two antioxidants, vitamin C and beta-carotene, play an important role in brain aging and memory.

OSTEOPOROSIS

Salt Intake

Matkovic and colleagues (1995) evaluated 381 girls age 8 to 13 years, during early puberty, for urinary calcium levels and bone mineral density. Excess intakes of calcium were excreted in the urine, and the more salt the girls ate, the more calcium they excreted and the lower their bone density levels.

Based on diets and bone changes over 2 years, a similar study of 124 postmenopausal women showed that for sodium levels beyond 2,600 mg/day, as much as 891 mg of calcium was lost. Switching to fresh vegetable condiments (slices of tomato instead of ketchup or salsa) can reduce sodium intake by 175 mg or more.

PARKINSON'S DISEASE

Up to two million older Americans are estimated to be affected by Parkinson's disease (PD), a chronic, progressive neurological disorder. Classic symptoms include tremors (intensified by stress or fatigue that disappear during sleep or concentrated effort), muscular stiffness or rigidity, slowing of body motion, and a characteristic shuffle.

Schneider and colleagues (1997) used a case-controlled study to examine the possible role of long-term dietary antioxidant intake in PD etiology. Participants included 57 men age 45 to 79 with at least two cardinal signs of PD and age-matched friend controls chosen from lists provided by participants. Antioxidant intake, except for lycopene (primarily tomatoes and related products), was not associated with reduced PD risk. Intakes of sweet foods, including fruit, were associated with higher PD risk. The researchers theorized that pesticide residues in the fruits and vegetables may have contributed to the development of PD.

De Rijk and colleagues (1997) investigated whether high dietary intake of antioxidants decreased the risk of PD in 5,342 individuals living independently without dementia between the ages of 55 and 95 years of age. The data suggested that a high intake of dietary vitamin E may protect against the occurrence of PD (de Rijk et al., 1997).

PMS: FOOD AND SUPPLEMENTS

Calcium Supplementation Relieves PMS Symptoms

Thys-Jacobs and colleagues (1989) used a randomized crossover trial to study the efficacy of calcium supplementation in women with PMS. Thirty-three women in a clinic at a large hospital completed the trial. Seventy-three percent of the women reported fewer symptoms while taking calcium supplements. Calcium significantly alleviated water retention, pain, and negative affect.

Carbohydrate Beverage Relieves Symptoms

Sayegh and colleagues (1995) used a specially formulated carbohydrate-rich beverage known to increase the serum ratio of tryptophan to test its effect on PMS symptoms. Twenty-four women with confirmed PMS participated in a double-blind, crossover study that compared the special formula with two other isocaloric products. The carbohydrate-rich beverage significantly decreased self-reported depression, anger, confusion, and carbohydrate crav-

ing 90 and 180 minutes after ingestion. Memory word recognition was also improved significantly.

Flavonoids May Reduce PMS Congestion

Serfaty and Magneron (1997) reported a national multicenter study evaluating the use of micronized purified flavonoid to treat PMS symptoms. Daily assessment diaries and weight and circumferential measurements (twice per cycle) were taken on all 1,473 women who completed the trial. The duration of PMS decreased on average by 2.6 days, and symptoms of congestion and weight gain gradually lessened in both frequency and severity by approximately 60%.

Magnesium Used for Negative Mood Changes

Rosenstein and colleagues (1994) demonstrated decreased red blood cell concentrations of magnesium in women with PMS. Facchinetti and associates (1991) used a double-blind, randomized design with 32 women with PMS. The data suggested that magnesium supplementation could be an effective treatment for negative mood changes during PMS.

Stewart (1987) reported on the effect of a double-blind, placebo-controlled study at high and low dosages of supplementation. Laboratory evidence showed significant deficiencies in vitamin B_6 and magnesium, among other nutrients. The multivitamin/multimineral supplement used in the study corrected the deficiencies and improved the symptoms of PMS.

Using a double-blind, randomized design, Facchinetti and colleagues (1991) evaluated the effects of oral magnesium on a sample of 32 women age 23 to 39 years with confirmed PMS (Moos Menstrual Distress Questionnaire). The score of cluster "pain" was significantly reduced during the second month in both groups (baseline recording). Magnesium treatment significantly affected both the total Menstrual Distress score and the negative affect subscale rating.

Vitamin E May Prove Helpful

London, Sundaram, Murphy, and Goldstein (1983) used a double-blind, randomized dose-response design with 75 women with benign breast disease before and after two months of treatment with placebo or alpha-tocopherol (vitamin E) of 150, 300, or 600 IU per day. After age and pretreatment were controlled for, vitamin E had a significantly greater effect than placebo, improving three of four classes of PMS symptoms, suggesting that vitamin E supplementation can be of value to women with severe PMS symptoms.

London, Murphy, Kitlowski, and Reynolds (1987) repeated their study to confirm their findings. A significant improvement in certain affective and physical symptoms was noted in women treated with vitamin E.

Zinc Levels Low in PMS Sufferers

Chuong and Dawson (1994) studied the effect of zinc and copper levels on symptoms of premenstrual syndrome. Ten women with PMS and 10 controls gave blood at 2- or 3-day intervals through three menstrual cycles. The researchers concluded that zinc deficiency occurs in PMS during the luteal phase and is further reduced by an elevation in copper.

STRESS

Deficiencies in vitamin E, vitamin B_6, and riboflavin reduce cell numbers in lymphoid tissue and produce abnormalities in immune function. Vitamins C and E exert anti-inflammatory effects in studies in humans and animals. Dietary supplementation in humans with vitamins C, E, and B_6 enhances lymphocyte function especially in older adults (Grimble, 1997).

Martin and colleagues (1996) studied the effect of vitamin E on oxidative stress in human aortic endothelial cells. Vitamin E treatment significantly reduced interleukin production after AAPH exposure, showing the vitamin's antioxidant protection against lipid peroxidation.

Sen and colleagues (1997) also studied vitamin E's effect on lipid peroxidation in rats. The liver appeared to be relatively less susceptible to exercise-induced oxidative stress in the fish oil and vitamin E group.

STROKE

Strokes occur when brain tissue is deprived of blood supply due to an arterial obstruction. The stroke mortality rate in the United States increased for the first time in four decades in 1993, from 26.2 deaths per 100,000 events to 26.4 per 100,000. This increase may correspond to the aging of the population.

Protective Effect of Flavonoids

Some flavonoids are better platelet inhibitors than aspirin and better antioxidants than vitamin E. One recent study examined a cohort of 552 men age 50 to 69. Keli, Hertog, Feskens, and Kromhout (1996) cross-checked and calculated mean nutrient and food intake on dietary histories for

15 years. Dietary flavonoids, mainly quercetin, were inversely associated with stroke incidence. Vitamins C and E were not associated with stroke risk, whereas black tea and apples were. The researchers concluded that habitual intake of flavonoids and their major source (tea) may protect against stroke. Men who drank more than 4.7 cups of tea a day had a 69% reduced risk of stroke compared with those who drank less than 2.6 cups a day.

Fruits and Vegetables

Gillman and colleagues (1995) examined the effect of fruit and vegetable intake on risk of stroke among 832 middle-aged men. The estimated total number of servings per day of fruits and vegetables was the variable used for analysis. Age-adjusted risk of stroke decreased across increasing quintile of servings per day. Manson and colleagues (1994) found similar results for women.

Milk

Abbott and colleagues (1996) found that men who were nondrinkers of milk experienced stroke at twice the rate of men who consumed 16 oz or more. Intake of dietary calcium was also associated with a reduced risk of stroke, although its association was confounded with milk consumption. Calcium from nondairy sources was not related to stroke. This suggests that other covariates or constituents related to milk ingestion may be important. For example, milk drinkers tended to be leaner and more physically active and to consume healthier foods.

ULCERS

Peptic ulcer sufferers complain of a severe burning, gnawing epigastric pain beginning an hour or two after eating and are frequently addicted to antacids.

Cayenne

Kang and colleagues (1995) studied 103 Chinese with peptic ulcers and a control group of 87 using a standardized questionnaire. The median amount of chile used per month was 312 units in the ulcer group compared to 834 units in the control group. The data support the hypothesis that chile use has a protective effect against peptic ulcer disease.

Licorice

Baker (1994) reported studies since the 1950s, showing that licorice-derived compounds had antiulcer effects raising the local concentration of prostaglandins that promote mucous secretion and cell proliferation in the stomach. This action leads to the healing of ulcers. Dehpour, Zolfaghari, Samadian, and Vahedi (1994) found the same result when using licorice to reduce the number and size of ulcers in gastric ulcers induced by aspirin in rats.

Vitamin E

Aldori and colleagues (1997) examined the effect of vitamin A and fiber on risk for developing a duodenal ulcer. The nearly 48,000 men with the highest intake of vitamin A had a 54% lower risk of a duodenal ulcer than those ingesting small amounts of vitamin A–rich foods. Men who had the highest intake of fiber had a 45% lower risk for duodenal ulcer than those who followed a low-fiber diet. Eating vitamin A–rich yams and liver and fiber-rich apples provided special protection.

WEIGHT LOSS: RECOMMENDATIONS

Factors that help people include:

- an emphasis on changing behavior through keeping food diaries of types and amount of food eaten, time of eating, location, position, mood, and companions
- a review of the diary with a helping person
- setting specific behavior change goals
- rewards for changing are designated: tokens, money, prizes, participant-identified rewards
- a combination of mass media approaches and one-on-one counseling
- a design for creating ways of keeping participants in the program; less than half of the participants remain in a program long enough to achieve their weight loss goals
- emphasis on the immediate benefits of good nutritional practices such as attractiveness and self-confidence.

The National Center for Health Education in San Francisco (1982) released a report identifying various approaches that have worked with individuals:

- Identify why weight loss is important, listing the reasons in as specific a way as possible.
- Write down the advantages and disadvantages of becoming thinner.
- Record each incident of eating and the circumstances surrounding it for a week.
- Set goals for becoming thinner and formalize them in a contract; have a trusted other person sign it.
- Set up a reward system; praise or other pleasant happening if weight is lost;

forfeit money (or another reward) if pledged weight is not lost.
- Find a buddy or a small group of weight losers with whom to discuss the weight loss process and from whom to garner support; keep the support going after desired weight has been reached to avoid slippage.
- Use imagery to picture oneself as fat as currently or as thin as desired.
- Role play with a buddy how to handle pressure from others to eat.
- Learn relaxation techniques and diversionary tactics (drink a glass of water, take a walk, deep breathe) when eating urges overwhelm.
- Get at least one family member involved in the process to offer support and to help change family eating patterns.

Other common weight loss recommendations found helpful by the author in her work with clients include:

- Analyze eating in detail in an individual or group setting, including:
  —Why do I want to change?
  —What are the advantages and disadvantages of changing?
  —Exactly how do I sabotage my eating plan now?
  —What skills do I need to learn to resist pressure from others to maintain old eating patterns? (saying no, refraining from getting defensive)
  —What kind of support do I need from others to attain my goals? (phone calls, or written reminders when I feel I'm slipping)
- Eat only at specified meal times and only while sitting down in the one household spot identified for eating; eating while cooking and eating while watching television increase chances of inappropriate eating.

- Slow down eating pace by putting down the fork after each bite, taking a break during the meal, and concentrating on the taste and texture of food; when food is eaten quickly there is insufficient time for body/mind to identify satiation.
- Never do anything else while eating.
- Set goals guaranteed to bring success; start small and gradually increase expectations as success is achieved.
- Develop an exercise program to increase lean body mass, tone the body, increase fitness, and moderate hunger urges.
- Eat whole foods (e.g., a baked potato rather than french fries) to increase satiety.
- Cut down on appetite stimulants such as coffee, spices, chocolate, sugar, colas, and salt.
- Say or write the following affirmation 25 times each day until it is believed: It is getting easier and easier to eat food that is healthy and that enhances my wellness.
- Stay away from fad diets, monodiets, and other quick loss ideas that end in quick loss and quick weight regain; such a syndrome can result in hypertension, frustration, and reduced wellness.
- To lose body fat, emphasize whole grain cereals, rice, bread and pasta, include plenty of fresh fruits and vegetables and legumes such as dried beans, peas, and lentils. Stick to appetizer-sized portions (three to four ounces) of low or nonfat dairy products, fish, chicken, or turkey, or soy products.
- Use a measuring tape or the way your clothes fit as measures of success. Lost inches are a more tangible sign of a lean body than lost pounds.
- Calories don't always count. You can eat a low-fat diet and unlimited complex carbohydrates. If you're hungry, eat a piece of bread, a rice cracker, an apple or some steamed vegetables topped with lemon and a dash of olive oil. Never allow yourself to feel deprived. Eat something, just be sure it's a grain, legume, fruit or vegetable and you'll still lose weight (Shaw, 1994).
- To add taste to your food, put a thin coat of olive oil in the pan, wipe away the excess, then cook your food.
- Before eating, ask yourself: Do I really want this food? If yes, visualize yourself eating it, savoring the taste, and then picturing how you'll feel one-half hour later. If the experience is positive, eat the food. If not, don't.
- Avoid being negative if you don't follow your plan for a day or two once in a while. Give yourself permission to be human, then resume your program the next day with a positive attitude.

Dr. Roland Weinsier (1985) of the University of Alabama has investigated another method of weight management called the *"Time Calorie Displacement" (TCD) method.* It features high-bulk, low-calorie foods such as fruits, vegetables, and unrefined starches. These foods take longer to consume than high calorie, less bulky foods such as meats, fats and oil, and sugar products. The longer the dieter spends in eating, the greater the satisfaction and the fewer calories consumed. Some of the recommended foods are rice pudding made with small amounts of honey and fiber-rich brown rice and mock pizza sandwiches made with whole wheat English muffins, part skim milk cheese, and tomatoes.

Clinical studies with obese participants at the University of Alabama show that the TCD food plan keeps people satisfied on about 1,500 calories a day, is nutritionally balanced, and is effective in loss of fatty tissue. Thirty-five percent of the participants lost more than 20 lb. and 7% lost more than 40 lb. over an average of 26 weeks. Steady but small weight loss allows participants to establish new eating patterns so that excess weight does not reappear.

Weinsier tested 20 people: 10 were obese and 10 were of normal weight. Given as much food as they wanted, all reached the same degree of fullness while eating half the number of calories from the high-bulk, low-calorie meals as from the high-calorie meals and rated both meal plans as equally enjoyable. A separate study showed that skinfold thickness (a measure of body fat) fell significantly while muscle mass was maintained. Blood levels of all essential vitamins and minerals were also maintained without vitamin supplementation.

Theories concerning weight maintenance have changed radically over the years. A newer explanation, *set point theory*, holds that fatness is not an accident of fat. According to the theory, the body does not know the difference between dieting and starvation. In an effort to protect the individual, the body goes into starvation practices, requiring fewer calories to do the work of the metabolic processes. Thus, when individuals attempt to diet, their setpoint rises and fat is held on to, making weight loss difficult when rich foods, inactivity, and short-term fad diets reign. Studies of animals under starvation conditions and force fed humans support setpoint theory (Bennett & Gurin, 1982, pp. 64–84).

Recurrent dieting may be an important variable affecting weight gain. Dieting leads to a lower metabolic rate; when "normal" eating is resumed, weight is regained. Repeated dieting may be leading many to weight gain after dieting. Bennett and Gurin (1982) suggest alternatives to dieting; change food plan to reduce intake of fat, sugar, and artificial sweeteners; and increase physical activity.

A number of studies have demonstrated that the setpoint can be countered by physical activity. Working at the University of California at Davis, Judith Stern, a nutritionist, collaborated with two exercise physiologists to study six people placed on a low-calorie food plan. As expected, metabolic rates fell after 2 weeks (starvation reaction). The subjects then began an exercise program and metabolic rates returned to normal in half the dieters; one dieter lost 30 lb. that month.

Basal metabolism decreases at a rate of 2 to 5% with every decade past the age of 30, so activity may be the only safe way to diminish the accumulation of fat that is normal with aging (Bennett & Gurin, 1982, p. 252). Studies of populations who are vigorously active also lend credence to the argument that exercise lowers set point. For example, Norwegian woodcutters do not grow fat with age; they maintain about 15% body fat for 40 years (Skobak-Kaczynski & Andersen, 1975).

A recent study comparing lean to obese men and women found that both groups consumed the same number of calories. What differed was the amount of fat, added sugar, and fiber. Obese people derived a greater part of their energy intake from fat, a greater percentage of their sugar intake from added sugar, and a lower intake of fiber than lean people (Miller et al., 1994). Alterations in diet composition rather than number of calories ingested may have been an important weight control strategy for overweight adults.

The following visualization exercise in Box 10.1 gives information useful for attaining ideal weight.

TIPS FOR EATING AWAY FROM HOME

When working with clients who eat out, you might suggest the following tips from the

---

Box 10.1   Getting to Your Ideal Weight

The idea that your mind controls your body is not new, but how many of us tap our considerable mind power to enhance our wellness? Positive affirmation and visualization can be combined to obtain your ideal weight. Before each meal, try the following exercise:

Step One: Find a quiet, peaceful spot and spend 5 minutes relaxing your body. Keep your eyes closed throughout the exercise.

Step Two: Say, "I see and feel my body as I want it to look and feel." Repeat this sentence 10 times very slowly while picturing your body at your ideal weight.

Step Three: Say, "I am able to move toward my ideal weight with increasing comfort." Repeat this statement 10 times while picturing yourself looking and feeling more comfortable.

Step Four: Say, "I *am* able to move toward higher levels of wellness and positive energy." Repeat this statement slowly five times while visualizing yourself moving to increased states of wellness and becoming filled with positive energy.

Step Five: Slowly open your eyes and prepare to eat, carrying with you the image of yourself at your ideal weight.

National Center for Nutrition and Dietetics:

The Choice is Yours

- The type of restaurant you select affects the amount of control you will have over food choices. A full service restaurant offers the most flexibility. Cafeterias allow you to control portion sizes and toppings like gravy, sauce, and salad dressing.
- Do not be afraid to ask questions about how a dish is prepared and whether lower fat substitutions are available.

Less Fat, Still Fast

- Fast food chains are jumping on the low fat bandwagon—look for low fat dairy products and hearty healthy grilled chicken or lean meat entrees.

- Although most chains have converted to all-vegetable fat for frying, fried foods still are among the highest in fat and calories.
- Take a trip to the salad bar for a lower fat sidedish alternative to fries and onion rings. Keep your salad lean by going easy on the bacon bits, croutons, regular salad dressing, and prepared salads, and by choosing low calorie or yogurt-based dressings.

Plan Ahead

- Make up for the extra calories and possible lack of variety in the meal you eat out by having lower calorie, nutrient-rich foods at home. Low or nonfat dairy products, fresh fruits and vegetables, and high fiber breads and cereals provide a lot of the nutrients in shorter supply in meals away from home.

- Healthy choices for snacks at home that you can prepare ahead of time include pita wedges with a cottage cheese and vegetable dip, high fiber muffins, a low fat yogurt parfait made with fruit and dry cereal, or a mixed fruit cup.

Eating on the Road

- Feel like you and your family live in the car? Be sure to take along individually portioned juices, raw vegetables, low fat cheese or peanut butter and whole grain crackers, snack boxes or bags of dried fruits, and seasoned, air-popped popcorn.
- Your best breakfast bets on the road are cereal with milk, waffles or pancakes with fresh fruit toppings, a bagel or toast with preserves, fruits and juices.
- If you are at a convention, buffet, or party, fill up first on raw vegetables and seltzer. Then survey the scene to decide what else to eat.
- Watch out for foods that sound healthier than they are: teriyaki dishes are low in fat but high in sodium, potato skins often are fried and with high fat toppings, pasta primavera can be made with cream, and light menu items may be nothing more than high fat appetizers.

REFERENCES

Abbott, R. D., Curb, J. D., Rodriguez, B. L., Sharp, D. S., Burshfield, C. M., & Yano, K. (1996). Effect of dietary calcium and milk consumption on risk of thromboembolic stroke in older middle-aged men: The Honolulu Heart Program. *Stroke, 27*(5), 813–818.

Adler, A. J., & Holub, B. J. (1997). Effect of garlic and fish-oil supplementation on serum lipid and lipoprotein concentration in hypercholesterolemic men. *American Journal of Clinical Nutrition, 65*(2), 445–450.

Alabaster, O., Tang, Z., & Shivapurkar, N. (1997). Dietary fiber and the chemopreventive modulation of colon carcinogenesis. *Mutation Research, 350*(1), 185–197.

Aldori, W. H., Giovannucci, E. L., & Rimm, E. G. (1997). Association between dietary fiber, sources of fiber, other nutrients, and the diagnosis of symptomatic diverticular disease. *American Journal of Clinical Nutrition, 60*(5), 757–764.

Aloisi, P., Marrelli, A., & Porto, C. (1997). Visual evoked potentials and serum magnesium levels in juvenile migraine patients. *Headache, 37*(6), 383–385.

Anderson, R. A. (1997). Chromium as an essential nutrient for humans. *Regulated Toxicology and Pharmacology, 26*(1), 46, 48.

Appel, L. J., Moore, T. J., Obarzanek, E., Vollmer, W. M., Svetkey, L. P., Sacks, E. M., Bray, G. A., Vogt, T. M., Cutler, I. A., Windhauser, M. M., Lin, P. H., & Karanja, N. (1997). A clinical trial of the effects of dietary patterns on blood pressure. DASH Collaborative Research Group. *New England Journal of Medicine, 336*(16), 117–1124.

Augusti, K. T. (1996). Therapeutic values of onion and garlic. *Indian Journal of Experimental Biology, 34*(7), 634–640.

Avon, J., Monane, M., Gurwitz, J. H., Glynn, R. J., Choodnovsky, I., & Lipsitz, L. A. (1994). Reduction of bacteriuria and pyuria after ingestion of cranberry juice. *Journal of American Medical Association, 271*(10), 751–754.

Azen, S. P., Qian, D., Mack, W. J., Sevanian, A., Selzer, R. H., Liu, C. R., & Hodis, H. (1996). Effect of supplementary antioxidant vitamin intake on carotid arterial wall intima-media thickness in a controlled clinical trial of cholesterol lowering. *Circulation, 94*, 2369–2372.

Bagga, D., Capone, S., & Wang, H. (1997). Dietary modulation of Omega-3/Omega-6 poly-unsaturated fatty acid ratios in patients with breast cancer. *Journal of the National Cancer Institute, 89*(15), 1123–1131.

Baker, M. E. (1994). Licorice and enzymes other than 11 beta-hydroxysteroid dehydrogenase: An evolutionary perspective. *Steroids, 59*(2), 136–141.

Barnard, R. J., Jung, T., & Inkebs, S. B. (1994). Diet and exercise in the treatment of NIDDM. *Diabetes Care, 17*(12), 1469–1472.

Bennett, W., & Gurin, J. (1982). *The dieter's dilemma: Eating less and weighing more.* New York: Basic Books.

Blot, W. J., Li, J., Taylor, P. R., Guo, W., Dawsey, S., Wang, C., & Yang, C. S. (1993). Nutrition intervention trials in Linxian, China: Supplementation with specific vitamin/mineral combinations, cancer incidence, and disease-specific mortality in the general population. *Journal of the National Cancer Institute, 85*(18), 1483–1492.

Boik, J. (1996). *Cancer and natural medicine.* Princeton, MN: Oregon Medical Press.

Bonjour, J. P., Schurch, M. A., & Rizzoli, R. (1996). Nutritional aspects of hip fractures. *Bone, 18*(Suppl. 3), 139S–144S.

Botterweck, A. A., van den Brandt, P. A., & Goldbohm, R. A. (2000). Vitamins, carotenoids, dietary fiber, and the risk of gastric carcinoma: Results from a prospective study after 6.3 years of follow-up. *Cancer, 88*(4), 737–748.

Britton, J., Pavord, I., Richards, K., Wisniewski, A., Knox, A., Lewis, S., Tattersfield, A., & Weiss, S. (1994). Dietary magnesium, lung function, wheezing, and airway hyperreactivity in a random adult population. *Lancet, 344*(8919), 357–362.

Brodsky, M. A. (1994). Magnesium therapy in a new-onset atrial fibrillation. *American Journal of Cardiology, 73*, 1227–1229.

Bucher, H. C., Guyatt, C. H., Cooke, R. J., Hatala, R., Cook, D. J., Lang, J. D., & Hunt, D. (1996). Effect of calcium supplementation on pregnancy-induced hypertension and preeclampsia. A meta-analysis of randomized controlled trials. *Journal of the American Medical Association, 275*(14), 1113–1117.

Bunout, D., Garrido, A., Suazo, M., Kauffman, R., Venegas, P., de la Maza, P., Petermann,

M., & Hirsch, S. (2000). Effects of supplementation with folic acid and antioxidant vitamins on homocysteine levels and LDL oxidation in coronary patients. *Nutrition, 16*(2), 107–110.

Carey, O. J., Locke, C., & Cookson, J. B. (1993). Effect of alterations of dietary sodium on the severity of asthma in men. *Thorax, 48*(7), 714–718.

Cerda, J. (1996). Florida nutrition research advocates cholesterol-lowering foods instead of drugs. Press Release, University of Florida, Health Science Center, PO Box 100253, Gainesville, FL 32610-0253.

Ceremuzynski, L., Chamiec, T., & Herbaczynski-Cedre, K. (1997). Effect of supplemental oral L-arginine on exercise capacity in patients with stable angina pectoris. *American Journal of Cardiology, 80*(3), 331–333.

Chasan-Taber, L., Selhub, J., & Rosenberg, E. (1996). A prospective study of folate and vitamin B6 and risk of myocardial infarction in U.S. physicians. *Journal of the American College of Nutrition, 15*(2), 136–143.

Chuong, C. J., & Dawson, E. G. (1994). Zing and copper levels in premenstrual syndrome. *Fertility and Sterility, 62*(2), 313–320.

Dalery, K., Lussier-Cacan, S., & Selhub, J. (1995). Homocysteine and coronary artery disease in French Canadian subjects: Relation with vitamins B_{12}, B_6, pyridoxal phosphate, and folate. *American Journal of Cardiology, 75*(16), 1107–1111.

Dehpour, A. R., Zolfaghari, M. E., Samadian, T., & Vahedi, Y. (1994). The protective effect of liquorice components and their derivatives against gastric ulcer induced by aspirin in rats. *Journal of Pharmaceutical Pharmacology, 46*(2), 148–149.

Deneo-Pellegrini, H., DeStafani, E., Boffetta, P., Ronco, A., & Mendilaharsu, M. (1999). Dietary iron and cancer of the rectum: A case-control study in Uruguay. *European Journal of Cancer Prevention, 8*(6), 501–508.

de Rijk, M. C., Breteler, M. M., den Breeijen, J. H., Launer, L. J., Grobbee, D. E., Van der Meche, F. G., & Hoffman, A. (1997). Dietary antioxidants and Parkinson's disease: The Rotterdam Study. *Archives of Neurology, 54*(6), 762–765.

Dirshl, D. R., Henderson, R. C., & Oakley, W. S., Jr. (1995). Correlation of bone mineral density in elderly patients with hip fractures. *Journal of Orthopaedic Trauma, 9*(6), 470–475.

Dow, I., Tracey, M., Villar, A., Coggon, D., Margettes, B. M., Campbell, M. J., & Holgate, S. T. (1996). Does dietary intake of vitamins C and E influence lung function in older people? *American Journal of Respiratory and Critical Care Medicine, 154*(5), 1401–1404.

Facchinetti, F., Borella, P., & Sances, G. (1991). Oral magnesium successfully relieves premenstrual mood changes. *Obstetrics and Gynecology, 78*(2), 177–181.

Facchini, F., Coulston, A. M., & Reaven, G. M. (1996). Relationship between dietary vitamin intake and resistance to insulin-mediated glucose disposal in healthy volunteers. *American Journal of Clinical Nutrition, 63*(6), 946–949.

Fawzi, W. W., Herrera, M. G., Willett, W. C., Nestel, P., el Amin, A., Lipstiz, S., & Mohamed, K. A. (1994). Dietary vitamin A intake and the risk of mortality among children. *American Journal of Clinical Nutrition, 59*(2), 401–408.

Fleet, J. C. (1994). New support for a folk remedy: Cranberry juice reduces bacteriuria and pyuria in elderly women. *Nutrition Reviews, 5*(2), 168–170.

Flynn, M. A., Irvin, W., & Krause, G. (1994). The effect of folate and cobalamin on osteoarthritic hands. *Journal of American College of Nutrition, 13*(4), 351–356.

Fotherby, M. D., & Potter, J. F. (1997). Long-term potassium supplementation lowers blood pressure in elderly hypertensive subjects. *International Journal of Clinical Practice, 51*(4), 219–222.

Franceschi, S., Bidoli, E., & La Vecchia, C. (1994). Tomatoes and risk of digestive-tract cancers. *International Journal of Cancer, 59*(2), 181–184.

Franceschi, S., Favero, A., & La Vecchia, R. (1995). Influence of food groups and food diversity on breast cancer risk in Italy. *International Journal of Cancer, 63*(6), 785–789.

Fraser, G. E., Lindsted, K. D., & Beeson, W. L. (1995). Effect of risk factor values on lifetime risk of and age at first coronary event. The Adventist Health Study. *American Journal of Epidemiology, 142*(7), 746–758.

Freudenheim, J. L., Marshall, J. R., & Vena, J. E. (1996). Premenopausal breast cancer risk and intake of vegetables, fruits and related nutrients. *Journal of the National Cancer Institute, 88*(6), 340–348.

Gallai, V. (1994). Magnesium content of mononuclear blood cells in migraine patients. *Headache, 34,* 160–165.

Galland, L. D., Baker, S. M., & McLellan, R. K. (1986). Magnesium deficiency in the pathogenesis of mitral prolapse. *Magnesium, 5,* 165–174.

Garland, C. F., Garland, F. C., & Gorham, E. D. (1999). Calcium and vitamin D: Their potential roles in colon and breast cancer prevention. *Annals of the New York Academy of Science, 889,* 107–119.

Garg, A., Bonanome, S. A., & Grundy, S. (1988). Comparison of a high-carbohydrate diet with a high-monosaturated diet in patients with non-insulin-dependent diabetes mellitus. *New England Journal of Medicine, 319,* 829–934.

Gerster, H. (1997). The potential role of lycopene for human health. *Journal of the American College of Nutrition, 16*(2), 109–126.

Gillman, M. W., Belanger, A., D'Agostino, R. B., Ellison, R. C., & Posner, B. M. (1994). Protective effect of calcium intake on development of hypertension. Presented at the 34th Annual Conference on Cardiovascular Disease Epidemiology and Prevention, March 16–17, Hyatt Regency Westshore, Tampa, Florida, p. 10.

Gillman, M. W., Cupples, L. A., & Gagnon, D. (1995). Protective effect of fruits and vegetables on development of stroke in men. *Journal of the American Medical Association, 273*(14), 1113–1117.

Giovannuci, E., Rimme, E. G., & Colditz, G. A. (1993). A prospective study of dietary fat and risk of prostate cancer. *Journal of the National Cancer Institute, 85,* 1571–1579.

Giovannuci, E., Ascherio, A., & Rimmie, E. G. (1995). Intake of carotenoids and retinol in relation to risk of prostate cancer. *Journal of the National Cancer Institute, 87*(2), 1767–1776.

Goodman, M. T., Wilkens, L. R., & Hankin, J. H. (1997). Association of soy and fiber consumption with the risk of endometrial cancer. *American Journal of Epidemiology, 146*(4), 294–306.

Grimble, R. F. (1997). Effect of antioxidative vitamins on immune function with clinical applications. *International Journal of Vitamin and Nutrition Research, 67*(5), 312–320.

Grundman, M. (2000). Vitamin E and Alzheimer's disease: The basis for additional clinical trials. *American Journal of Clinical Nutrition, 71*(2), 630S–636S.

Guttormsen, A. B., Ueland, P. M., & Nesthus, I. (1996). Determinants and vitamin responsiveness of intermediate hyper-homocysteinemia: The Hordaland Homocysteine Study. *Journal of Clinical Investigation, 98*(9), 2174–2183.

Hallfrish, J., Singh, V. N., & Muller, D. C. (1994). High plasma vitamin C associated with high plasma HDL- and HD12 Cholesterol. *American Journal of Clinical Nutrition, 60*(1), 100–105.

Hansen, G. V., Nielsen, L., & Kluger, E. (1996). Nutritional status of Danish rheumatoid arthritis patients and effects of a diet adjusted in energy intake, fish-meal, and antioxidants. *Scandinavian Journal of Rheumatology, 25*(5), 325–330.

Hasselmark, L., Malmgren, R., & Zetterstrom, O. (1993). Selenium supplementation in intrinsic asthma. *Allergy, 48*, 30–36.

Haugen, M. A., Kjeldsen-Kragh, J., Bjerve, K. S., Hostmark, A. T., & Fone, O. (1994). Changes in plasma phospholipid fatty acids and their relationship to disease activity in rheumatoid arthritis patients treated with a vegetarian diet. *British Journal of Nutrition, 72*(4), 555–566.

Hee, J., Klag, M. J., Whelton, P. K., Chen, J. Y., Qian, M. C., & He, G. Q. (1995). Dietary micronutrients and blood pressure in southwestern China. *Journal of Hypertension, 13*(11), 1267–1274.

Humphrey, J. H., Agoestina, T., Wu, L., Usman, A., Nurachim, M., Subardja, D., Hidayat, S.,

Tielsch, J., West, K. P., & Sommer, A. (1996). Impact of neonatal vitamin A supplementation on infant morbidity and mortality. *Journal of Pediatrics, 128*(4), 489–496.

Ishihara, N., Yuzawa, M., & Tamakoshi, A. (1997). Antioxidants and angiogenetic factor associated with age-related macular degeneration. *Nippon Ganka Gakkai Zasshi, 101*(3), 248–251.

Ji, L., Stratment, F., & Lardy, H. (1992). Antioxidant enzyme response to selenium deficiency in rat myocardium. *Journal of the American College of Nutrition, 11*, 79–86.

John, E. (1997). Sunlight may guard against breast cancer. Paper presented to a scientific meeting of breast cancer oncologists, Washington, DC: November 3.

Kang, J. K., Yelh, K. G., & Chin, H. P. (1995). Chili-protective factor against peptic ulcer? *Digestive Diseases and Sciences, 40*(3), 576–579.

Kang, J. X., & Leaf, A. (1996). The cardiac antiarrhythmic effects of polyunsaturated fatty acid. *Lipids, 31*, A41–A44.

Katiyar, S. K., Korman, N. J., Mukhtar, H., & Agarwal, R. (1997). Protective effects of silymarin against photocarcinogenesis in a mouse skin model. *Journal of the National Cancer Institute, 89*(8), 556–566.

Keli, S. O., Hertog, M. G., Feskens, E. J., & Kromhout, D. (1996). Dietary flavonoids, antioxidant vitamins, and incidence of stroke: The Zutphen study. *Archives of Internal Medicine, 156*(6), 637–642.

Kendler, B. S. (1997). Recent nutritional approaches to the prevention and therapy of cardiovascular disease. *Progress in Cardiovascular Nursing, 12*(3), 3–23.

Key, T. J., Silcocks, P. B., & Davey, G. K. (1997). A case-control study of diet and prostate cancer. *British Journal of Cancer, 76*(5), 678–687.

Kiecolt-Glaser, J. K., Glaser, R., Cacioppo, J. T., MacCallum, R. C., Snydersmith, M., Kim, & Malarkey, W. B. (1997). Marital conflict in older adults: Endocrinological and immunological correlates. *Psychosomatic Medicine, 59*(4), 339–349.

Kjeldsen-Kragh, I., Haugen, M., Borchgrevink, C. F., & Forre, O. (1994). Vegetarian diet for patients with rheumatoid arthritis. Two years after introduction of the diet. *Clinical Rheumatology, 13*(3), 475–482.

Knight, D. C., & Eden, J. A. (1996). A review of the clinical effects of phytoestrogens. *Obstetrics and Gynecology, 87*(5, Pt. 2), 897–904.

Kremer, J. M., & Bigaouette, J. (1996). Nutrient intake of patients with rheumatoid arthritis is deficient in pyridoxine, zinc, copper and magnesium. *Journal of Rheumatology, 23*(6), 990–994.

Krishna, G. G. (1994). Role of potassium in the pathogenesis of hypertension. *American Journal of Medical Science, 307*(Suppl. 1), S21–S25.

Kurzer, M. S., Lampe, J. W., Martini, M. C., & Adlercreutz, H. (1995). Fecal lignan and isolfavonoid excretion in premenopausal women consuming flaxseed powder. *Cancer Epidemiology, Biomarkers and Prevention, 4*(4), 353–358.

Kushi, L. H., Folsom, A. R., & Prineas, R. J. (1996). Dietary antioxidant vitamins and death from coronary heart disease in postmenopausal women. *New England Journal of Medicine, 334*(18), 1156–1162.

Lampertico, M., & Comis, S. (1993). Italian multicenter study on the efficacy of Coenzyme Q10 as an adjuvant therapy in heart failure. *Clinical Investigator, 71,* S129–S133.

Landon, R. A., & Young, E. A. (1993). The role of magnesium in regulation of lung function. *Journal of the American Dietetic Association, 93*(6), 674–677.

Le Marchand, L., Hankin, J. H., & Wilkens, L. R. (1997). Dietary fiber and colorectal cancer risk. *Epidemiology, 8*(6), 658–665.

LeMarchand, L., Murphy, S. P., Hankin, J. H., Wilkens, L. R., & Kolonel, L. N. (2000). Intake of flavonoids and lung cancer. *Journal of the National Cancer Institute, 92*(2), 154–160.

Leventhal, L. J., Boyce, E. G., & Zurier, R. B. (1994a). Treatment of rheumatoid arthritis with gammalinolenic acid. *Annals of Internal Medicine, 119*(9), 867–873.

Leventhal, L. J., Boyce, E. G., & Zurier, R. B. (1994b). Treatment of rheumatoid arthritis with gammalinolenic acid. *British Journal of Rheumatology, 33*(9), 847–852.

London, R. S., Murphy, L., Kitlowski, K. E., & Reynolds, M. A. (1987). Efficacy of alpha-tocopherol in the treatment of premenstrual syndrome. *Journal of Reproductive Medicine, 32*(6), 400–404.

London, R. S., Sundaram, G. S., Murphy, L., & Goldstein, P. J. (1983). The effect of alpha-tocopherol on premenstrual symptomatology: A double-blind study. *Journal of the American College of Nutrition, 2*(2), 115–122.

Losonczy, K. G., Harris, T. B., & Haulik, R. J. (1996). Vitamin E and vitamin C supplement use and risk of all-cause and coronary heart disease mortality in older persons: The Established Populations for Epidemiologic Studies of the Elderly. *American Journal of Clinical Nutrition, 64*(2), 190–196.

Manson, J. E., Willett, W. C., & Stampfer, M. J. (1994). Vegetable and fruit consumption and incidence of stroke in women. 34th Annual Conference on Cardiovascular Disease Epidemiology and Prevention. March 16–17. Tampa, Florida.

Mares-Perlman, J. A. (1995). Serum antioxidants and age-related macular degeneration in a population-based case-control study. *Archives of Ophthalmology, 113*(2), 1518–1523.

Mares-Perlman, J. A., Klein, R., & Klein, B. E. (1996). Association of zinc and antioxidant nutrients with age-related maculopathy. *Archives of Ophthalmology, 114*(2), 991–997.

Martin, A., Wu, D., Baur, W., Meydani, S. N., Blumberg, J. B., & Meydani, M. (1996). Effect of vitamin E on human aortic endothelial cell responses to oxidative injury. *Free Radical Biological Medicine, 21*(4), 505–511.

Martin, A., Foxall, T., Blumberg, J. B., & Meydani, M. (1997). Vitamin E inhibits low-density lipoprotein-induced adhesion of monocytes to human aortic endothelial cells in vitro. *Arteriosclerosis, Thrombosis and Vascular Biology, 17*(3), 429–436.

Martin-Moreno, J. M. (1994). Dietary fat, olive oil intake and breast cancer risk. *International Journal of Cancer, 58*(6), 774–780.

Matkovic, V. (1995). Urinary calcium, sodium, and bone mass of young females. *American Journal of Clinical Nutrition, 62,* 417–425.

McAlindon, T., Zhang, Y., & Hannan, M. (1996). Are risk factors for patellofemoral and tibiofemoral knee osteoarthritis different? *Journal of Rheumatology*, *23*(2), 332–337.

McAlindon, T. E. (1997). Nutrition: Risk factors for osteoarthritis. *Annals of Rheumatic Disease*, *56*(7), 397–400.

McCarty, M. F. (1996). Magnesium taurate and fish oil for prevention of migraine. *Medical Hypotheses*, *47*(6), 461–466.

Meunier, P. (1996). Prevention of hip fractures by correcting calcium and vitamin D insufficiencies in elderly people. *Scandinavian Journal of Rheumatology*(Supp. 103), 75–78.

Meydani, S. N., Meydani, M., & Blumberg, J. B. (1997). Vitamin E supplementation and in vivo immune response in healthy elderly subjects: A randomized controlled trial. *Journal of the American Medical Association*, *277*, 1380–1386.

Meyer, F. (1994). Ischemic heart disease incidence and mortality in relation to vitamin supplement use in a cohort of 2,226 men. Presented at the American Heart Association's 34th Annual Conference on Cardiovascular Disease Epidemiology and Prevention, March 16–19, Tampa, Florida.

Meyer, H. E., Tverdal, A., & Henriksen, C. (1996). Risk factors of femoral neck fractures in Oslo. *Tidsskrift for Den Norske Laegeforening*, *116*(2), 2656–2659.

Meyer, H. E., Pedersen, J. I., Loken, E. G., & Tverdal, A. (1997). Dietary factors and the incidence of hip fracture in middle-aged Norwegians: A prospective study. *American Journal of Epidemiology*, *145*(2), 117–123.

Miller, W. C., Niederpruem, M. G., Wallace, J. P., & Lindeman, A. K. (1994). Dietary fat, sugar, and fiber predict body fat content. *Journal of the American Dietetic Association*, *94*(6), 612–615.

Moerman, C. J. (1993). Dietary sugar intake in the etiology of biliary tract cancer. *International Journal of Epidemiology*, *22*, 207–214.

Moon, T. E., Levine, N., Cartmel, B., & Bangert, J. L. (1997). Retinoids in prevention of skin cancer. *Cancer Letters*, *114*(1–2), 203–205.

Morcos, N. C. (1997). Modulation of lipid profile by fish oil and garlic combination. *Journal of the National Medical Association*, *89*(10), 673–678.

Mortensen, S. A. (1993). Prospectives on therapy of cardiovascular disease with coenzyme Q10 (Ubiquinone). *Clinical Investigation*, *71*, S116–S123.

Muntzel, M., & Drueke, T. (1992). A comprehensive review of the salt and blood pressure relationship. *American Journal of Hypertension*, *5*(4), 1s–4s.

Murray, M. (1994). Dietary and life-style factors in treating asthma, hay fever and allergies. *Natural Alternatives to Over-the-Counter and Prescription Drugs* (pp. 91–99). New York: William Morrow and Company, Inc.

National Center for Health Education. (1982). *Recommendations for weight loss*. San Francisco, CA: National Center for Health Education.

Nelson, L. M., Matkin, C., Longstreh, W. T., & McGuire, V. (2000). Population-based case-control study of amyotrophic lateral sclerosis in western Washington State: II. Diet. *American Journal of Epidemiology*, *151*(2), 164–173.

Ness, A. R., Chee, D., & Elliott, P. (1997). Vitamin C and blood pressure—an overview. *Journal of Human Hypertension*, *11*(6), 343–350.

Nygard, O., Refsum, H., & Ueland, R. M. (1997). Coffee consumption and plasma total homocysteine: The Hordaland Homocysteine Study. *American Journal of Clinical Nutrition*, *65*(1), 136–143.

Patrick, L. (2000). Nutrients and HIV: Part two—Vitamins A and F. *Alternative Medical Review*, *5*(1), 39–51.

Pauletto, P., Puato, M., & Angeli, M. T. (1996). Blood pressure, serum lipids, and fatty acids in populations on a lake-fish diet or on a vegetarian diet in Tanzania. *Lipids*, *31*, S309–S312.

Peretz, A., Neve, J., & Famaey, J. (1991). Selenium in rheumatic disease. *Seminars in Arthritis and Rheumatism*, *20*, 305–316.

Perrig, W. J., Perrig, P., & Stahelin, H. B. (1997). The relation between antioxidants and memory performance in the old and very old. *Journal of the American Geriatrics Society*, *45*(6), 718–724.

Peters, E. M., Goetzsche, J. M., Grobbelaar, B., & Noakes, T. D. (1993). Vitamin C supplementation reduces the incidence of post-race symptoms of upper-respiratory-tract infection in ultra-marathon runners. *American Journal of Clinical Nutrition, 57*, 170–174.

Pienta, K. J., Naik, H., & Alchtar, A. (1995). Inhibition of spontaneous metastasis in rat prostate cancer model by oral administration of modified citrus pectin. *Journal of the National Cancer Institute, 87*(5), 348–353.

Pinto, J. T., Qiao, C., & Xing, J. (1997). Effects of garlic thioallyl derivatives on growth, glutathione concentration, and polyamine formation of human prostate carcinoma cells in culture. *American Journal of Clinical Nutrition, 66*(2), 398–405.

Potter, J. D. (1996). Nutrition and colorectal cancer. *Cancer Causes and Control, 7*(1), 127–146.

Rahman, M. M., Mahalanabis, D., Alvarez, J. O., Wahed, M. A., Islam, M. A., Habte, D., & Khaled, M. A. (1996). Acute respiratory infections prevent improvement of vitamin A status in young infants supplemented with vitamin A. *Journal of Nutrition, 126*(3), 628–633.

Ramadan, N. M., Halvorson, H., & Vonde-Linde, A. (1989). Low brain magnesium in migraine. *Headache, 29*, 590–593.

Reis, J. G. (1995, June 26). A Parkinson's primer. *Nursing Spectrum*, 12–14.

Ren, S., & Lien, E. J. (1997). Natural products and their derivatives as cancer chemopreventive agents. In E. Jucker (Ed.), *Progress in Drug Research Volume 48* (pp. 147–170). Basek, Switzerland: Birkhauser Verlag.

Richer, S. (1996). Multicenter ophthalmic and nutritional age-related macular degeneration study: 2. Antioxidant intervention and conclusions. *Journal of the American Optometric Association, 67*(1), 30–49.

Riggs, D. R., DeHaven, J. I., & Lamm, D. (1997). Allium sativum (garlic) treatment for murine transitional cell carcinoma. *Cancer, 79*(10), 1987–1994.

Risch, H. A., Jain, M., & Marrett, L. D. (1994). Dietary fat intake and risk of epithelial ovarian cancer. *Journal of the National Cancer Institute, 86*, 1409–1415.

Rosenstein, D. L., Elin, R. J., & Hosseini, J. M. (1994). Magnesium measures across the menstrual cycle in premenstrual syndrome. *Biological Psychiatry, 35*(8), 557–561.

Rozen, F., Yang, X. F., Huynh, H., & Pollak, M. K. (1997). Antiproliferative action of vitamin D-related compounds and insulin-like growth factor-binding protein 5 accumulation. *Journal of the National Cancer Institute, 89*, 652–656.

Sabate, J., Fraser, G. E., & Burke, K. (1993). Effects of walnuts on serum lipid levels and blood pressure in normal men. *New England Journal of Medicine, 328*(9), 603–607.

Salmeron, J., Manson, J. E., & Stampfer, M. J. (1997). Dietary fiber, glycemic load, and risk of non-insulin-dependent diabetes mellitus in women. *Journal of the American Medical Association, 277*(6), 472–477.

Salonen, J., Salonen, R., & Seppanen, K. (1991). Effects of antioxidant supplementation on platelet function: A randomized pair-matched, placebo-controlled, double-blind trial in men with low antioxidant status. *American Journal of Clinical Nutrition, 53*, 1222–1229.

Sayegh, R., Schiff, I., & Wurtman, J. (1995). The effect of a carbohydrate-rich beverage on mood, appetite and cognitive function in women with premenstrual syndrome. *Obstetrics and Gynecology, 86*(part 1), 520–528.

Scheider, W. L., Hershey, L. A., & Vena, J. E. (1997). Dietary antioxidants and other dietary factors in the etiology of Parkinson's disease. *Movement Disorders, 12*(2), 190–196.

Schoenthaler, S. J., & Bier, I. D. (2000). The effect of vitamin-mineral supplementation on juvenile delinquency among American schoolchildren: A randomized, double-blind placebo-controlled trial. *Journal of Alternative Complementary Medicine, 6*(1), 7–17.

Seddon, J. M., Ajani, U. A., & Sperduto, R. D. (1994). Dietary carotenoids, vitamins A, C and E, and advanced age-related macular degeneration. *Journal of the American Medical Association, 272*, 1413–1420.

Seelig, M. S. (1994). Consequences of magnesium deficiency on the enhancement of stress reactions: Preventive and therapeutic implications. *Journal of the American College of Nutrition, 13*(5), 429–446.

Sempertegui, F., Estrella, B., Correa, E., Aguirre, L., Saa, B., Torres, M., Navarrete, Fl., Alarcon, C., Carrion, J., Rodriguez, G., & Griffiths, J. K. (1996). Effects of short-term zinc supplementation on cellular immunity, respiratory symptoms, and growth of malnourished Equadorian children. *European Journal of Clinical Nutrition, 50*(1), 42–46.

Sen, C. K., Atalay, M., Agren, J., Laaksonen, D. E., Roy, S., & Hanninen, O. (1997). Fish oil and vitamin E supplementation in oxidative stress at rest and after physical exercise. *Journal of Applied Physiology, 83*(1), 189–195.

Serfaty, D., & Magneron, A. C. (1997). Premenstrual syndrome in France. Epidemiology and therapeutic effectiveness of 1000 mg of micronized purified flavonoid fraction in 1473 gynecological patients. *Contraception, Fertility and Sex, 25*(1), 85–90.

Serraino, M., & Thompson, L. (1992). The effect of flaxseed supplementation on the initiation and promotional stages of mammary tumorigenesis. *Nutrition in Cancer, 17,* 153–159.

Shapiro, D., Goldstein, I. B., & Jamner, L. D. (1996). Effects of cynical hostility, anger out, anxiety, and defensiveness on ambulatory blood pressure in black and white college students. *Psychosomatic Medicine, 58*(4), 354–364.

Sharma, R. D., Raghuram, T. C., & Rao, N. S. (1990). Effect of fenugreek seeds on blood glucose and serum lipids in type I diabetes. *European Journal of Clinical Nutrition, 44,* 301–306.

Sheela, C. G., & Augusti, K. T. (1992). Antidiabetic effects of S-ayyl cysteine suphoxide isolated from garlic. *Indian Journal of Experimental Biology, 30,* 523–526.

Singh, R. B., Niaz, M. A., Rastogi, S. S., & Rastogi, S. (1996). Usefulness of anti-oxidant vitamins in suspected acute myocardial infarction (the Indian experiment of infarct survival—3). *American Journal of Cardiology, 77*(4), 232–236.

Sivam, G. P., Lampe, J. W., & Ulness, B. (1997). Helicobacter pylori—in vitro susceptibility to garlic (Allium sativum) extract. *Nutrition in Cancer, 27*(2), 118–121.

Skobak-Kaczynski, J., & Andersen, L. (1975). The effect of a high level of habitual physical activity in the regulation of fatness during aging. *International Archives of Occupational and Environmental Health, 36,* 41–46.

Smith, S. R., Klotman, P. E., & Svetkey, L. P. (1992). Potassium chloride lowers blood pressure and causes natriuresis in older patients with hypertension. *Journal of the American Society of Nephrology, 2*(8), 1302, 1309.

Snodderly, D. M. (1995). Evidence for protection against age-related macular degeneration by carotenoids and antioxidant vitamins. *American Journal of Clinical Nutrition, 62*(Suppl. 6), 1448S–1461S.

Srivastava, Y. (1993). Antidiabetic and adaptogenic properties of Momordica charantia extract: An experimental and clinical evaluation. *Phytotherapy Research, 2,* 285–289.

Stamler, J., Ruth, K. J., Lui, D., & Shekelle, R. B. (1994). Dietary antioxidants and blood pressure change in the Western Electric Study. Presented at the 34th Annual Conference on Cardiovascular disease Epidemiology and Prevention. Tampa, FL, March 16 and 17.

Stephens, N. G., Parsons, A., & Schofield, P. M. (1996). Randomized controlled trial of vitamin E in patients with coronary disease: Cambridge Heart Antioxidant Study. *Lancet, 347*(9004), 781–786.

Stewart, A. (1987). Clinical and biochemical effects of nutritional supplementation on the premenstrual syndrome. *Journal of Reproductive Medicine, 32*(6), 435–441.

Stoll, B. A. (1997). Macronutrient supplements may reduce breast cancer risk: How, when and which? *European Journal of Clinical Nutrition, 51*(9), 573–577.

Suadicani, P., Hein, H., & Gyntelberg, F. (1992). Serum selenium concentration and risk of ischemic heart disease in a prospective cohort study of 3000 males. *Atherosclerosis, 96,* 33–42.

Swanson, D. R. (1988). Migraine and magnesium: Eleven neglected conditions. *Perspectives in Biological Medicine, 31,* 526–527.

Temple, M. E., Luzier, A. B., & Kazierad, D. J. (2000). Homocysteine as a risk factor for atherosclerosis. *Annals of Pharmacotherapy, 34*(1), 57–65.

Thys-Jacobs, Jacobs, S., Ceccarelli, S., & Bierman, A. (1989). Calcium supplementation in premenstrual syndrome: A randomized crossover trial. *Journal of General Internal Medicine, 4*(3), 183–189.

Ting, H. H., Timini, F. K., & Boles, K. S. (1996). Vitamin C improves endothelium-dependent vasocilation in patients with non-insulin-dependent diabetes mellitus. *Journal of Clinical Investigation, 97*(1), 22–28.

Trevisanato, S. I., & Kim, Y. I. (2000). Tea and health. *Health Reviews, 58*(1), 1–10.

Trichopoulou, A., Katsouyanni, K., & Stuver, S. (1995). Consumption of olive oil and specific food groups in relation to breast cancer risk in Greece. *Journal of the National Cancer Institute, 87*(2), 110–116.

Troisi, R. J., Willett, W. C., & Weiss, S. T. (1995). A prospective study of diet and adult-onset asthma. *American Journal of Respiratory and Critical Care Medicine, 151*(5), 1401–1408.

Tucker, K. L., Selhub, J., Wilson, P. W., & Rosenberg, I. H. (1996). Dietary intake pattern relates to plasma folate and homocysteine concentrations in the Framingham Heart Study. *Journal of Nutrition, 126*(12), 3025–3031.

Vachon, C. M., Kushi, I. H., Cerhan, J. R., Kuni, C. C., & Sellers, T. A. (2000). Association of diet mammographic breast density in the Minnesota breast cancer family cohort. *Cancer and Epidemiological Biomarkers and Prevention, 9*(2), 151–160.

Vermeulen, E. G., Stehouwer, C. D., Twisk, J. W., vanden Berg, M., de Jong, S. C., Mackay, A. J., van Campen, C. M., Visser, F. C., Jakobs, C. A., Bulterjis, E. J., & Rauwerda, J. A. (2000). Effect of homocysteine-lowering treatment with folic acid plus vitamin B6 on progression of subclinical atherosclerosis: A randomised, placebo-controlled trial. *Lancet, 355*(9203), 517–522.

Welihinda, J. (1982). The insulin-releasing activity of the tropical plant Momordica charantia. *Acta Biology Medicine Germany, 41,* 1229–1240.

West, S., Vitale, S., Hallfrisch, J., Munoz, B., Muller, D., Bressler, S., & Bressler, N. M. (1994). Are antioxidants or supplements protective for age-related macular degeneration? *Archives of Ophthalmology, 112*(2), 222–227.

Weinsier, R. (1985). News release from Media Relations Director, Masnning, Selvage and Lee, 1250 Eye St., N.W., Washington, DC 20005.

Whelton, P. K., He, J., & Culter, J. A. (1997). Effects of oral potassium on blood pressure. Meta-analysis of randomized controlled clinical trials. *Journal of the American Medical Association, 277*(20), 1624–1632.

Wu, A. H., Ziegler, R. G., & Horn-Ross, P. L. (1996). Tofu and risk of breast cancer in Asian-Americans. *Cancer Epidemiology Biomarkers Prevention, 5*(11), 901–906.

Wu, A. H., Yu, M. C., & Mack, T. M. (1997). Smoking, alcohol use, dietary factors and risk of small intestinal adenocarcinoma. *International Journal of Cancer, 70*(5), 512–517.

Yo, A. (1997). Diet and stomach cancer in Korea. *International Journal of Cancer*(Suppl. 10), 7–9.

Yong, L. C., Brown, C. C., & Schatzkin, A. (1997). Intakes of vitamins E, C, and A and risk of lung cancer. The NHANES I epidemiologic followup study. First National Health and Nutrition Examination Survey. *American Journal of Epidemiology, 146*(3), 231–243.

Zava, D. R., Blen, M., & Duwe, G. (1997). Estrogenic activity of natural and synthetic hormones in human breast cancer cells in culture. *Environmental Health Perspectives, 105*(Suppl. 3), 637–645.

Zheng, W., Sellers, T. A., & Doyle, T. J. (1995a). Retinol, antioxidant vitamins, and cancers of the upper digestive tract in a prospective cohort study of postmenopausal women. *American Journal of Epidemiology, 142*(9), 955–960.

Zheng, W., Kushi, L. H., & Potter, J. C. (1995b). Dietary intake of energy and animal foods and endometrial cancer incidence. The Iowa women's health study. *American Journal of Epidemiology, 142*(4), 388–394.

Ziegler, J. (1994). Just the flax, ma'am: Researchers testing linseed. *Journal of the National Cancer Institute, 86*(23), 1746–1748.

CHAPTER 11

Fitness and Flexible Movement

Barbara Resnick

BENEFITS OF EXERCISE

Despite the generally accepted belief that exercise is good for health and that inactivity is associated with many of the leading causes of death and disability in the United States, only a small percentage of the adult population actually engages in regular exercise. The 1996 Surgeon General's Report on Physical Activity and Health reported that only 15% of American adults engaged in exercise at least three times a week for at least 20 minutes. Moreover, approximately 25% of adults report engaging in no physical activity at all during their leisure time. Physical inactivity is more prevalent in women, African Americans, Latinos, and those with lower social and economic status. Working with clients on physical activity goals can be a real challenge, but it can be rewarding also. One way to encourage clients to increase their activity is to promote the specific benefits of physical activity and exercise, including: decreasing cardiovascular disease, disability, osteoporosis, and psychological problems. That is, teach these individuals that participating in a regular exercise program can reduce blood pressure, cholesterol levels, improve heart function, strengthen bones, keep muscles strong and flexible, improve balance, and give an overall sense of well-being.

HOW MUCH EXERCISE IS NEEDED

It is not uncommon for clients to ask how much exercise is needed to achieve these benefits. The National Institutes of Health Consensus Development Conference (1995), "Physical Activity and Cardiovascular Health," focused on this question and concluded that the majority of benefits of physical activity can be gained by performing a moderate-intensity activity other than exercise. Encourage clients to participate in 30 minutes of moderate-intensity physical activity such as walking, climbing the stairs, or washing the floor daily to help them achieve the positive health benefits described.

Fitness Training

Fitness training, which focuses on increasing strength and endurance, is different than simply doing some type of activity to achieve positive health benefits (an overall sense of well-being, for example). Aerobic exercise is physical activity with oxygen. It includes exercise that uses repetitive movement of large muscle groups (such as the thigh muscles) but does not cause an accumulation of lactic acid. Examples include walking, cycling, swimming, or jogging. The physiological effects of fitness or aerobic exercise training include: (a) cardiovascular improvements such as a decrease in heart rate and an increase in the efficiency of heart function (DeVito, Hernandez, Gonzalez, Felici, & Figura, 1994; Larson & Bruce, 1996); (b) overall increase in maximum aerobic capacity (called VO_2 Max), or the amount of oxygen consumed by the body (Larson & Bruce, 1996); (c) using oxygen more efficiently so that less oxygen is required by the skeletal muscles (Larson & Bruce, 1996); and (d) an increase in brain serotonin (a neurotransmitter in the brain that evokes feelings of well-being) (Chaouloft, 1997).

Achieving a Targeted Heart Rate

To become physically fit, encourage clients to begin training at low levels and gradually increase to the training zone, or *targeted heart rate* (THR). THR is 60% to 80% of the individual's maximum heart rate (MHR), or 220 minus one's age (American College of Sports Medicine, 1995). Table 11.1 provides examples of target heart rates. Exertion within the training zone of 60% to 80% of the MHR for 20 to 40 minutes three times per week for several weeks is needed for conditioning (Green & Crouse, 1995). Evidence of conditioning can be measured by (a) calculating VO_2 Max (maximum amount of oxygen consumption in the body); (b) the ability to

TABLE 11.1   Maximum and Target Heart Rate

Age	Maximum Heart Rate (220 minus age)	Target Heart Rate (60%–80% Maximum Heart Rate)
40	180	108–144
50	170	102–136
60	160	96–128
70	150	90–120
80	140	84–112
90	130	78–104

achieve and sustain THR during exercise; or (c) the ability to walk or run faster. Evidence of conditioning should occur within 2 weeks of initiating an exercise program, if performed regularly.

RECOMMENDATIONS FOR SCREENING PRIOR TO STARTING AN EXERCISE PROGRAM

The degree of screening recommended for clients prior to starting an exercise program can range from a self-administered questionnaire to expensive and sophisticated diagnostic tests. The Physical Activity Readiness Questionnaire (PAR-Q) (Thomas, Reading, & Shephard, 1992) is recommended as a minimal screening standard for starting low-to-moderate intensity exercise programs for adults ages 15 to 69 and is shown in Box 11.1.

If your clients are 70 years of age and above and have not previously been active, recommend that they check with their health care provider prior to starting an exercise program. (This could be you or someone you refer them to.) The American College of Sports Medicine (1995) guidelines help place clients into one of the following categories to determine what

---

Box 11.1   Physical Activity Readiness Questionnaire (PAR-Q)

Regular physical activity is fun and healthy, and more people are becoming more active every day. Although being more active is very safe for most people, some should check with their doctors before becoming much more physically active. The PAR-Q will indicate if you should check with a health care provider before you start to exercise.

Question   Yes   No

1. Has your health care provider ever said that you have a heart condition and that you should only do physical activity as recommended by a health care provider?

2. Do you feel pain in your chest when you perform physical activity?

3. In the past month, have you had chest pain when you were *not* performing physical activity?

4. Do you lose your balance because of dizziness or do you ever lose consciousness?

5. Do you have a bone or joint problem that could be worsened by a change in your physical activity?

6. Is your doctor currently prescribing drugs for your blood pressure or heart condition?

7. Do you know of any other reason why you should not perform physical activity?

Answer Guide:

1. If you answered yes to one or more questions: Talk with your health care provider by phone or in person before you start become more physically active.

2. If you answered no to all questions: You can become more physically active. Begin slowly and build up gradually.

---

screening tests are needed to exercise safely:

1. Low risk, or healthy with no more than one of the risk factors for coronary heart disease (high blood cholesterol, high blood pressure, diabetes, cigarette smoking, obesity, or a sedentary lifestyle);

2. Moderate risk, or individuals who have two or more of the risk factors for coronary heart disease. This category is further broken down into those with symptoms (e.g., chest pain or shortness of breath), and those without symptoms;

3. High risk, or individuals with chronic disease such as heart, lung, or metabolic disease. Once you have categorized a client, a decision can be made about whether there is a need for a complete medical evaluation or stress test prior to starting an exercise program. Table 11.2 shows exercise prescreening of older adults.

TABLE 11.2   Prescreening of Older Adults for Safe Exercise

Type of Activity	Low-risk Healthy Individual	High-risk No Symptoms	High-risk Symptoms	Chronic Disease
Low intensity < 60% MHR	no	no	no	no
Moderate intensity < 60–80% MHR	no	no	yes	yes
Vigorous activity > 80% MHR	yes	yes	yes	yes

No matter their age and physical condition, clients can safely begin a moderate exercise program. Healthy young individuals can initiate more vigorous activity or exercise intense enough to tire them in 20 minutes. Older adults who are considering vigorous exercise activity should have an examination and clinical exercise test prior to starting an intensive exercise program.

ESTABLISHING AN EXERCISE PROGRAM

The general recommendation of the consensus conference was that all children and adults should attempt at least 30 minutes or more of cumulative moderate-intensity physical activity on most (preferably all) days of the week. Box 11.2 contains definitions of exercises and activities. Help clients achieve this by letting them know that the activity can be spread out through the day. For example, walking a dog for 10 minutes three times a day would meet the required 30 minutes of moderate-intensity physical activity. The exercise prescription you work out with clients should consist of four interrelated components: mode of activity, intensity, duration, and frequency. The optimal exercise program for clients is determined by their response to exercise such as their heart rate or their *ratings of perceived exertion* (Borg, 1982). Ratings of perceived exertion (RPE) is a subjective report by the participant of how hard they are exercising (see Box 11.3).

Mode of Activity

The *mode* or type of exercise chosen is based on the goals you and the client agree on. For example, if your client is interested in improving cardiorespiratory endurance then it is important to do activities that involve the use of large muscle groups over prolonged periods and that is rhythmic and aerobic in nature (walking, jogging, hiking, or running). Other activities such as swimming, skiing, or dancing are also considered excellent forms of exercise activity; however, skill level must also be considered. Resistive exercise such as weight training is more appropriate for improving strength and balance.

Intensity

The choice of exercise intensity or degree of energy (work) required to perform an activity also depends on client goals. To gauge how clients perceive their exercise,

---

Box 11.2   Definitions of Exercise

Wisdom Box

Definitions:

Physical activity: Bodily movement produced by the skeletal muscles that requires energy expenditure and produces progressive health benefits.

Exercise: A type of physical activity defined as a planned, structured, and repetitive bodily movement to improve or maintain one or more components of physical fitness.

Aerobic exercise: Physical activity that stimulates mitochondrial oxidative metabolism. It is typified by repetitive movement of large muscle groups that does not result in progressive blood-stream lactic acid accumulation (i.e., walking, cycling, running).

Resistive exercise: Training with resistance to movement to increase muscle strength. It includes the use of weights, bands, air pressure, or one's own body weight (e.g., push-ups).

Isometric exercise: Exertion during which the muscle does not change length (i.e., pushing against immovable object).

Moderate activity: Activity that results in maintaining a heart rate of 60% to 80% of targeted heart rate. Examples include:
    Washing windows or floors for 45–60 minutes
    Gardening for 40 minutes
    Wheeling self in wheelchair for 40 minutes
    Walking 1 3/4 mile in 35 minutes
    Bicycling 4 miles in 15 minutes
    Running 1 3/4 miles in 15 minutes

---

ask them to rate their efforts either during or after exercise on a scale of 6 (for very, very light exertion) to 20 (for very, very hard exertion). Another way to evaluate exercise intensity is based on heart rate and is shown in Box 11.4.

Low intensity exercise is at a heart rate of less than 60% of the individual's maximum heart rate, and moderate intensity exercise is at 60% to 80% of the maximum heart rate. The goal during any exercise session is to maintain an average heart rate close to the midpoint of the prescribed range. An RPE score between 12 and 16 on the Borg measure is indicative of moderate exercise.

Duration

Recommend that clients get at least 20 to 30 minutes of daily exercise, excluding time spent warming up and cooling down. It was believed previously that this should be done in a continuous time frame; however, short spurts of exercise throughout the day that add up to the 30 minutes daily have been found to be just as beneficial. The duration of an exercise period refers to the amount

Box 11.3   Perceived Exertion Scale: Assessment Corner

Numerical Scale	Ratings
6	
7	Very, very light
8	
9	Very light
10	
11	Fairly light
12	
13	Somewhat hard
14	
15	Hard
16	
17	Very hard
18	
19	Very, very hard
20	
Hard	

Frequency

Frequency of exercise refers to the number of times the activity is performed. When exercise intensity levels are low, encourage clients to increase the frequency of the exercise. Again, the goal is to have your clients add up these short spurts of activity to total 30 minutes of activity every day of the week.

RATE OF PROGRESSION OF EXERCISE ACTIVITY

The rate of progression of an exercise program depends on the client's exercise goals. In the initial stage of starting to exercise, encourage clients to do light muscular endurance exercise and low-level aerobic activities that will not cause muscle soreness. The amount of time these exercises are done depends on the endurance of the client, but encourage them to progress to a full 20 minutes and to do this at least three times per week. These activities should be

Box 11.4   Evaluation of Exercise Using Heart Rate: Assessment Corner

Type of Activity	Heart Rate
Low intensity	< 60% maximum heart rate*
Moderate intensity	< 60%–80% maximum heart rate
Vigorous activity	> 80% maximum heart rate

*Maximum heart rate is 220 minus age

of time involved in the activity. By increasing the frequency and duration of a low- to moderate-intensity activity, health benefits can be realized without risking injury. The duration of a single activity is far less important than the accumulation or volume of activities. Use this new information when working with clients to plan fitness activities; it will encourage those who resist to get involved in structured exercise plans.

continued for 4 to 6 weeks prior to increasing the exercise intensity and duration of time. Duration of the exercise activity can then be increased every 2 to 3 weeks until the client is able to exercise for 20 to 30 minutes continuously. By approximately 6 months clients should reach their exercise goals in terms of intensity and duration of activity and will be encouraged to maintain this level of activity.

MUSCULOSKELETAL FLEXIBILITY

Musculoskeletal function and flexibility is essential to maintain adequate balance, decrease the risk for chronic back pain, and improve overall function. There are basically three types of stretching activities (Box 11.5). Encourage clients to perform these stretching exercises in the warm-up and cool-down periods prior to and following their aerobic activity. Stretching should include all major muscle groups with a special focus on the lower back and thighs. Ask clients to stretch to the point of mild discomfort and hold the stretch for 10 to 30 seconds and repeat this three to five times. Stretching should be done at least three times per week.

RESISTIVE EXERCISE FOR MUSCULAR FITNESS

Resistance exercise is training with resistance to movement to increase muscle strength and is an important part of adult exercise programs. In addition to the development and maintenance of muscle strength and mass, resistance training will also increase bone mass, strengthen connective tissue, reduce body fat, improve glucose tolerance, and improve balance and performance of specific activities such as walking or climbing stairs (Morris et al., 1999). Muscular strength is best achieved by using weights that develop maximal or nearly maximal muscle tension with relatively few repetitions. Muscular endurance is built by using lighter weights with a greater number of repetitions. To have a combined effect, recommend that clients do 8 to 12 repetitions of an activity. You can alter the intensity of resistance training by varying the weight, the number of repetitions, the length of interval between exercises, and the number of sets (groups) of

exercises completed. Resistance training for the average adult should be rhythmical, should be performed at moderate-to-slow speeds, should involve a full range of motion, and should not interfere with breathing. Box 11.6 provides guidelines for resistance training in adults and a series of resistive exercises that cover all the major muscle groups.

RISKS THAT COMMONLY OCCUR DURING EXERCISE

Although the benefits of regular exercise clearly outweigh the risks, there are some common risks that can occur and that clients should be familiar with. Box 11.7 lists the signs and symptoms that clients should recognize as warning or danger signs. Tell clients to stop whatever exercise activity they are doing if these warning signs occur.

Cardiovascular Risks

Heart attacks and sudden cardiac death during exercise do occur, although it is very rare. Clients are at greatest risk for cardiovascular problems during exercise if they have been sedentary. To minimize this risk begin with low-intensity exercise and slowly build up. Pay attention to client complaints of chest pain, shortness of breath that does not go away in 30 minutes, leg pain, or dizziness when exercising, and warn them to stop the exercise activity they were doing when these symptoms occurred and to visit their primary health care provider for further evaluation.

Musculoskeletal Injuries

Musculoskeletal complaints and injuries commonly occur in adults who exercise. In

Box 11.5   Definition and Examples of Stretching Activities

Types of Stretching Activities

Static stretching: Slowly stretching a muscle to the point of mild discomfort and then holding that position for 10–30 seconds

Ballistic stretching: Repetitive bouncing movements to produce muscle stretch

Proprioceptive neuromuscular facilitation: A combination of alternating contraction and relaxation of both agonist and antagonist muscles

Warm-up/cool-down exercises that cover all major muscle groups (try to do these standing if you can, otherwise you may sit):

1. Deep breathing
    Raise your arms slowly above your head while taking a deep breath. Lower your arms slowly while exhaling. Repeat 3 times.
2. Shoulder rolls
    Roll your shoulders forward 5 times and backward 5 times.
3. Arm swings
    Swing your right arm forward in small circles 5 times and then backward 5 times. Do this with your right and then left arm.
4. Body side stretch
    Place your left hand on your hip and extend your right arm over your head with your palm down (or palm up for a challenge) and bend toward the left. Repeat 3 times. Repeat this on the opposite side by placing your right hand on your hip and extending your left arm over your head with your palm down and bending to the right.
5. Lower back stretch
    Sit up in a chair and tighten your stomach muscles while pushing your lower back into the chair. Hold this for 3 seconds. Repeat 3 times.
6. Ankle stretch
    While seated, lift your right leg straight in front of you about 2 inches off the floor. Point your toes to the ceiling and then to the floor. Repeat 5 times. Now rotate your foot clockwise 10 times and counterclockwise 10 times. Repeat the same exercise using your left leg.
7. Shoulder stretch
    While seated, lift your shoulders up and down slowly 10 times.
8. Chest stretch
    Stretch your arms out in front of you and cross them giving yourself a big hug. Reach for your shoulder blades and hold this for 3 seconds. Now uncross your arms and stretch those elbows out to the sides trying to jab someone with your elbows! Repeat 5 times.

Box 11.5　*(continued)*

9. Knee extension

   Sit with both feet on the floor. Raise your right leg 45 degrees (not quite as high as straight out in front of you). Keep your toes pointed to the ceiling. Repeat 10 times alternating the right and left leg.

10. Calf stretch

    Place your hands on the grab bar of the stairstep or against the wall. Put your right heel on the floor about 4 inches in front of your left foot and lean forward slightly so you feel a stretch in your left calf. Hold this for 3 seconds and repeat it 3 times. Now switch legs and lean forward on your left leg, stretching your right calf.

11. Leg stretch

    Standing up, hold the grab bar of your stairstep and bend forward slowly at the waist to no more than 90 degrees. Repeat 3 times.

Box 11.6　Guidelines for Resistance Training in Adults

- Include 8 to 10 different muscle groups
- Perform one set of 8 to 12 repetitions for each muscle
- Perform resistance exercise 2 days per week
- Move each muscle through a full range of motion
- Perform both the lifting (concentric phase) and lowering (eccentric phase) of the exercise slowly
- Breath normally during the exercises

Box 11.7　Warning Signs to Recognize During Exercise

- Pale, clammy, cool skin
- Change in cognition, confusion, or disorientation
- Nausea or vomiting
- Shortness of breath that does not resolve in 30 minutes
- Chest pain
- Dizziness
- Unusual fatigue
- A change in balance or unsteadiness

order to decrease the risk of injury, monitor your clients' frequency or duration of exercise. Initially they should exercise three times per week, and alternate high-intensity and low-intensity training sessions. If they are overweight or have arthritis they should stick to low-impact exercise such as cycling, swimming, or walking. Avoiding excessive fatigue and warming up and stretching prior to starting any type of exercise activity is an effective way to reduce the risk of injury. Remaining well hydrated during exercise also preserves muscle function, reducing the reliance on muscle glycogen as a fuel source. Carbohydrate ingestion also improves exercise performance, an effect that is independent of and additive to preventing dehydration. Encourage clients to replace any fluid lost during exercise. This is particularly important for older adults who may not feel thirsty.

Injuries Related to the Environment

The weather and condition of the environment can influence safety during exercise. Heat and heat stress are particularly dangerous. During exercise, large amounts of heat are generated by active muscles. When it is hot and humid outside the body is less able to dissipate the heat created by the muscles and that puts clients at risk for heat exhaustion. Heat exhaustion involves progressive weakness, fatigue, frontal headache, hypotension (a drop in blood pressure), tachycardia (increased heart rate to above 120 beats per minute), and can eventually cause a change in thinking and ability to stay awake. Provide information for clients about the dangers of exercising, including heat exhaustion. If they think they are experiencing heat exhaustion, tell them to immediately stop exercising and drink a lot of fluids, especially water. If un-

treated, heat exhaustion can progress to heatstroke. The classic findings in heatstroke include hypotension, tachycardia, vomiting, diarrhea, impaired thinking, and ultimately coma. If clients have heatstroke they will have a high core body temperature, and treatment will focus on lowering body temperature and on fluid replacement.

To prevent heat-related injuries, ask clients to wear loose clothing, to maintain adequate hydration before and after exercising, and to avoid scheduling exercise at the hottest time of the day. Preventing dehydration by encouraging adequate fluid replacement during exercise enables the cardiovascular system to maintain blood pressure and cardiac output, thereby sustaining the increase in skin blood flow and sweating that are essential for optimal temperature regulation. In addition to replacing fluids, it is important to replace essential vitamins and minerals that are lost in perspiration. Review chapter 10 which describes the foods that would be the best sources of vitamins and minerals.

FACTORS THAT INFLUENCE EXERCISE BEHAVIOR AND BARRIERS TO EXERCISE

There are a number of reasons that adults don't exercise regularly. These include time constraints, environmental barriers and lack of appropriate exercise facilities, unpleasant consequences from exercise, and a dislike of the activity or boredom. There are also some unique barriers to physical activity in older adults including: (a) a lack of knowledge about the benefits of exercise at an advanced age (Dishman, 1994); (b) impaired health (Blair et al., 1996); (c) lack of access to appropriate facilities (Boyette, Sharon, & Brandon,

1997; King et al., 1992); (d) fear of injury (Dishman, 1994); and (e) unpleasant sensations associated with exercise (Resnick, 1996; Resnick & Spellbring, in press). There are many steps you can take to increase the likelihood that clients will begin an exercise program and stick to it.

MOTIVATING YOUR CLIENTS TO EXERCISE: THE SEVEN-STEP APPROACH

Based on prior research, and using the theory of self-efficacy, a seven-step approach was developed and has been used as a safe and successful way to help adults initiate and adhere to regular exercise programs. The seven steps combine education, assessment, and motivational interventions all geared toward helping clients increase their beliefs about their ability to exercise and the positive benefits of exercise. Strengthening these beliefs motivates them to exercise regularly.

Step 1: Education

Provide clients with written information about the many benefits of exercise (see Table 11.3). Knowing as much as possible about exercising regularly for their physical as well as mental health is a wonderful way to help clients recognize the need to exercise initially and to keep them exercising. There may be classes in the community about exercise, or local health care providers may have information about this.

Step 2: Exercise Prescreening

From a motivational perspective, screening is important to help clients believe they will be able to succeed safely in an exercise program. Moreover, successfully "passing" a screening evaluation for exercise will give them the assurance that they are capable of exercising regularly, and it should lower the barrier that the fear of dying or experiencing a cardiac event during exercise can pose.

Step 3: Facing Barriers

There may be a number of reasons clients tell themselves they can't exercise: time, money, opportunities, fatigue, pain, or boredom. Ask clients to make a list of each of their excuses and go over them together, pointing out positive ways to overcome these barriers (see Box 11.8). For example, if the lack of time is an issue have the client keep a log of his or her activities during the week and see if there aren't small blocks of time in which walking could be inserted. If clients believe that pain prevents them from exercising, address this so that the pain can be managed and clients can exercise comfortably. If clients worry about falling or getting hurt during exercise, these issues should also be explored so that appropriate precautions can be taken. Moreover, with regard to pain and fear of falling, educate clients that exercise itself is the best way to reduce the pain of arthritis and osteoporosis and to decrease the risk of falling. Point these facts out to clients. You may have to say it more than once to be heard.

Step 4: Setting Goals

Setting short- and long-term goals related to exercise is a great way to motivate clients to exercise. Goals should be clear, specific, and attainable. The goal you set together should realistically fit into the client's daily schedule, it should be an enjoyable activity

TABLE 11.3   Exercise/Activity Resources

Resource	Contact Information	Cost
Fit Over 40	Advil Forum on Health Education 1500 Broadway New York, NY 10036	Free
Living with Exercise: Improving Your Health Through Moderate Physical Activity	The LEARN Education Center 1555 W. Mockingbird La., Ste. 203 Dallas, TX 75235	$18.50
American College of Sports Medicine Fitness Book	Human Kinetics Box 5076 Champaign, IL 61825-5076	11.96
Shape Up America	Shape Up America 6707 Democracy Blvd. Ste. 107 Bethesda, MD 20817	Free
The Walking and Jogging Kit	Health Promotion Resource Center 1000 Welch Rd. Palo Alto, CA 94304-1885	$2.75 each
Web page	American College of Sports Medicine *http://www.acsm.org/sportsmed*	Free

and one the client feels capable of doing (such as walking). Set goals that are moderately difficult. Relatively easy goals are not challenging enough to arouse much interest or effort, and goals set well beyond one's reach can be discouraging. Initially it is helpful to set a goal that focuses on the amount of time the individual is expected to participate in exercise, rather than the extent of exertion. This decreases the pressure to perform a more challenging task.

Examples of specific short-term goals are to walk three times a week for 20 minutes at one's own pace, to take the dog for three 10-minute walks daily, to park at the farthest parking space wherever you go, or to exercise at the gym or in a community exercise room three times per week for 20 to 30 minutes performing both resistive and aerobic exercise in divided time frames. Examples of long-term goals include: being able to walk faster, losing weight, walking farther

before becoming short of breath, walking without an assisting device, or going away on a vacation that requires a certain level of physical activity. Review client goals with them weekly so that the focus is on the wonderful reward of goal achievement, or revise the goal so that it is more appropriate.

Step 5: Exposure to Exercise

Getting out there and exercising is the best way to show clients they are capable of exercising and can do so safely. It may take repeated attempts to help them get started. Keep reviewing the benefits of exercising, go over the goals you have developed together and make sure the client really wants to achieve, and keep telling clients that they need to at least give it a try. Tell clients to give themselves a reward once the first

Box 11.8   Facing Your Barriers

Barrier	Suggested Ways to Overcome the Barrier
Not enough time	Incorporate activity into your daily life: park as far as possible from you destination; walk to work; walk up the stairs; skip a TV show and spend 20 minutes walking after work.
Exercise causes pain	Use appropriate pain-relieving medications such as Tylenol, or ice joints prior to exercise. Remember that exercise is the best way to decrease pain from osteoarthritis or osteoporosis.
Exercise is boring	Do an activity you enjoy. Listen to a book on tape, a radio, or music. Exercise with a friend and walk and talk.
Exercise is too tiring	Take a rest prior to exercising. Remember that exercise will actually increase your energy level.
I am afraid of falling.	Choose a safe, well-lit level area to walk and remember that exercise is the best way to strengthen muscles, improve balance, and reduce the risk of falling.
I am afraid of getting hurt.	Walking and swimming are very safe exercises that will not put stress on joints or muscles.
I am too old to exercise.	You will benefit from regular exercise no matter what age you are and can improve your strength, balance, and cardiovascular health, as well as overall mood and well being by exercising when you are older.
I am too fat to exercise.	Being overweight is a good reason to exercise. It is safe as long as you follow the right guidelines and begin with a low- to moderate-intensity activity such as walking.
There is no place to exercise.	Pick an activity you can do in a convenient place; walk outside if it is safe or in the hallways of an apartment building. Another option is to pick a stair and do some stair walking and stepping.
I don't see any reason to exercise; I don't want to live forever!	Exercise may not dramatically increase the length of your life but it will increase the quality by helping you stay as healthy and independent as possible.

exercise session is completed. This will build in success and help make exercise fun. That first session should be used to remind your client that he or she is quite capable of doing this every day.

Step 6: Provide Peer Support

Encourage clients to find an exercise partner; or, if they would rather exercise alone, help them identify a friend who is also interested in exercise. Ask clients to agree to do the following to provide their own peer support network: Make plans to meet with that partner regularly to exercise, or at least talk with them about whether they exercised that day or not. Be accountable to another person for their exercise. (It can help adherence to exercise.) Surround themselves with people who believe in exercise and in the benefits of exercising regularly. Notice other people who are exercising and recognize that these individuals face the same barriers to exercise that they do but are exercising anyway. Reinforce the notion that if others can exercise so can they!

Step 7: Rewards

Rewards are an important tool for motivating clients to exercise. The rewards they plan for themselves will vary according to their own interests. These rewards might simply be attaining the goals, getting an extra hour of sleep one morning, a special night out, or a new piece of jewelry. Other rewards may be the physical benefits of exercise such as a decrease in weight, blood pressure, and pulse. These rewards, whether external (such as buying some jewelry) or based on the benefits client's experience from regular exercise, will help them "keep up the good work."

CASE STUDY: WORKING WITH A CLIENT TO DEVELOP AND IMPLEMENT A FITNESS PROGRAM

Mrs. P, an 82-year-old white female, expressed concern to her nurse practitioner about a consistent weight gain over the past few years, 15 to 20 pounds despite no changes in her diet. She believed that she was actually eating fewer calories than when she was younger. Mrs. P had never exercised regularly, just "always kept busy" with her daily activities. She didn't see much need for more than that and had heard that some people actually died during exercise. Prior to developing an appropriate exercise program for Mrs. P, her geriatric nurse practitioner used the American College of Sports Medicine (1995) guidelines to establish Mrs. P's degree of risk with exercise (see Box 11.2).

With the exception of a history of cystic breasts and hypercholesteremia (elevated cholesterol), Mrs. P had no major health problems and was placed in a low-risk category. It was explained to her that there was no need for any further testing prior to starting an exercise program because she was low risk.

As Mrs. P was not particularly interested in exercising and didn't see the benefits of regular exercise activity, the first step in developing her exercise program was to educate her. This was done using a printed booklet that was developed by the nurse practitioner, which reviewed the physical and mental health benefits of exercise such as increased strength and balance, lowered cholesterol, improved blood pressure, and an overall sense of well-being. Mrs. P was reminded of her low-risk status relative to exercise and was assured that a life-threatening event during exercise was extremely unlikely.

She was asked to make a list of all the reasons she hadn't exercised previously and of the things that might stop her from exercising now. Her list included doubts about the benefits of exercise, and the fear of falling, getting hurt, or dying during exercise.

Mrs. P was assured that it was safe to exercise in the ways that were recommended to her and, even more important, that exercise was the best way to reduce her risk of falling, fracturing a bone, or dying from a cardiac event. In fact, not exercising increased her risk for all of these unpleasant possibilities.

Mrs. P was introduced to several other women her age who had successfully started exercise programs. These women further reinforced the health benefits of exercise for them—which for one included some weight loss and the ability to carry her groceries with less difficulty—as well as the positive psychological benefits of feeling better in general.

The exercise mode, intensity, duration, and frequency for Mrs. P were established. She was familiar and comfortable with walking and so was more willing to engage in this form of exercise. Ultimately, the goal was for her to walk at an intensity that would achieve her targeted heart rate (60% to 80% of her maximum heart rate). Initially, however, she would need to exercise at a lower intensity (less than 60% of her maximum heart rate). Her maximum heart rate was 138 (220 minus her age), and her targeted heart rate ranged from 83 to 110. Although the ultimate duration of exercise for Mrs. P was to reach 30 minutes daily, she was started at more reasonable length for her, which was 10 minutes daily. Goals were identified with Mrs. P based on these recommendations. Her short-term goal: To walk for 10 minutes daily so that her heart rate is around 83 beats per minute when she is walking. Her long-term goal: To maintain her weight or lose weight over the next 6 months.

Mrs. P received a calendar to record her exercise activity daily and was asked to come back to the office in 1 week to report on what she had done. Her nurse practitioner called to encourage Mrs. P and to be sure that she did begin her exercise program. Mrs. P was praised for her intentions and encouraged to adhere to their scheduled goal.

The following week Mrs. P came back to the office and brought her calendar showing that she had walked on 5 of 7 days for 10 minutes each day. She was praised for her work, and her short-term goal to walk daily for 10 minutes was reviewed. The positive benefits of exercise were discussed, and Mrs. P was asked to describe how she felt about her achievements. She was quite proud, feeling as if she had truly accomplished something, and actually found that the walk was easier each day. These benefits were reinforced and she was asked to return to the office in another week.

Mrs. P continued to adhere to the exercise plan as recommended and eventually increased her activity level to the recommended 30 minutes daily. She also achieved her long-term goal and was hoping to maintain or lose weight by incorporating exercise into her daily life.

SUMMARY

There is general consensus that adults can exercise safely and that regular exercise will improve physical fitness (Fiatarone et al., 1994; Green & Crouse, 1995; Pate, Pratt, & Blair, 1995; Bravo et al., 1996); prevent injury and disease (LaCroix et al., 1993; Province et al., 1995); and improve quality of life (King et al., 1997; Sharpe et al., 1997; Larson & Bruce, 1996). The seven steps outlined here provide a useful guide for helping clients implement an appropriate exercise program and helping them stick to this program once it is initiated.

REFERENCES

American College of Sports Medicine. (1995). *Guidelines for exercise testing and prescription* (5th ed.). Baltimore: Williams & Wilkins.

Blair, S., Horton, E., Leon, A., Lee, I., Drinkwater, B., Dishman, R., Mackey, M., & Kienholz, M. (1996). Physical activity, nutrition, and chronic disease. *Medicine and Science in Sports and Exercise, 28,* 335–349.

Boyette, L., Sharon, B., & Brandon, L. (1997). Exercise adherence for a strength training program in older adults. *The Journal of Nutrition, Health & Aging, 1,* 93–97.

Bravo, G., Gauthier, P., Roy, P., Payette, H., Gaulin, P., Harvey, M., Peloquin, L., & Dubois, M. (1996). Impact of a 12-month exercise program on the physic and psychological health of osteopenic women. *Journal of the American Geriatrics Society, 44,* 756–762.

Borg, G. (1982). Psychosocial bases of perceived exertion. *Medicine Science Sports and Exercise, 472,* 194–381.

Chaouloft, F. (1997). Effects of acute physical exercise on central serotonergic systems. *Medicine and Science in Sports and Exercise, 29,* 58–62.

De Vito, G., Hernandez, R., Gonzalez, V., Felici, F., & Figura, F. (1994). Low-intensity physical training in older subjects. *The Journal of Sports Medicine and Physical Fitness, 37,* 72–77.

Dishman, R. (1994). Motivating older adults to exercise. *Southern Medical Journal, 87,* s79–s82.

Fiatarone, M., O'Neill, E., Ryan, N., Clements, K., Solares, G., Nelson, M., Roberts, S., Kehayias, J., Lipsitz, L., & Evans, W. (1994). Exercise training and nutritional supplementation for physical frailty in very elderly people. *The New England Journal of Medicine, 330,* 1769–1775.

Green, J., & Crouse, S. (1995). The effects of endurance training on functional capacity in the elderly: A meta-analyses. *Medicine and Science in Sports and Exercise, 27,* 920–926.

King, A., Blair, S., Bild, D., Dishman, R., Dubbert, P., Marcus, B., Oldridge, N., Paffenbarger, R., Powell, K., & Yeager, K. (1992). Determinants of physical activity and interventions in adults. *Medicine and Science in Sports and Exercise, 24,* 3221–s223.

King, A., Oman, R., Brassington, G., Bliwise, D., & Haskell, W. (1997). Moderate-intensity exercise and self-rated quality of sleep in older adults. *Journal of the American Medical Association, 277,* 32–37.

LaCroix, A., Guralnik, J., Berkman, L., Wallace, R., & Satterfield, S. (1993). Maintaining mobility in late life. *American Journal of Epidemiology, 137,* 858–868.

Larson, E., & Bruce, R. (1996). Exercise. In C. Cassell et al. (Eds.), *Geriatric medicine* (pp. 815–832). Springer: New York.

National Institutes of Health Consensus Development Conference Statement. (1995). *Physical Activity and Cardiovascular Health.* December 18–20, pp. 1–20.

Pate, R., Pratt, M., & Blair, S. (1995). Physical activity and public health: A recommendation from the centers for disease control and prevention and the American college of sports medicine. *Journal of the American Medical Association, 273,* 402–407.

Province, M., Hadley, E., Hornbrook, M., Lipsitz, L., Miller, J., Mulrow, C., Ory, M., Sattin, R., Tinetti, M., & Wolf, S. (1995). The effects of exercise on falls in elderly patients. *Journal of the American Medical Association, 273,* 1341–1347.

Resnick, B. (1996). Motivation in geriatric rehabilitation. *Image, 28,* 41–47.

Resnick, B., & Spellbring, A. (in press). Who wants to live to be 100? Understanding what motivates older adults to exercise. *Journal of Gerontological Nursing.*

Sharpe, P., Jackson, K., White, C., Vaca, V., Hickey, T., Gu, J., & Otterness, C. (1997). Effects of a one-year physical activity intervention for older adults at congregate nutrition sites. *The Gerontologist, 37,* 208–215.

Thomas, S., Reading, J., & Shephard, R. (1992). Revision of the physical activity readiness questionnaire (PAR-Q). *Canadian Journal of Sport Science, 17,* 338–345.

CHAPTER 12

Typical Childhood Communicable Diseases: Promoting Community Resiliency

Margo A. Drohan

In addition to a detailed section on the epidemiology of typical childhood communicable diseases, this chapter examines the following:

1. communicable-disease prevention from the broader perspective of an ecological health paradigm, allowing a view of communicable diseases in the physical world as well as in the psychosocial and spiritual developing world of the individual in relationship to the community;

2. the development of immunization policies from consumer and community health practitioner perspectives and the development of informed consent and legislative efforts to tackle both the needs of the community and the needs of the individual;

3. the public's growing concern about holistic-wellness perspectives and interventions to promote health and resiliency;

4. a philosophical explanatory model for why some families choose not to immunize their children;

5. the ethical issues raised by this practice for the community health practitioner;

6. specific interventions to promote respiratory resiliency with an emphasis on children.

The communicable diseases discussed in detail in this chapter are limited to typical childhood illnesses: measles, mumps, rubella, varicella (chicken pox), and pertussis, which are likely to be seen in your community in both child and adult populations despite immunization rates being at an all-time high. Although each of these diseases and their treatments are separate entities, they do have "group" characteristics that allow them to be discussed together.

Effective health teaching is still the most significant intervention you can contribute to communicable-disease prevention. You can empower families and communities to make informed decisions and support options for self care as an integrative approach to communicable-disease prevention.

EPIDEMIOLOGY, SYMPTOMS, AND COMPLICATIONS OF CHILDHOOD COMMUNICABLE DISEASES

A *communicable disease* occurs when an infectious agent is transmitted from one person to another by direct transmission or by indirect transmission through interaction with a contaminated object that causes an illness or disease. Typical childhood communicable diseases such as measles, mumps, rubella, varicella (chicken pox), and pertussis (whooping cough) are spread via the respiratory tract, cause a fever, skin eruption, or respiratory symptoms and are highly contagious. Children are the primary reservoir for these illnesses. They often have devastating results when adults get them. It is necessary for you to be aware of the common signs and symptoms of these illnesses for prompt referral and early treatment, including reporting the disease to the appropriate public health department to contribute to surveillance and data analysis.

Box 12.1 briefly outlines the epidemiology of these common childhood communicable diseases. It is only an overview meant to illustrate that each illness has its own distinctive pathogenic epidemiology. For more detailed information, please consult the references at the end of Box 12.1, your local or state department of health, or the Centers for Diseases Control in Atlanta, Georgia.

Epidemiology

The *epidemiology of a disease* is the description of the sum of knowledge gained in the study and science concerned with the factors that determine and influence the frequency and distribution of the disease and its causes in a defined human population for the purpose of establishing pro-grams to prevent and control its development and spread. Epidemiology is based on the pathogenic paradigm that includes the transmission, or how the germ, virus, or causative agent is spread; the incubation period, which is how long it takes to develop symptoms of the diseases from the time one was first exposed; the infectious period, which describes the time that a person with the illness can spread it to others; and the immunity status conferred for that disease, which is the protection against getting that disease.

Symptoms

The symptoms of a communicable disease are those that are evidenced by the person during the disease process. There are subjective symptoms—what the person may perceive to be happening—such as fatigue or dizziness, and there are objective signs such as a clearly defined rash, fever, or respiratory congestion. Observations about the illness process have identified standard symptoms for each communicable disease for diagnostic purposes. It is possible to contract the illness even after being immunized. Symptoms are generally less severe and may be different from the standard identified symptoms, making the diagnosis more difficult.

Complications from Communicable Diseases

The most serious complications from communicable disease include pneumonia, which is the most common cause of death from measles and pertusis, and encephalitis, an inflammation of the brain that can lead to permanent brain damage or death from chicken pox, mumps, or measles. Well children rarely experience devastating ill-

Box 12.1   Sample Epidemiology of Communicable Diseases*

Measles (rubeola, paramyxovirus, "hard" measles, "regular" measles)
Transmission: contact, air
Incubation period: 8–12 days
Infectious period: From 7 days after exposure until 5 days after rash appears
Immunity: Lifelong immunity at this time is thought to be conferred after completion
  of two doses, begun at 12 months and completed by school-age. Given with mumps
  and rubella vaccine (MMR). Permanent immunity conferred from having the
  disease
Symptoms: Begins with fever and cold symptoms, conjunctivitis, nasal congestion,
  hacking cough. Koplik spots (white spots circumscribed in red in mouth). Fever
  increases to about 103° F. Acute phase begins with rash as fever fades. Dark red,
  dry, maculapapular rash usually begins behind hairline and spreads from head to
  feet. Lasts 10–15 days. Rash turns red and scaly after 5–6 days.
Complications: otitis media, pneumonia, encephalitis, appendicitis

Mumps (paramyxovirus, "parotitis")
Transmission: contact, air
Incubation period: 12–25 days
Infectious period: immediately before and after swelling occurs
Immunity: Considered lifelong immunity from clinical or subclinical infections; perma-
  nent immunity thought to be conferred with two doses (see measles)
Symptoms: May start with fever, muscular pain, headache, malaise. Active phase characterized by unilateral or bilateral parotid glands, and/or salivary glands. Two thirds
  of cases symptomatic, one third subclinical. Swelling peaks by 3rd day, returns to
  normal by 10th day. Chewing and sour liquids or hot foods aggravate the earlike pain
Complications: meningoencephalitis, orchitis, epididymitis, atrophy of affected testes,
  pancreatitis, nephritis, thyroiditis, myocarditis, mastitis, deafness, visual complications, arthritis

Rubella (rubella virus, "3-day measles," "German measles")
Transmission; air, transplacental (from mother to fetus)
Incubation period: 14–21 days
Infectious period: From up to 7 days before rash until rash disappears
Immunity: Permanent immunity from disease; permanent immunity thought to be
  conferred from two doses (see Measles)
Symptoms: In young children may start with lymphadenopathy; older children may
  start with low-grade fever, anorexia, mild conjunctivitis, runny nose, sore throat
Complications: Postinfectious encephalitis, arthritis, thrombocytopenia; virus crosses
  placenta, causing birth defects, such as deafness, visual anomalies, congenital heart
  defects, musculoskeletal defects, central nervous system defects, and immunological
  defects, especially if mother is exposed in first trimester

(continued)

Box 12.1   (continued)

Varicella (chicken pox, herpesvirus)
Transmission: contact, air
Incubation period: 10–21 days
Infectious period: From 1–2 days before lesions appear until all lesions are crusted, usually 5–6 days from onset
Immunity: Usually lifelong after illness, but second infections have been reported; vaccine now available for general use; passive immunity globulin within 3 days of exposure to children at high risk for serious complications.
Symptoms: Starts with low-grade fever, malaise, anorexia, sometimes scarlet unified rash; acute phase characterized by red maculapapular rash that turns to vesicles that ooze and crust; new crops continue to form for 3–5 days, spreading from the trunk to the extremities; disease course varies from mild with a few lesions to severe with several hundreds lesions and high fever.
Complications: Secondary skin infections, postinfectious encephalitis, aseptic meningitis, Reye's syndrome

Pertussis (bordetella pertussis, "whooping cough")
Transmission: contact, air; children under 5 are usually infected by adults
Incubation period: 5–35 days
Infectious period: Not exactly known; may extend 4 weeks past the coughing stage
Immunity: Newborns to 6 months have no immunity; immunity thought to be conferred by 4 or 5 doses, started at 2 months of age and completed by school age; immunity from immunization wanes in some people after 10 years of completing the series; permanent immunity conferred from having the disease
Symptoms: Starts with cold symptoms, irritating cough that lasts up to 2 weeks, followed by the paroxysmal cough; characterized by the "whooping" sound that lasts 4–6 weeks; patient often appears to be choking during the cough, followed by vomiting; the third stage may last 1–2 weeks, although the cough may linger for 3 months; this stage is characterized by less frequent coughing attacks, and appetite and strength return
Complications: pneumonia, atelectasis, otitis media, central nervous system dysfunction, hemorrhage, weight loss, dehydration, hernia, prolapsed rectum

*Data from: *Nelson Textbook of Pediatrics* (14th ed.), by R. E. Behrmann and C. Vaughan (Eds.), 1992, Philadelphia: W. B. Saunders. Adapted with permission. *Infectious Disease*, by A. Ball and J. Gray, 1993, Edinburgh, Scotland: Churchill Livingston. Reprinted with permission. *Report on the Committee on Infectious Diseases* (25th ed.), by American Academy of Pediatrics, 1994, Elk Grove, IL: American Academy of Pediatrics. Reprinted with permission. *Manual of Pediatric Therapeutics*, by J. Graef (Ed.), 1997, Philadelphia: Lippincott-Raven. Reprinted with permission. *Primary Health Care of Children*, by J. Fox, 1997, St. Louis, MO: Mosby. Reprinted with permission.

ness or complications from these infections (Wong, 1995; Feroli, 1994). The groups recognized as highest risk for developing these complications are those with preexisting conditions, those who are immunocompromised, the very young who do not have fully developed immune systems, and the very old or those in debilitated states of health.

Spiritual Distress

In a holistic paradigm, debilitated states of health may be extended to include those experiencing spiritual distress. This describes an individual or a group that is experiencing a disturbance in a belief or value system that provides strength, hope, and meaning to their lives. Spiritual support has long been recognized as a source of energy that enables people to cope with stress and illness (Carpenito, 1993). Lack of spiritual strength can be described as a risk factor in contracting an illness, especially when considering respiratory mode of transmission in communicable diseases.

Spiritual distress in the community may be used to describe those who may be disenfranchised from their culture, family, religious, or community ties. This may include those who are newly immigrated, homeless, runaways, or those who are institutionalized and separated from the groups that offer them strength. Physical or emotional exhaustion weakens the immune response on a cellular level and places one at risk for despair and hopelessness, which is a characteristic of spiritual distress. Community interventions that strengthen ties and collective spirituality provide another source of interventions for you to consider.

Immunity

Immunity is the protection against a specific infectious disease conferred by the immune response generated either by immunizations, previous infection, or other nonimmunological factors. Immunity is not necessarily a long-lasting phenomenon and is a significant limitation of the pathogenic paradigm. The only permanent immunity is natural active immunity, achieved by having had the disease. This does not occur in all types of communicable diseases. Of the group of diseases discussed here, it is only true for rubella and pertussis.

Maternal antibodies for pertussis do not cross the placenta so newborns do not receive their mothers' immunity for pertussis through natural passive immunity as they do for measles. There is also no test or titer that can measure the immune status of an individual against pertussis as there is with other communicable diseases such as rubella. Immune status is conferred against pertussis upon completion of the currently recommended series of dosages.

From studying the outbreaks of pertussis in communities, it has become evident that immunity wanes after about 10 years of completing the series (Larson, 1994). Looking at the immune status of pertussis in the community indicates that infants under 6 months, children under 4, and adolescents are at highest risk for contracting pertussis in immunized populations. Permanent immunity is only achieved by actively having pertussis.

THE DEVELOPMENT OF IMMUNIZATION POLICY

Initial immunization public health policy followed the principles of "herd immunity." The use of the term is probably related to the origins of the word vaccine, which is from *vacca*, Latin for cow. The first vaccination in 1796 was for smallpox, and it was made from cowpox sores. Underlying the policy of herd immunity is the belief that the greater good is to provide immunity for all community members through vaccinations. Side effects were believed to be such a rare occurrence that the community was willing to take the individual risk for the overall good. However, national reporting of side effects or adverse events was not mandated to be recorded in this country until 1986 so there was really no way of knowing what the incidence of side effects were.

The National Childhood Vaccine Injury Act of 1986

In 1962, the Centers for Disease Control and Prevention (CDC) began keeping immunization records as with any other pharmacological agent, and statistical data on side effects and risks began to emerge. The term benefit-to-risk began being applied to immunization policy, the result of statistical data that weighed the risks of an individual's getting the disease against the possibility of being permanently harmed from the immunization itself and under what circumstances it might likely occur. After several successful and costly personal lawsuits against providers and manufacturers of immunizations for harm incurred as a result of some immunization, the National Childhood Vaccine Injury Act was passed in 1988. Its purpose was to reduce the associated costs of litigation and malpractice insurance related to the administration of immunizations, to develop a data collection system, and to provide standardized information about vaccines to the public.

For additional information about the current standards and guidelines for immunizations in your state, contact the Office of Health and Human Services through your

state board of health. Information is also available for downloading from the Internet, and providers are required to utilize this source for updated information.

True Contraindications and Precautions

In the past providers based immunization on their own assessments. For example, if a child had a fever the provider may have withheld the immunization; or if a child had a severe reaction to one vaccine, the provider may have broken dosages in half to minimize the severity of future reactions. Review of the data by the CDC and other agencies involved with setting guidelines indicates that these are not effective practices. Withholding the immunization because of a low-grade fever is not contraindicated and leads to parents not returning their children in the future just for an immunization, resulting in a higher risk of not completing the series. Divided dosages lessen the chance of immunity being conferred. As more data became available for analysis, the CDC developed the *Guide to Contraindications to Childhood Vaccinations*, which medical practitioners are legally bound to use in determining whether a vaccine should be given, based on the benefit-to-risk data (see Table 12.1, Sample True Contraindications). The CDC periodically updates these immunization guidelines to indicate when the risk to the individual's health is greater than that to the community and to designate those for whom immunizations are not appropriate, according to current available data analysis.

Vaccines Can Cause Injury

Because vaccination can result in damage to those immunized, the Federal Vaccine

TABLE 12.1 Sample True Contraindications and Precautions*

Vaccine	True Contraindications and Precautions
Measles, mumps, rubella (e.g., MMR, MR, M, R)	anaphylactic reaction to eggs, neomycin, gelatin, pregnancy or possible pregnancy in 3 months; known altered immunodeficiency; encephalopathy within 7 days of previous dose; history of thrombocytopenic purpura
Varicella (chicken pox)	HIV or immunodeficiency in recipient; unknown immune status of household members; anaphylaxis to gelatin
Vaccines containing pertussis (e.g., DTaP, DTP, P, DTP-Hib)	anaphylaxis within 4 hours of administration of previous dose encephalopathy within 7 days of previous dose; fever above 105° F within 48 hours of previous dose; collapse into shocklike state within 48 hours of previous dose; seizure within 3 days of previous dose; persistent inconsolable crying within 48 hours of previous dose; Guillian-Barré syndrome within 6 weeks of previous dose; underlying neurological disorder

Note: *This sample is not inclusive of all contraindications. Providers should consult current resources for updated information. Table adapted from the *Guide to Contraindications to Childhood Vaccines*, 1998, U.S. Department of Health and Human Services.

Injury Compensation Program (VICP) was established. This program streamlined injury claims so parents did not have to prove the vaccine caused the injury through litigation if it occurred within a specific time frame and was a recognized event. Providers and immunization manufacturers were no longer accountable for injuries that occurred as a result of an immunization when policies were followed. The federal government accepts a "presumption of causation" and awards monetary compensation to the family based on the degree of damage. By 1996, more than $755 million has been paid out in more than 2,300 cases (The Berkshire Eagle, 1997).

The data from these events and other side effects noted by the provider are supplied to the Centers for Disease Control for inclusion in "Epidemiological Studies and Surveillance of Disease Problems." While this surveillance data is needed to identify who is at risk and for what, and statistically

at what rate events and side effects occur, some studies have indicated a provider noncompliance rate in reporting mandated events as high as 89% (Larson, 1994).

Standardized Benefit-Risk Statements: Vaccine Information Sheets (VIS)

Since 1996, providers who administer immunizations are required to use standardized information forms called vaccine information sheets (VIS) developed by the American Academy of Pediatrics and distributed by the Centers for Diseases Control. These are periodically updated and available from the CDC on the Internet. They include information on what true contraindications are, possible side effects such as temperature and irritability, and what to do for each vaccine if an adverse event occurs. It lists Web sites where additional and updated information can be obtained. Providers are required to use the most recent statements issued.

The signature of the parent or guardian on the pediatric immunization record implies informed consent, that they agree to treatment for their child, and that they have been educated about that particular vaccine and understand the ramifications of their agreement. However, parents do not have the right to refuse an immunization for their child although some states do accept refusal based on religious grounds. The vaccine information sheet also legally dictates what the provider must say about a particular vaccine based on information released from the Advisory Committee on Immunization Practices (ACIP), whose members include the CDC, the American Academy of Pediatrics, and the American Academy of Family Physicians.

Provider Accountability

Once unheard of, an out-of-court settlement for $650,000 against an individual provider has brought home the reality of provider accountability. This provider did not discuss all the known risks of serious side effects of live oral polio vaccine (OPV) listed on the VIS. The vaccination resulted in the child's father contracting polio, a rare but known documented risk (Starr, 2000). As of January 2000, OPV is no longer recommended by ACIP for general use because of this very serious side effect. A different form of the vaccine, IPV (inactivated polio vaccine), has been shown in numerous studies to be just as effective as OPV but to have 50% fewer serious receptions and is now recommended for use (Contemporary Pediatrics, 2000).

Provider accountability also includes full documentation in the medical record of an appropriate immunization history and

physical: previous adverse reactions, existing conditions, food and drug allergies, immunization status of family and household contacts, use of chemotherapy and blood products, pregnancy and anticipated pregnancy, and a written summary of questions asked and answered.

The development of an immunizations policy in recent years does not minimize their importance as a proven means to protect the public from the morbidity and mortality of communicable diseases. It does demonstrate that there are acknowledged risks to individuals and a growing recognition that community well-being may not be best served by mandated routine immunizations, as had been previously thought. Currently, medical contraindications are the only acceptable reason in most communities for not immunizing.

ECOLOGICAL HEALTH PARADIGM FOR COMMUNICABLE-DISEASE PREVENTION

An ecological health paradigm offers a view of communicable diseases that is comprehensive and holistic in scope. It extends the environmental realm beyond the agent-disease relationship. The root of the word ecology comes from the Greek *oikos*, which means household. All household members in their various stages of development continuously interact and form a co-creative whole. This is especially true in the relationship to communicable diseases, how we resist it, how we get it, how we respond to the infectious process, how we treat it, how we do or do not develop complications, and how what we do as individuals affects the household at large and its future development. It connects the individual's health status to that of the community as a co-created environment.

Holistic and wellness interventions avoid focusing on risks and disease and focus on client strengths, resilience, and the healing process. While complementary therapies can promote resiliency and improve the total health of the community, they do not replace the role of immunizations in community health. The process of healing as the body forms antibodies to develop immunity after an immunization includes balancing and integrating the physical, emotional, and spiritual aspects of oneself to achieve high level wellness just as when a body may be infected with a disease. An ecological health paradigm places this within the context of the whole household maintaining homeostasis and balance while trying to achieve a collective higher level of wellness.

A Holistic View of Immunization

An ecological paradigm offers a view of the physical, psychosocial, emotional, and spiritual components of health in time and the individual in relationship to the whole. Some may not feel that immunization as the primary preventive of communicable disease is the "right" choice to promote harmony and balance in the functioning of the whole.

What is important for you to understand as a community health practitioner is that some parents chose not to immunize their children, not because they are ignorant of the risks from communicable diseases, nor because they have just not gotten around to it. Their beliefs in the ecological balance in the physical world or religious reasons about the balance in the spiritual world may prevent their interfering with "God's will." Also, as previously stated, some states allow parents to refuse immunizations for their children based on religious beliefs.

Some parents may decide the merits and risks of each immunization on an individual basis and believe that the risk from the specific disease does not justify the risk from the specific immunization for their child or for their community. Additionally, some parents and community members may know and question you about the long-term side effect of neurological damage from immunizations that has been suggested by research completed outside this country. These considerations are not recognized or dealt with in our public health laws or immunization policies. The National Institute of Medicine (IOM), which authorizes our immunization policy, does not recognize damage that occurs beyond 7 days of administrating the immunization because the relationship of immunizations to neurological injury is not clearly understood (Larson, 1994). It is beyond the scope of this chapter to present or critique this research or the IOM's position. There is, however, recent recognition by the members of the IOM—The American Academy of Pediatrics, the Advisory Committee on Immunization Practices, and the U.S. Public Health Service—of a possible link between thimerosal, a preservative used in some vaccines that contains mercury (thimerosal has never been used in measles, mumps, or IPV vaccines) and neurological, developmental, or renal disorders. As a result, drug manufacturers are eliminating or reducing thimerosal content in their products (Clinician Reviews, 2000).

Immunization: Ethical Considerations

The issue of the community perspective versus the individual perspective may create an ethical dilemma for you as a community health practitioner. Many may argue that this is all just ignorance, considering the contributions immunizations have made to improving community health, while others may argue that this is informed consent. Some may argue that the community's right to health protection takes precedence over the individual's right. Communities have the right to take parents to court to obtain guardianship *ad lite*, wherein the community grants itself guardianship of the child. It may then authorize the immunization over the will of the parent if the court orders it, just as communities may do when a parent withholds perceived necessary medical treatment for a child.

All communities have public health laws that refuse a child's admittance to school without immunization, unless the school superintendent recognizes exception for religious reasons. Parents may opt for home schooling if they are denied this. However, no child is denied admittance to school if they are not immunized for medical reasons.

Community members may question you if another parent chooses not to have a child immunized and then the child contracts measles and infects an entire school. In answer to the question, "How is the overall quality of the community affected by these issues?", your responsibility is to be aware of the ethical issues and to address them as knowledgeably and objectively as possible. Community health practitioners need to examine their own thoughts and actions on these issues. The following are some perspectives to consider:

Whether for medical or religious reasons, the issue of the unimmunized child's spreading the disease in a community becomes less evident when the epidemiology of the illness and the immunization process is reviewed. The unimmunized child is at greater risk of contracting than of spreading a communicable disease in an immunized population. The source of infection is frequently from a recently immunized child or an immunized child who has a subclinical case of the disease. The child who has received an immunization against rubella can actively spread that disease for approximately 2 weeks. An immunized population assumes that they will not contract rubella because of the immunization. It is known that the immunization does not necessarily confer immunity and that subclinical cases may emerge—that is, the symptoms may be milder and the illness may not be properly diagnosed, although it may still be spread. This is frequently used as an argument to encourage parents to immunize their child because not doing so increases the child's risk of contracting a more severe case of the disease. School policy is that if an outbreak occurs, parents are required to keep their child home until the disease subsides because of the increased risk to their child and the increased risk this child's spreading it.

The *Standards for Pediatric Immunization Practices* (U.S. Department of Health and Human Services, 1996), endorsed by more than 10 professional organizations, are recommended for use by all health professionals who are involved with immunizations, although the *Standards* recognize that not all providers are in compliance. The goal of these standards was to immunize 90% of all 2-year olds with mandated vaccines. As a community health provider, professional compliance and ethics are a consideration. Some primary care providers such as physicians and nurse practitioners have the professional and legal right to deny a client services because of unresolvable differences in treatment opinions, as when the provider recommends immunizations and the client refuses to so. Although this practice is declining, it leaves the emergency room or practitioners outside the traditional medical community to provide care for these families.

The practice of excluding families who do not immunize their children from primary care potentially excludes large populations and leaves them and the community at higher risk for complications not only from communicable but from other diseases as well. For example, consider the risk of complications for a child with diabetes in a medically unattended ketoacidosis versus the risk to the community from rubella. Does the parents' refusal to immunize justify refusal of the benefits of primary health care services?

These are issues that need to be addressed openly, recognizing that it is not only the child whose parent opted against immunizations, but also the immunized child and adult, the medically contraindicated nonimmunized child, and the medically frail, immunized or not, who are all potential reservoirs. So why immunize at all?

The data speaks for itself in support of immunizations as a successful means to decrease the morbidity and mortality from communicable diseases. What it cannot do is speak to the individual with confidence. Statistics do not mean very much if your child develops a permanent disability or dies as a result of a communicable disease or as a result of an immunization. The possibilities of either event need to be explored fully. This is the difference in the immunization policies that have developed over the last 10 years. In the past, parents blindly took their children to the clinic for immunizations, and community health practitioners believed that immunizations would stop the spread of communicable diseases permanently without significant risk to the individual. Neither of these approaches have worked very well for the individual. The strongest limitation of the pathogenic paradigm is that it does not leave many options for individualism, self-determination, or self care.

HOLISTIC WELLNESS MEASURES FOR COMMUNICABLE DISEASE PREVENTION

Whether a child is immunized or not, holistic wellness interventions can serve as an adjunctive protection against the morbidity and mortality of communicable diseases. Practicing a healthy lifestyle increases resistance to all illnesses and one's ability to recover more effectively if an illness does occur. The choice of a combination of arts is an individualized one, which generally includes nutrition or the use of herbs, body work or massage, psychosynthesis techniques, and a form of meditation.

Promoting Resiliency

In communicable diseases when the means of transmission is within communities from person to person via air transmission (the respiratory system), the significance of putting an ecological health paradigm into operation to look for household remedies is of paramount significance. Proper handwashing is still the most effective barrier to the transmission of diseases. Children can be taught quite young the importance of handwashing, especially after touching other people or other people's belongings.

Exposure to environmental pollutants in the home due to modern building techniques (as opposed to poor sanitary conditions) continues to contribute to respiratory vulnerability. Promoting resiliency in children and adults can serve as guide to interventions for you to choose in order to support community wellness, decrease communicable diseases transmission, and minimize its consequences.

Children are not mini-adults. They require careful consideration of their physical, emotional, and spiritual development when adults intervene. Promote resiliency in children by supporting their autonomy and their integration into the community by advocating for a healthy environment at all times. Choose your interventions well, not only in the context of what is best for the developing child, but also in the context of what will be best for the health of the community at large, now and in the future. In terms of communicable disease prevention, the question to ask yourself is: What will yield the greatest good for the child within the context of the future health of the community?

Promoting Respiratory Resilience

A healthy lifestyle, regular exercise, and healthy breathing promote respiratory resiliency. For healthy children who naturally breathe correctly, this means providing an environment that is oxygen-rich and as user-friendly as possible. Irritants such as smoke, chemicals, dryness, or high humidity should be avoided. Cigarette smoke, harsh cleaning agents, odors, and dry heat are common irritants.

Household mold, dust mites, cockroaches, animal dander, and endotoxins created by man-made materials can contribute to respiratory problems. Good household hygiene, limited use of carpeting, adequate natural air, light, and living space for each member can eliminate some problems. Reducing household humidity to less than 50%, encasing bedding in impermeable covers, and using vacuum cleaners in good working order can reduce mold and mite allergens in the home (Codina & Lockey, 2000). An environment that is supplemented with plants will help supply oxygen in crowded situations. Open windows in good weather, exposure to fresh air, and proper breathing techniques will promote respiratory resilience.

In children with respiratory weakness such as asthma, or adults who have weaknesses from chronic diseases or from sedentary lifestyles, breathing exercises are extremely effective. Breathing patterns often reflect the harmony or disharmony we are experiencing in life. The goal of respiratory exercise is to develop a relaxed, fully functional balanced breath that can be accomplished by practicing a few minutes a few times a day. There are many recommendations available for breathing techniques, often as part of a meditative exercise program.

One method that can be used for adults and modified for children is based upon Michael Grant's *The Breath Wave and the Speed Bump of Life* (White, 1997), described in Box 12.2. It is a combination of imagery and breathing techniques that can be used to promote relaxation as well. The goal of this exercise is to promote deep, relaxed abdominal breathing at approximately 12 or fewer breaths per minute, with the abdomen and chest rising during inhalation, falling during expiration in a slightly faster and longer pattern, with a slight pause at the end of exhalation. The imagery of the rise and fall of waves mimics a healthy breathing pattern. Clients need to start at their own pace, in their own rhythm, discover their own "speed bumps" that impede natural, healthy breathing, and work toward overcoming them.

Another way to promote respiratory resiliency is through nutrition and the use of herbs. Ask clients to avoid foods that cause congestion or that they have allergies to. For some people these are milk and dairy products, red meats, and the gluten in wheat. Not all people react the same. What is a good nutritional tonic for one may be a pollutant for another. Ayurveda is a system of health, healing, and a philosophy of life. Health is thought to be obtained

---

Box 12.2   Breathing Exercise

1.   Have client lie down and close eyes for best results, although this exercise may be done sitting up with eyes opened.

2.   Ask the client to imagine that she is at the beach and to recall pleasant sensory memories they associate with being there: the sound of the waves, the feel of the air, the color of the sky, etc.

3.   Ask the client to breathe slowly and deeply, inhaling through the nose and exhaling through the mouth, focusing on the sound of the waves on the beach. Allow her a few moments to experience this. Observe the client's breathing pattern as she does this, and continue when it is rhythmic.

4.   Ask the client to observe the wave starting about 50 yards from the shore, as she inhales.

5.   Ask the client to imagine her chin as a raft that is gently raised as the water approaches the shore.

6.   Ask the client to exhale and imagine the water receding along the shore and to note that the expiration is slightly faster and longer in duration than inspiration.

7.   Ask the client to note the pause in sound between the end of one wave and the beginning of another, as she notes the pause in her own breathing pattern.

8.   Ask the client to note any impediments to her breathing patterns.

9.   Encourage the client to practice this exercise a few times a day for a few minutes.

---

through maintaining harmony and balance through diet, meditation, and lifestyle changes. Ayurveda may offer further insights into what may be appropriate for you or your clients (Credit, Hartunian, & Nowak, 1998).

Many different herbs are recommended for use as a respiratory tonic when a tendency toward an illness may be recognized but no overt disease is present. *Mullein Verbascum thapus* rates high because it can be safely used over long periods of time and has several medicinal properties that are effective for promoting respiratory resiliency. It is an expectorant, which helps loosen and thin secretions; a demulcent, which soothes and relieves inflamed membranes; a mild diuretic and a mild sedative. Mullein is offered as an example of a respiratory tonic to promote resiliency (Hoffman, 1996). If overt signs of an illness

are apparent, a health care practitioner should be consulted before beginning any treatment.

SUMMARY: EMPOWERING FAMILIES AND GROUPS THROUGH HEALTH TEACHING

Empowering families and groups through health teaching to prevent communicable diseases includes: being knowledgeable about the individual disease processes and their complications and about immunization benefit-to-risk factors; and being aware of and contributing to this body of knowledge. A holistic wellness approach acknowledges your clients' ability to make informed health decisions that are right for them, even if they are different from your own, and offers adjunctive interventions, including ones to strengthen community ties and collective spirituality that promote resiliency.

By law, parents may be limited in what decisions they may make for their children. Informed consent is a right for adults *only*. There are many who believe that when clients and practitioners are in harmony, though not necessarily in agreement, there is less of a risk of serious complications. Whether that be a parent's truly informed consent to immunize their child or the parent's informed denial, or if the immunization is contraindicated for that child, the parent's right to advocate for what they believe to be best for their child can be supported. When communicable disease outbreaks occur, they offer an opportunity to teach lay members and refresh medical members about what is currently known, and as a community to collectively ask, What interventions will lead to the greater good for this child and for the community?

REFERENCES

American Academy of Pediatrics. (1994). *Report of the committee on infectious diseases* (The Redbook 25th ed.). Elk Grove, IL: American Academy of Pediatrics.

Ball, A., & Gray, J. (1993). *Color guide: Infectious diseases.* Edinburgh, Scotland: Churchill Livingston.

Behrman, R. E., & Vaughan, C. (Eds.). (1992). *Nelson's textbook of pediatrics* (14th ed.). Philadelphia: W. B. Saunders.

Berkshire Eagle. (1997). *Parents want more say in vaccinations.* April 12, A5.

Carpenito, L. (1993). *Nursing diagnosis: Application to clinical practice* (pp. 746–748). Philadelphia: J. B. Lippincott.

Clinician Reviews. (2000). Thimerosal-free vaccines: A progress report. *Clinician Reviews, 10*(8), 95–96.

Codina, R., & Lockey, R. (2000). Environmental asthma: Nine questions physicians often ask. *Consultants in Primary Care, 40*(1), 66–70.

Credit, L., Hartunian, S., & Nowak, M. (1998). *Your guide to complementary medicine.* Garden City Park, NY: Avery.

Feroli, K. L. (1994). Infectious disease. In C. L. Betz, M. M. Hunsberger, & S. Wright (Eds.), *Family-centered nursing care of children* (2nd ed., pp. 1678–1684). Philadelphia, PA: W. B. Saunders.

Fox, J. (1997). *Primary health care of children.* St. Louis, MO: Mosby.

Graef, J. (Ed.). (1997). *Manual of pediatric therapeutics* (4th ed.). Philadelphia: Lippincott-Raven.

Haupt, L. (1996). An ecology of the body. *Massage, 60,* 42–46.

Hoffman, D. (1996). *The new holistic herbal.* Rockport, MA: Element Books.

Larson, L. (1994). Report: Vaccine might trigger reactions. *American Academy of Pediatrics News, 10,* 1, 16.

Livingston, R., Adam, B., & Bracha, S. (1994). Season of birth and neuro developmental disorders: Summer birth is associated with dyslexia. *Pediatrics, 94*(2), 212.

Special Report: What's new in the 2000 immunization schedule. *Contemporary Pediatrics, 17*(1), 32–34.

Starr, D. (2000). The smallest details. *The Clinical Advisor, 3*(1), 88–89.

U.S. Department of Health and Human Services. (1996). *Standards for pediatric immunization practices* (7th printing). Atlanta, GA: Centers for Disease Control and Prevention.

U.S. Department of Health and Human Services. (1998). *Guide to contraindications to childhood vaccinations.* Atlanta, GA: Centers for Disease Control and Prevention.

White, M. G. (1997). The breath wave and the speed bump of life. *Massage Magazine,* 83–87.

Wong, D. L. (1995). Health problems of early childhood. In *Whaley and Wong's nursing care of infants and children* (5th ed., pp. 677–682). St. Louis, MO: Mosby.

CHAPTER 13

Stress Management

Carolyn Chambers Clark

STRESS: PHYSIOLOGICAL AND IMMUNE SYSTEM EFFECTS

Stress can be experienced as a result of the interactions of one or more of the wellness dimensions. For example, it is possible to experience stress due to under- or overnutrition, negative interpersonal relationships or nagging thoughts about others or situations, insufficient exercise or ineffective body movement, negative environmental factors or conflicting values or beliefs.

In 1914 Cannon described the *fight or flight response* or "emergency reaction" that prepares the individual to fight or run. Physiological changes include: increase in blood pressure, heart rate, respiration, metabolism, epinephrine, blood glucose, peripheral vascular constriction, dilation of the pupils, and decreased testosterone levels (Benson & Klipper, 1976; Cannon, 1914; Selye, 1956). If stress is chronic, the immune system weakens, lowering resistance to disease (Zeagans, 1982). With chronic stress, temporary conditions can become permanent, turning transient high blood pressure into hypertension, stomach upset into colitis or ulcers, and so forth. Stress has been related to many diseases

and ailments including headaches, peptic ulcers, arthritis, colitis, diarrhea, asthma, cardiac arrhythmias, sexual problems, circulatory problems, muscle tension, and cancer (Davis, McKay, & Eshelman, 1995, p. 6).

A large body of literature has evolved documenting the relationship between stress and illness (Halley, 1991). Evidence points toward stress-induced immunosuppression (Ben-Eliyahu, 1991) though bidirectional effects may be more likely. Knowledge of the relationship between body and mind is rapidly expanding, having spawned the new discipline *psychoneuroimmunology*. Research suggests that measurable immune system parameters can be influenced by relaxation and imagery techniques, biofeedback, assisted strategies, the use of humor, social support, journalling, therapeutic touch, hypnosis, and conditioning (Kiecolt-Glaser et al., 1986; Acterberg & Rider, 1989; Basmajian, 1989; Houldin, McCorkle, & Lowery, 1993; Levy et al., 1990; Post-White & Johnson, 1991; Quinn & Strelkaukas, 1993).

ASSESSING STRESS SYMPTOMS

It is not possible or even wise to turn off innate fight or flight responses to threats.

Adapted from *Wellness Practitioner: Concepts, Research and Strategies*, by C. C. Clark (1996), NY: Springer.

It is possible and wise to learn to interpret and label experiences differently, thereby lessening negative stressor impact.

The first step in reducing stress is to assess the major sources of stress. The Holmes "Schedule of Recent Experience" was developed by Thomas Holmes at the University of Washington School of Medicine in Seattle, Washington. It gives a value for each life event (such as divorce, change in financial state, sexual difficulties, death of a spouse, vacation, etc.) and allows the respondent to obtain a total score. The assumption is that the more change an individual has to adjust to, the more likely he or she is to get sick. Holmes found that 80% of the persons he studied who had a score over 300 were apt to get sick in the near future.

A major controversy about the Holmes scale concerns the idea that some changes are not stressful and may even be pleasant. For example, although Holmes claims that a job change is stressful, it may be less stressful to take a new job in pleasanter surroundings than it is to stay in a job that is dead-end, draining, and results in ongoing resentment. Table 13.1 presents information for assessing and reducing stressful life changes.

Symptom relief can be a powerful motivator for clients to begin stress management procedures. Table 13.2 offers a Stress Symptom Assessment.

Physical symptoms may have physiological sources, so it is unwise to proceed on the assumption that all symptoms are completely stress-related. Stress management procedures are generally of two types: those that focus on relaxing the body and those that focus on handling stress differently. Often it is useful to use at least one approach from each broad category. For example, breathing exercises and progressive relaxation may be used to calm the body and refuting irrational ideas may be used to reduce perspectives on events that increase stress (Davis, McKay, & Eshelman, 1995).

It is useful to keep a *Stress Awareness Diary* to make note of times that a stressful event occurs and the time a physical or emotional symptom could be related to stress. In time, it is possible to recognize where the body scores muscular tension. With increased awareness, specific procedures for releasing tension in those areas can he practiced. Keeping a record of progress will assist in the change process because it reinforces success and points out what needs further focus.

STRESS MANAGEMENT INTERVENTIONS

Breathing

Breathing is essential for life, yet many breathe in the upper part of the chest, not allowing sufficient blood to reach the lungs, brain, and other tissues. Under stress, many people restrict their breathing even further, increasing fatigue, muscular tension, irritability, and anxiety (Davis, McKay, & Eshelman, 1995).

While breathing exercises can be learned readily, it is important to maintain continued practice of them in a nonstressful, relaxing environment to attain the full benefits. The first step in enhancing breathing is breathing awareness.

Breathing Awareness

Wellness practitioners are best able to teach the client the procedure if they practice it first. The first step is to lie on a rug or blanket on the floor with legs straight and slightly apart and toes pointed comfortably out, with arms at sides, not touching the body, and with palms up and eyes closed.

Attention is brought to breathing and one hand is placed on the spot that seems to rise and fall during inhalation and exhalation. The other hand is placed on the

TABLE 13.1   Assessing and Reducing Stressful Life Changes

1. Identity sources of stress by listing changes in the following areas in the past 2 years.

    - school
    - work
    - close relationship with friends, family, and significant other people or pets
    - living arrangements or place of residence
    - life style
    - financial matters
    - sudden challenges
    - amount of worry about the future

2. Identify which changes were negative (−) and which were positive (+) by placing a + in front of positive changes and a − in front of negative ones.

3. For the negative changes, decide on a procedure for limiting the effects of unresolved stress.* (See Table 13.2)

Source of Continued Stress   Stress Management Procedure

4. List changes anticipated in the next year and identify at least two procedures to use to reduce the effects of the change on the level of stress.

*Read the rest of this chapter for ideas.

abdomen and breathing is very gently brought to the abdominal area.

The Relaxation Sigh

The relaxing sigh can be used by practitioners prior to approaching a client or can be taught to clients who want to reduce tension levels. The relaxing sigh can be completed in the standing or sitting position. Upon exhalation, a deep sigh is used to let out a sound of deep relief as the air rushes out of the lungs. Inhalation is allowed to occur automatically. The procedure is repeated as necessary, as many times as necessary.

Breathing and Imagery

Breathing can be combined with imagery to provide a powerful healing stimulus. The breath is accomplished in a comfortable position while sitting or lying. The hands are placed on the abdomen; upon inhalation, energy is pictured rushing into the lungs and moving into the solar plexus for storage. Upon exhalation, energy is pictured flowing to all parts of the body. In the case of an injury or illness, energy can be pictured flowing to the injured or ill part.

Alternate Breath

The alternate breath has been found useful for general relaxation and to alleviate tension or sinus headaches (Davis, McKay, & Eshelman, 1995). The procedure is accomplished while sitting in a comfortable position using good posture. The index and second finger of the right hand rest on the forehead, and the right nostril is held closed gently by the thumb. Inhalation occurs through the left nostril. The left nostril

TABLE 13.2   Stress Symptom Assessment

Rate the stress-related symptom for degree of discomfort on a scale of 1 (slight discomfort) to 10 (extreme discomfort). After ensuring the symptom does not have a purely physiological source, choose the appropriate procedure from the list of codes and proceed to use it. After the procedure has been mastered, reevaluate degree of discomfort for each symptom experienced; this will provide a measure of the effectiveness of the procedure.

	Pre-practice degree of discomfort (1–10)	Procedure*	Post-practice degree of discomfort (1–10)
Anxiety in specific situations		PR, B, M, I, SH, TS, RII, CS, TM	
Test anxiety	———		———
Deadline anxiety	———		———
Interview anxiety	———		———
Other performance anxiety	———		———
Anxiety in personal relationships		PR, BR, SN, AS, AF	
with spouse/date	———		———
with parents	———		———
with children	———		———
other	———		———
Generalized anxiety	———	PR, BR, M, I, A, TS, RII, CS, E, B, AF	———
Depression	———	PR, BR, M, TS, AF, RII, CS, AS, N, E	———
Hopelessness	———		———
Powerlessness	———		———
Low self-esteem	———		———
Hostility	———	BR, M, A, RII, I, B, N, E	———
Resentment	———		———
Anger	———		———
Irritability	———		———
Phobias	———	PR, TS, CS, I, BR, AF	———
Fears	———		———
Unwanted thoughts	———	BR, M, TS, I, AF	———
High blood pressure	———	PR, M, A, BN, E, I, AF	———
Headaches	———	PR, I, SH, A, B, N, E, AF	———
Neckaches	———		———
Backaches	———		———
Indigestion	———	PR, SH, A, B, N, E, AF	———
Irritable bowel	———		———
Ulcers	———		———

TABLE 13.2 *(continued)*

Rate the stress-related symptom for degree of discomfort on a scale of 1 (slight discomfort) to 10 (extreme discomfort). After ensuring the symptom does not have a purely physiological source, choose the appropriate procedure from the list of codes and proceed to use it. After the procedure has been mastered, reevaluate degree of discomfort for each symptom experienced; this will provide a measure of the effectiveness of the procedure.

	Pre-practice degree of discomfort (1–10)	Procedure*	Post-practice degree of discomfort (1–10)
Chronic constipation	_____		_____
Muscle spasms	_____	PR, I, SH, B, E	_____
Tics	_____		_____
Tremors	_____		_____
Fatigue, chronic	_____	PR, BR, SH, I, A, TS, N, E	_____
Insomnia	_____	PR, SH, A, TS, B, N, E, I, AF	_____
Obesity	_____	N, E	_____
Weakness	_____	E, N, I, AF	_____

Codes

A	=	Autogenics	CS	=	Coping Skills	PR	=	Progressive relaxation
AF	=	Affirmation	E	=	Exercise	RII	=	Refusing irrational ideas
AS	=	Assertiveness	I	=	Imagery	SH	=	Self-hypnosis
B	=	Biofeedback	M	=	Medication	TS	=	Thought stopping
BR	=	Breathing	N	=	Nutrition	TM	=	Time management

is then gently closed with the ring finger and the right thumb is simultaneously removed from the right nostril. Air is exhaled slowly and soundlessly through the right nostril. The cycle is continued in a slow and even manner: inhale through right nostril, close right nostril with thumb and open the left nostril; exhale through the left nostril; inhale through the left nostril. Five cycles are suggested for beginners, slowly working up to 10 or 25 cycles.

Biofeedback

Biofeedback means getting feedback from the body about internal processes. Thus, breathing with awareness, imagery, and any intervention that allows feedback about the body is biofeedback.

More specifically, the term is used to refer to the use of instrumentation to develop the ability to read tension in various body systems. Instruments are especially useful when the client is unable to identify signs of stress, such as decreased hand temperature, increased muscle tension, or increased blood pressure. However, reading the signs of tension is only the first step in reducing stress. Once the clues have been identified, the client will still need assistance in learning to let go of the physical tension.

According to Davis, McKay, and Eshelman (1995), biofeedback works as follows:

Biofeedback instruments monitor selected body systems that can be picked up by electrodes and transformed into visual or auditory signals. Any internal change instantly triggers an external signal, such as a sound, a flickering light, or readings on a meter.

The following symptoms have been treated with biofeedback: tension headache, migraine, hypertension, insomnia, spastic colon, muscle spasm or pain, epilepsy, anxiety, phobic reactions, asthma, stuttering, and teeth grinding (Davis, McKay, & Eshelman, 1995).

Clients may come to a sophisticated biofeedback center for treatment, or they can purchase inexpensive monitoring equipment for home use. Levels of in-home equipment vary. Sometimes measures are broadly calibrated and may not be completely accurate. Treatment will probably be most effective when the client works with a professional who has high quality equipment and who can assist in overcoming roadblocks that might interrupt progress. A directory of certified biofeedback practitioners is available from The Biofeedback Society of America, 4301 Owen Street, Wheat Ridge, CO 80030.

Progressive Relaxation as a Wellness Measure

Progressive relaxation was developed by Jacobson in 1938 and involves tightening and relaxing the muscle groups of the body, beginning with the hand and moving to the upper and then the lower arm, the forehead, eyes and nose, mouth, neck, upper back, abdomen, buttocks, thigh, calf, and foot for 5 to 7 seconds. The client is encouraged to cheek for relaxation prior to moving to the next major muscle group. If the practitioner is working directly with the cli-

ent in a relaxation session, the practitioner and client can agree that if the client is tense, the index finger of the right or left hand will be raised when the practitioner checks for relaxation.

Scandrett and Uecker (1985, p. 33) suggest that a careful assessment of the client is essential prior to employing relaxation techniques. Symptoms need to be identified and an anxiety scale or anxiety symptom checklist may prove useful. Baseline and posttreatment vital sign measures will validate physiological changes associated with relaxation. Essential components of the pretreatment interview include assessing:

- a report of the client's identification of the most bothersome symptom
- onset, duration, and full description of symptoms
- family history of similar complaints
- client interventions and a description of the results
- an investigation of why the client now seeks help for this symptom
- current and recent medications, including over-the-counter drugs
- physical limitations or illnesses
- previous experience with relaxation training
- use of alcohol or mind-altering drugs
- dietary patterns, especially use of caffeine, sugar, and daily alcohol intake
- sleep patterns
- exercise patterns
- overview of daily routine, including stressors
- psychiatric history, including screening for major depressive or psychotic disorders
- willingness to learn and practice at home

Scandrett and Uecker (1985, p. 34) include self-hypnosis, biofeedback, autogenics, and meditation under the rubric of relaxation therapy and suggest the following nursing diagnoses as appropriate for intervention with it: anxiety, sleep disturbance, activity intolerance, powerlessness, ineffective breathing pattern, comfort alterations in pain, ineffectual coping, impaired physical mobility, and fear.

Although progressive relaxation has proven effective in most studies, some precautions for its use include the following (Snyder, 1984, p. 57):

- In persons who are depressed, relaxation may precipitate further withdrawal.
- In persons experiencing hallucinations and delusions, loss-of-reality-contact reactions may occur.
- The toxic effects of medications can be increased by the relaxation state.
- Tightly tensing muscles can increase blood pressure; those with cardiac conditions should use nontensing relaxation exercises.
- Some clients may experience heightened pain by focusing their attention on body functions; for these clients, imagery may be the treatment of choice.

Self-Hypnosis

Hypnosis is a wakeful state of deep relaxation; there is an alteration in the conscious level of thinking and remembering, and an increase in the ability to focus in on a particular situation. Hypnosis is a heightened state of awareness during which people are more open to suggestion; most people have experienced a trance state at one time or another, e.g., while daydreaming, or when concentrating intently on a book, movie, television program, or work project. All hypnosis is really self-hypnosis because no one will accept a suggestion unless he or she really wants to; thus, the "self" is always in control.

When using self-hypnosis as an intervention, the client usually begins by listening to a taped relaxation and suggestion session or works with a health care professional skilled in the maneuver. With practice, clients can learn quite quickly to relax and put themselves in a trance state. Table 13.3 gives basic instructions for self-hypnosis. As with all procedures in the book, the practitioner should try it out first to understand what the experience is like and to anticipate any difficulties clients might have with the procedure.

For hypnosis to be effective, positive suggestions must be used. Suggestions are used all the time by lay and professional people, but often they are in a negative form. Both negative and positive suggestions affect the subconscious mind even when asleep or unconscious. Adverse suggestions, such as "She'll never recover from this," or "It's malignant, the patient doesn't have a chance," or "You can't be helped, you will have to learn to live with the condition" are heard and acted upon by the hearer. The last comment seems innocuous, but taken literally it means the client will die if the symptom is lost (LeCron, 1964).

Table 13.4 gives suggestions for coaching clients in self-hypnosis.

Suggestions are most effective and wellness-enhancing when phrased in a positive form, e.g., "I will feel comfortable and confident during the interview tomorrow" (as opposed to "I will not feel tension tomorrow"). Formulating suggestions in the becoming mode is often most effective, e.g., "My comfort is gradually increasing" (instead of "I am totally comfortable"). The best results are forthcoming when only one or two suggestions are focused on. Bombarding oneself with numerous suggestions dilutes the force of all of them.

TABLE 13.3   Basic Instructions for Self-Hypnosis

1. Sit or lie in a comfortable position. Remind yourself that whenever you want to come out of hypnosis you can.
2. Use a candle, picture, crack in the ceiling, fire in the fireplace, or some other object to encourage eye fixation.
3. While watching the object, suggest your eyes are getting heavier, are beginning to sting, or are starting to flutter (whichever works best) to induce eyelid heaviness.
4. Preselect a word or phrase to use at the moment your eyes close. The words "relax now," or a color or a place that is beautiful and has special meaning to you, can also be used.
5. With eyes closed, begin relaxing all your muscles, starting with forearms and biceps; first tighten, then relax them. Move to the face, neck, shoulders, chest, stomach, lower back, buttocks, thighs, calves, and toes.
6. Picture the top of an escalator with the steps moving down in front of you. As you step on, count back slowly from 10 to 0. Repeat counting back slowly for two more floors.
7. Begin to notice a feeling of heaviness in your right arm (if right-handed, or left arm if left-handed); then notice your arm getting lighter and lighter as if balloons are tied to it, lifting it higher and higher. Soon your hand will begin to move, imperceptibly at first, but then it will float, moving closer and closer to your face. When your hand touches your face, you will be in hypnosis.
8. When ready, return from hypnosis, feeling refreshed and relaxed.

TABLE 13.4   Coaching Clients in Self-Hypnosis

Directions to Give Clients:

1. If uncomfortable with the word "hypnosis," tell the client the experience will increase comfort and relaxation.
2. Encourage the client to practice self-hypnosis regularly; provide praise for a practice attempt; reinforce practice and success and reduce resistance to self-hypnosis by responding with "Good, you are beginning to learn the technique" to whatever they report as effects of their practice.
3. Tell clients they may feel tingling, warmth, or some other sensations, but whatever they experience will be relaxing; this suggestion will reduce resistance and assist clients to integrate transitory reactions.
4. Word suggestions positively and simply; try stating suggestions in a louder, firmer voice.
5. Use rhythm. repetition, and a monotone voice when coaching.
6. If there is a distracting noise during a practice session, give clients the suggestion, "The sounds you hear will tend to deepen your relaxation."
7. Assist the client in setting up a schedule for self-hypnosis practice and agree on a helpful (not nagging) way the practitioner can encourage practice and the client or practitioner can reward success or practice attempts.

Eighty to 90% of people can be hypnotized, but those who are severely emotionally disturbed, depressed, or suicidal respond more positively to psychotherapy than to hypnosis. Others who may not respond positively to hypnosis include: 1) people with psychosomatic illnesses—who deny any emotional component to their problems—and 2) those who are neurologically impaired or mentally retarded (LeCron, 1964), or who are in crisis (Hadley & Staudacher, 1989).

Clients expected to respond most favorably to hypnosis include those who are highly motivated to learn the technique, are optimistic, willing to try something new, able to concentrate easily, receptive to rather than afraid of hypnosis, and have a good imagination. Clients who do not possess all the above characteristics can learn self-hypnosis if they are willing to practice the technique more frequently.

Some people respond best to permissive suggestions ("I can feel more relaxed and refreshed") while others respond best to commands ("I will feel more relaxed and refreshed"). Experimentation is the best method of determining whether suggestions should be phrased in the permissive or the command mode.

Self-hypnosis can be used to reduce stress related to smoking, drinking, overeating, taking harmful drugs, destructive anger, timidity, anxiety, allergies, itching, asthma, anger, study problems, and pain. The basic self-hypnosis state is induced (see Table 13.4), but the suggestions used differ depending on the stressor. Suggestions can be said aloud, placed on an audiotape, or written and then read to oneself or the client. Bernhardt and Martin (1977, pp. 1–20) suggest the following suggestions be used:

> For my body, not for me, smoking (this harmful drug, destructive anger, anxiety, timidity, head symptom, drinking, overeating) is a poison. I need my body to live, I will protect my body as I would protect (name of loved one).

Suggestions for itching, allergies, and asthma would follow the same format with slight variation (Bernhardt & Martin, 1977, pp. 60–74).

> Not for me, but for my body, this itch is damaging; it means my body is out of balance. To live comfortably, I need my body in balance. To the point I wish to

live in comfort, I will itch when I choose to and at the body location I choose.

For allergies, asthma, or colds, the basic suggestion is used and the following is added:

> If I choose to live this day symptom-free, I can, because I have power over my body. I can tell my nose when to get stuffed up and when not to. I can declare myself master of my body.

Self-hypnosis is also useful in slowing the heart or breathing rate, using the suggestion: "My pulse is slowing down a few beats a minute, and I am relaxing" or "I am beginning to breathe more slowly and comfortably." Clients can be instructed to take their pulse after several minutes until it has slowed sufficiently; at this point, the following suggestion can be used: "This is the heart rate (or pulse) I am comfortable with and want to remain at."

When learning self-hypnosis, some people may not respond well to either muscle relaxation *or* visualization. Poems that use rhythm, repetition, and imagery can be used in that case, or children can be held and rocked rhythmically. Older children (age 4–16 years) can draw a clown face on their preferred thumbnail. They then place a quarter between that thumb and their forefinger while looking at the clown face. Children are told to look only at the clown face and as they do, the coin will slowly become heavy and slip down and fall. When the coin slips, the children are told their eyes will close and they will be very relaxed. Next, the children are told to place their hands on their legs and answer questions by raising their "yes" hand or their "no" hand. (Which hand is which is agreed on prior to the induction technique.) Questions are then asked that pertain to the problem at hand. For example, for bedwetters, the question is asked, "Would you like to have dry beds at night?" Before asking questions about the problem area, children are asked questions of a neutral type such as, "Do you like ice cream?" Those who answer "yes" to the bedwetting question are told they can learn a "trick" but they must practice it very hard every day, and then the "trick" will help them urinate only in the toilet. The children are asked to practice saying the following statement every time the quarter falls out of their hand:

> When I need to urinate, I will wake up all by myself, go to the bathroom all by myself, urinate in the toilet, and return to my nice dry bed. (Bricklin, 1976)

Dr. Karen Olness, Assistant Professor of Medicine at George Washington University, tried this with 20 girls and 20 boys. Within the first month, 20 were "cured" (and had no recurrence of bedwetting 6 months after the study), six others improved, one did not practice, one had a urinary tract operation, and one answered "no" when asked if he wanted a dry bed; this client was referred to psychiatric evaluation (Bricklin, 1976).

Self-Hypnosis and Pain

There are many advantages of using relaxation and self-hypnotic techniques with clients, particularly with those who are immobile due to physical or emotional difficulties. Those who are hospitalized may benefit from this approach because it can replace the sense of mastery and control they have lost due to the process of hospitalization. Being taught self-hypnosis techniques also provides a special experience for them when the health practitioner says, "I understand that you are having a lot of

pain (discomfort, trouble, etc.) and I'm going to teach you a special way to feel better."

Often, merely conveying a firm, clear message of intent to help with pain will provide relief. Some comments to use in this regard are: "I am here to help you relieve your pain," or "I want to work with you to reduce your pain." Other types of statements that are helpful are: "What is the pain?" "Describe the pain to me." "What do you do to relieve your pain?" This discussion is then followed by a decision by the client (if possible) regarding his or her choice of pain relief measure. Approximately 30 minutes after the choice and implementation, the wellness practitioner discusses the measure if necessary. Assuming clients have pain if they say they have pain, having confidence they can help, using measures other than medication, checking to ensure the relief measure works, finding out which warnings of pain people have and helping them intervene in the pain before it becomes intense are helpful wellness practitioner measures.

Individuals in chronic, ongoing pain tend to take on the pain as part of their identity. They can be encouraged to question, "What meaning does this pain have for me?" "Can I imagine myself without pain?" "Is it worth it to me to give up this pain?" while deeply relaxed in self-hypnosis. Clients with this kind of pain may require self-hypnosis sessions of 15 minutes or more twice a day. Practitioners working with these clients must be willing to spend additional time with them and realize that there may be times when hypnosis does not work. Clients may experience excruciating pain at meaningful times; for example, one person who had survived a fire that killed her daughter had a great deal of pain (despite hypnosis) at noon, the time the fire had occurred (Zahourek, 1976).

Clients who have ongoing pain begin to ask themselves, "Can I stand this pain indefinitely?" A suggestion to use with these people during self-hypnosis is "No pain lasts forever." Clients who have been through life-threatening situations may come to associate pain with being alive, since the feeling of pain may be the one thing that reassures them they are alive. This idea can remain in their subconscious as a self-given suggestion ("If I did not have this pain, I'd be dead"). These clients will often claim to have pain even while asleep. A suggestion that may be helpful in this case is: "When the other signs of life were missing, the pain was reassuring, but now it is preferable to be alive without this ongoing pain than to be alive with it." According to Ewin (1978), this type of psychic pain can be distinguished from the pain of cancer, arthritis, or fracture in that psychic pain is always present whereas pain from other afflictions is intermittent.

When using self-hypnosis, it is important to involve as many of the senses as possible (smelling odors, feeling ocean spray or warm sun, touching cool water, tasting salty spray, hearing waves on the beach, etc.). A relatively quick way to induce relaxation is to ask the client to picture him- or herself in a quiet, relaxing. comforting place and to hear, smell, taste, feel, and see everything associated with that place. The practitioner can remain with the client and ask that the index finger of the client's right hand be raised to indicate complete relaxation and the index finger of the left hand to indicate lack of relaxation. The practitioner can ask the client to indicate level of relaxation after a few minutes; if relaxation has not been attained, the practitioner can try progressive relaxation or some other method. For more information regarding the use of self-hypnosis, the reader can consult: Zahourek, Rothlyn P., *Clinical Hypnosis and Therapeutic Suggestion in Patient Care*, Brunner/Mazel, 1990.

Autogenics

Autogenics is a form of self-hypnosis that allows the participant to induce the feeling of warmth and heaviness associated with a trance state. Johannes H. Schultz, a Berlin psychiatrist, combined autosuggestion with some Yoga techniques and developed a system of autogenic training. The system has been found effective in the treatment of disorders of the respiratory tract, the gastrointestinal tract, the circulatory system, the endocrine system, as well as anxiety, irritability, and fatigue. The exercises can be used to increase resistance to stressors, reduce or eliminate sleep disorders, and modify pain reactions.

Autogenic therapy is not recommended for children under 5 years old, or for adults who lack motivation or have severe emotional disorders. Those with diabetes, hypoglycemic conditions, or heart conditions should discuss the use of the method with their physicians. Occasionally, a client may experience a sharp rise or drop in blood pressure when doing the exercises; those with high or low blood pressure should take or have their blood pressure taken to ensure the exercises are useful.

The exercises can be completed in a comfortable sitting or lying position. It may take up to 10 months to master the six exercises. Ninety-second sessions five to eight times a day are recommended for mastery. The client assumes an attitude of passive concentration; initially this will be difficult to attain, but a wandering mind can easily be brought back to concentration. Clients often experience some reactions that are normal but distracting, including a sensation of weight or temperature change, tingling, electric currents, involuntary movements, stiffness, some pain, anxiety, a desire to cry, irritability, headaches, nausea, or hallucinations. These discharges are transitory and will pass as the program is continued.

Each session is ended with a statement to oneself such as, "When I open my eyes I will feel refreshed and alert" and a few deep breaths and stretches until normal awakeness is achieved. Early exercises are focused on heaviness; this cues muscles to relax; the client repeats the following statements, working up from 90 seconds to 4 minutes four to seven times a day. "My right (dominant) arm is heavy." "My left (nondominant) arm is heavy." "Both my arms are heavy." "My right leg is heavy." "My left leg is heavy." "Both my legs are heavy."

Later exercises focus on warmth, which assists in attaining relaxation in blood vessels. The client repeats the following statements working up from 90 seconds to 10 minutes a day: "My right (dominant) arm is warm." "My left (nondominant) arm is warm." "Both my legs are warm." "My right leg is warm." "Both my legs are warm." "My arms and legs are warm."

Next, the client focuses on heartbeat and repeats the following statement: "My heartbeat is calm and regular." Clients who have difficulty becoming aware of their heartbeat can rest their hand over their heart. Those who experience any discomfort are counseled to move to the next three themes and return to the heartbeat following the forehead theme.

When focusing on the breathing theme, the client repeats, "It breathes me" or "My breathing is calm and relaxed." The client can picture him- or herself breathing easily to potentiate the effect of slow, deep respiration.

The solar plexus theme is not used for clients who have ulcers, diabetes, or any condition involving bleeding from the abdominal region. The statement that is focused on for other clients is: "My solar plexus (abdomen, stomach, or belly) is warm."

The forehead theme is best repeated while lying on the back since dizziness can result. The client repeats, "My forehead is cool."

Autogenics can also be used for organ-specific work. For example, for blushing, the client can repeat: "My feet are warm" or "My shoulders are warm." For coughs, the statements, "My throat is cool" and "My chest is warm" are helpful. For asthma, clients use, "It breathes me calm and regular."

Additional statements that can be interspersed with standard themes include: "I feel quiet." "My whole body feels quiet, heavy, comfortable, and relaxed." "My mind is quiet." "I withdraw my thoughts from the surroundings and I feel serene and still." "My thoughts are turned inward and I am at peace." "I feel an inward quietness." "Deep within my mind, I can visualize and experience myself as relaxed and comfortable and still" (Davis, McKay, & Eshelman, 1995, pp. 81–88).

Thought Stopping

Thought stopping is an approach that is especially useful when nagging, repetitive thoughts interfere with wellness. Unwanted thoughts are interrupted by the client with the command "stop," an image of the letters of the word stop, a loud noise (such as a buzzer or bell), or a negative stimulus, such as wearing a rubber band around the wrist and snapping it when the unwanted thought occurs.

Thought stopping may work because (a) distraction occurs, (b) the interruption behaviors serve as a punishment and what is punished consistently is apt to be inhibited, (c) it is an assertive response and can be followed by reassuring or self-accepting comments, and (d) it interrupts the chain of negative and frightening thoughts leading to negative and frightening feelings, thus reducing stress level.

For effective mastery, regular practice for 3 to 7 days is needed. The client chooses the problematic thought; if necessary, the client can be assisted to prioritize interfering thoughts and focus on the most bothersome one.

Next, the nagging thought is brought to attention. Clients are asked to close their eyes and imagine a situation during which the stressful thought is likely to occur. The next step is to interrupt the nagging thought with an egg timer, alarm clock, snap of the fingers, or an image or verbalization of the word, "STOP."

When clients are able to conjure up and dispense with the nagging thought at will, positive, assertive statements are used to replace the nonconstructive one, e.g.:

- fear of flying: "This is a beautiful view from up here."
- food obsession: "My body is using the food I have eaten to sustain me."
- fear of attack: "I am safe if I use the approaches I have learned to protect myself."
- inability to complete wellness behaviors: "I am confident in my ability to exercise (lose weight, stop smoking, etc.)."

Choosing the best extinguishing behavior and the best replacement statements involves an open discussion with clients; the practitioner enumerates the possible extinguishers and may hint at assertive replacement statements, but clients are encouraged to choose based on their knowledge of what is helpful to them.

Clients who experience failure with the approach can choose a less intrusive thought to begin with; once success is achieved, the more troublesome thought can be attempted. Clients need to know that distressful thoughts may return in the future, especially during times of stress; the procedure discussed above can be repeated in these cases.

Refuting Irrational Ideas

Human beings engage in almost continuous self-talk during their waking hours. *Self-talk* is the internal language we use to describe and interpret the world. When self-talk is accurate and realistic, wellness is enhanced; when irrational and untrue, stress and emotional disturbance occur.

Albert Ellis (*A Guide to Rational Living*, 1961) developed a system to attack irrational ideas or beliefs and replace them with more realistic interpretations and self-talk. At the root of irrational thought is the idea that something is being done *to* the person; rational thought is based on the idea that events occur and people experience these events. Irrational self-talk tends to lead to unpleasant emotions; rational self-talk is more likely to lead to pleasant feelings and a positive interpretation of experiences.

One common form of irrational self-talk is statements that "awfulize" experience by making catastrophic, nightmarish interpretations of events, e.g., interpreting a momentary chest pain as a heart attack, a grumpy word from a supervisor as intent to fire, or silence as negative criticism.

The kinds of statements Ellis considers irrational are:

1. External events cause most human misery—people simply react as events trigger their emotions.

2. Happiness can be achieved by inaction, passivity, and endless leisure.
3. People must be unfailingly competent and perfect in all endeavors.
4. It is easier to avoid than to face life's difficulties and responsibilities.
5. The past determines the present.
6. It is horrible when people and things are not the way they should be.
7. It is a necessity for adults to have love and approval from peers, family, and friends.
8. Unfamiliar or potentially dangerous situations always lead to fear and anxiety.
9. People are helpless and have no control over what they experience or feel.
10. People are fragile and cannot be told the truth.
11. Good relationships are built on sacrifice and giving.
12. Rejection and abandonment are the result if one does not always try to please others.
13. There is a perfect love and a perfect relationship.
14. A person's worth is dependent on achievement and production.
15. Anger is bad and destructive.
16. It is bad and wrong to go after what you want and need.

Goodman (1974) developed several guidelines for turning irrational thinking into rational thought, including:

1. The situation does not do anything to me; I say things to myself that produce anxiety and fear.
2. To say things should be other than they are is to believe in magic.
3. All humans are fallible and make mistakes.
4. It takes two to argue.

5. The original cause of a problem is often lost in antiquity; the best place to focus attention is on the present: what to do about the problem now.
6. People feel the way they think; the interpretation of events leads to emotions, not the events themselves.

Refuting irrational ideas is a skill and requires practice in the following five steps:

1. Write down the facts of the event, including only the observable behaviors.
2. Write down self-talk about the event, including all subjective value judgments, assumptions, beliefs, predictions, and worries.
3. Note which statements are classified by Ellis as irrational; a star or some other symbol can be used.
4. Focus on the emotional response to the event using one or two words, e.g., angry, hopeless, felt worthless, afraid.
5. Select *one* irrational idea to refute.
6. Write down all evidence that the idea is false.
7. Write down the worst thing that could happen if what is feared happens or what is desired is not attained.
8. Write down positive effects that might occur if what is feared happens or if what is desired is not attained.
9. Substitute alternative self-talk.

Table 13.5 provides an example of the use of Ellis's format for refuting irrational ideas.

Coping Skills Procedure

Coping skills training grew out of relaxation and systematic desensitization procedures

TABLE 13.5   Refuting Irrational Ideas

1. *Activating event:* Another employee complained about me to my supervisor.
2. *Rational ideas:* I know she's under a lot of pressure because she's new to the unit.
3. *Irrational ideas:* I can't stand being humiliated in public. Feelings of rage and wanting to kill her are taking over. I'm falling apart.
4. *Main feeling(s):* Rage, anger, humiliation.
5. *Refuting the irrational idea(s):* I'm falling apart.
   a.   Being put down in public is not pleasant, but I can handle it.
   b.   I'm mislabeling rage and anger as falling apart.
   c.   I usually get along O.K. with that employee and once I calm down, I will again.
6. *The worst thing that could happen:* The worst thing that could happen is that I could put down the employee in the future to get back at her.
7. *Good things that could occur as a result of this incident:* I can learn to handle put downs without feeling out of control.
8. *Alternate thoughts:* I'm O.K. It's O.K. to feel anger and rage and know I can still function. I can learn to handle this situation and feel good about myself for doing so.
9. *Alternate emotions:* I'm angry, but feel less out of control. The anger is starting to fade and I am feeling calmer.

that were expanded and refined by Meichenbaum and Cameron (1974). The procedures include a combination of progressive relaxation and stress coping self-statements that are used to replace the defeatist self-talk called forth in stressful situations.

Coping skills procedures can be used to rehearse via the imagination for real-life events deemed stressful. First, a stressful situation is called forth. Next, progressive relaxation is practiced. Finally, coping skills statements are repeated until the situation can be thoroughly completed in rehearsal without feeling stressed.

The procedures have been shown effective in the reduction of general anxiety and interview, speech, and test anxiety and appear to be effective in the treatment of phobias, especially the fear of heights. Davis, McKay, and Eshelman (1995) report the effects of 2-year follow-ups of hypertense, postcardiac clients showing that 89% were still able to achieve general relaxation using coping skills training, 79% could still generally control tension, and 79% were able to fall asleep sooner and sleep more deeply. According to Davis, McKay, and Eshelman (1995), coping skills procedures can be mastered in approximately 1 week, once progressive relaxation has been learned (1–2 weeks for mastery).

Coping thoughts can be divided into statements useful for different stages of the stressful situation: Preparatory, the situation, and reinforcing success. Examples of statements found effective for each stage follow; clients and practitioners can develop their own list and memorize them and/or carry a copy with them for use in stressful situations.

Preparatory Stage:

• I can handle this.
• There's nothing to worry about.
• I'll jump in and be all right.
• It will be easier once I get started.
• Soon this will be over.

The Situation:

• I will not allow this situation to upset me.
• Take a deep breath and relax.
• I can take it step by step.
• I can do this: I'm handling it now.

- I can keep my mind on the task at hand.
- It doesn't matter what others think; I will do it.
- Deep breathing really works.

Reinforcing Success:

- Situations don't have to overwhelm me anymore.
- I did it!
- I did well.
- I'm going to tell _____ about my success.
- By stopping thinking about being afraid, I wasn't afraid.

Time Management

According to Davis, McKay, and Eshelman (1995), symptoms of inappropriate time management include: rushing, fatigue, or listlessness with many slack hours of nonproductive activity, chronic vacillation between unpleasant alternatives, chronic missing of deadlines, insufficient time for rest or personal relationships, and the sense of being overwhelmed by demands and details.

Most methods of time management include three steps:

- establishing priorities
- eliminating low priority tasks
- learning to make decisions

Effective time management has been found effective in minimizing deadline anxiety, avoidance anxiety, and job fatigue (McKay, Davis, & Eshelman, 1995).

The first step in time management is exploring how time is currently being spent. An easy way to do this is to divide the day into three segments: waking through lunch, end of lunch through dinner, and end of dinner until bedtime. A small note-

book is carried and the number of minutes for each activity engaged in in each time segment is logged. The inventory is kept for 3 days. At the end of the time, the total amount of time spent in each of the following categories is noted: Table 13.6 provides a time management assessment for Eloise Strates, a wellness practitioner. Based on a review of the inventory, she made the following decisions:

1. Put out clothes for the next day prior to going to bed.

Table 13.6   Time Management Assessment

Activity	Time (minutes)
Waking Through Lunch	
Lying in bed and thinking about getting up	20
Shower	20
Decide what to wear and dress	25
Cook breakfast	15
Read paper/eat	30
Phone friend	15
Commute to work	30
Routine paperwork	30
Daydream	10
Nonmandatory meeting	60
Working with clients	120
Lunch	45
After Lunch Through Dinner	
Working with clients	90
Daydreaming while staring at paperwork	20
Shift report	20
Socializing	30
Commute	30
Shopping	45
Phone calls	30
Cooking	90
Eating	30
After Dinner Until Retiring	
Phone calls	60
Television	90
Study	90
Prepare for bed/read	30

2. Get up at the alarm and limit shower to 5 minutes.

3. Make breakfasts that don't require cooking, cut dinner preparation to 30 minutes, and enlist family to do food preparation 3 days/week.

4. Ask for a late lunch to take advantage of most productive work hours (11 a.m. to 2 p.m.).

5. Use thought stopping to limit daydreaming.

6. Stop attending nonmandatory, nonproductive meetings.

Eloise's next step was to set priorities. She began by making a list of things she most wanted to accomplish in the near future and comparing it to how she spent her time. She visualized herself being told she only had 6 months to live and began to imagine how she could best spend the time. She made the list without stopping to evaluate or judge what she wrote and suggested others might also find this the most helpful way to proceed.

Eloise's next step was to make a list of 1-month and 1-year goals she believed she could reasonably accomplish in terms of work, improvement, and recreation. Then she sat back and reflected that she now had long-, medium-, and short-range goals. Next, Eloise prioritized each list by deciding which were the top drawer items (most essential or desired), middle drawer items (can be put off for a while, but still important), and bottom drawer (can easily be put off indefinitely with no harm done).

Eloise then chose two top drawer goals for her lifetime goals, 1-year goals, and 1-month goals to begin working toward.

T-1: Buy a new car (1-year goal).

T-2: Write an article for a journal (lifetime goal to contribute to the profession).

T-3: Have dinner out with husband once a week (1-month goal).

T-4: Investigate ways of becoming a consultant (lifetime goal to communicate wellness knowledge).

T-5: Dance lessons with husband (1-year goal).

T-6: Complete old records pile at work (1-month goal).

Since Eloise was overwhelmed by the six goals, she decided to break each one down into manageable steps. For example, her goal of investigating ways of becoming a nursing consultant was divided into the following steps:

1. Borrow a friend's book on consultation and read a chapter a week.

2. Talk with other practitioners who are currently consultants; ask one or more to be my mentor.

3. Make a list of my wellness knowledge [and combine] to make a list of saleable consulting skills.

4. Purchase stationary, business cards, and brochures detailing my consulting skills.

Eloise found it so difficult to get started even after breaking down her priorities into manageable steps that she developed a daily "To Do" list including everything she wanted to accomplish that day. She rated each item top, middle, or bottom priority and worked only on the top priority items for the day.

This approach helped somewhat, but Eloise still had difficulty until she discovered the rules for making time (McKay, Davis, & Eshelman, 1995):

1. Learn to say "no": remind yourself this is your life and your time to spend as best befits you. Only when your boss asks should you spend time

on bottom priority items. Be prepared to say, "I don't have the time." If necessary, take an assertiveness training course.

2. Build time into your schedule for unscheduled events, interruptions, and unforeseen occurrences.

3. Set aside several time periods during the day for structured relaxation; being relaxed will allow you to use the time you have more efficiently.

4. Keep a list of short, 5-minute tasks that can be done any time you are waiting or are between other tasks.

5. Learn to do two things at once; plan dinner while driving home or organize an important letter or list while waiting in line at the bank.

6. Delegate bottom drawer tasks to sons, daughters, secretaries, or in-laws.

7. Get up 15 to 30 minutes earlier every day.

8. Allow no more than 1 hour of television-watching for yourself daily. Use it as a reward for working on your top drawer times.

Part of time management is the ability to make decisions. Procrastination is the great time robber. Procrastination can often be overcome by (Davis, McKay, & Eshelman, 1995):

1. Recognizing the unpleasantness of making some decisions versus the unpleasantness of putting it off; analyze the costs and risks of delay.

2. Examine the payoffs you receive for procrastinating, e.g., you won't have to face the possibility of failure, you can be taken care of by others, you can gain attention by being chronically unhappy.

3. Join the resistance you have created by exaggerating and intensifying whatever you are doing to put off the decision. Keep it up until you are bored and making the decision seems more attractive than whatever you are doing to procrastinate.

4. Take responsibility for your delaying tactics by writing down how long each delay took.

5. When making unimportant decisions, choose south or east over north or west; pick left over right; smooth over rough; pick the shortest; choose the closest; pick the one that comes first alphabetically.

6. Take small steps toward the decision: if you want to decide to sew on a button, take out the thread and materials and place them by you as a lead-in to the decision to begin.

7. Avoid beginning a new task until you have completed a predecided segment of the current one; allow yourself to fully experience the reward of finishing something, one of the great payoffs of decision making.

Music

Taped music has been studied and found effective for reducing the stress of anxiety in blood donors (Cameron, 1991), pain after surgery (Slyfield, 1992), and intensive care units (Johnson, 1991).

Hardiness

Dr. Suzanne Ouellette Kobasa has researched the ability of people to survive stress. She found that *psychological "hardiness"* or the ability to survive is composed of three ingredients: 1) Commitment to self, work, family, and other important values; 2) a sense of personal control over one's life; and 3) the ability to see change in one's life as a challenge to master.

Dr. Kobasa tested executives, lawyers, women in gynecologists' offices, telephone foremen, operator supervisors, U.S. Army officers, and college students; the results were the same: biology is not destiny. A hardy personality is more important than a strong constitution. It is possible to come from a family with chronic illness and do better under stress if one is hardy than to come from a "healthy" family but have few inner resources (Kobasa, 1984).

Exercise is a good antidote to stress but may be short-term. Jogging after an argument can help that evening, but the next morning stress levels can rise if the stress-provoking situation is re-encountered. Hardiness skills may be long-term inoculations against stressors.

Three techniques Dr. Kobasa found helpful for increasing hardiness skills are: focusing, restructuring stressful situations, and compensating through self-improvement. Focusing is a technique developed by Eugen Gendlin that can assist in recognizing signals from the body that stress is interfering with comfort. Dr. Kobasa found that executives are so used to pressure in their temples, tightened necks, or stomach knots that they have stopped noticing these signals that something is wrong. A beginning question might be: "Where is my tension located in my body'?" Those who have learned to tune out body signals can begin with a progressive relaxation tape; this will assist in identifying body locations of stress and tension. Another step is to make a list of "Things That Are Bothering Me Today." The list is then reviewed and the question, "What is keeping me from feeling terrific today?" can assist in the process. Using an affirmation such as, "This day is getting better and better" may help also.

The second technique (reconstruction of stressful situations) is accomplished by thinking about a recent episode of distress, writing down three ways it could have gone better, and three ways it could have gone worse. This exercise increases the ability to put the situation in perspective, a useful procedure for reducing stress.

The third technique (compensating through self-improvement) works most effectively with stressors that cannot be avoided: an illness, impending divorce, unexpected death or loss of a loved one, etc. The feeling of loss of control that results due to this kind of unexpected event can be balanced by taking on a new challenge. Learning to sew, knit, or scuba dive or teaching someone a skill can reassure that life can still be coped with adequately.

REFERENCES

Acterberg, J., & Rider, M. S. (1989). Effect of music-assisted imagery on neutrophils and lymphocytes. *Biofeedback and Self-Regulation, 14*(3), 247–257.

Basmajian, J. V. (Ed.). (1989). *Biofeedback: Principles and practice for clinicians* (3rd ed.). Baltimore: Williams & Wilkins.

Ben-Eliyahu, S., Yirmirya, R., Liebeskind, J. C., Taylor, A. N., & Gale, R. P. (1991). Stress increases metastatic spread of a mammary tumor in rats: Evidence for mediation by the immune system. *Brain, Behavior, and Immunity, 5,* 193–205.

Benson, H., & Klipper, M. (1976). *The relaxation response.* New York: Avon.

Bernhardt, R., & Martin, D. (1977). *Self-mastery through self hypnosis.* New York: Signet.

Bricklin, M. (1976). *The practical encyclopedia of natural healing.* Emmaus, PA: Rodale, pp. 289–290.

Cameron, K. (1991). The effect of music on vasovagal reactions and anxiety among first time blood donors. *Masters Abstracts International, 31-02,* 0758 #71 565.

Cannon, W. (1914). The emergency function of the medulla in pain and the major emotions. *American Journal of Physiology, 33,* 356–372.

Davis, M., McKay, M., & Eshelman, F. (1995). *The relaxation and stress reduction workload* (2nd ed.). Oakland, CA: New Harbinger.

Ellis, A., & Harper, R. (1961). *A guide to rational living.* North Hollywood, CA: Wilshire Books.

Ewin, D. (1978). Relieving suffering and pain with hypnosis. *Geriatrics, 33*(6), 87–89.

Goodman, D. (1974). *Emotional well-being through rational behavior training.* Springfield, IL: Charles C. Thomas.

Hadley, J., & Stauder sker, C. (1989). *Hypnosis for change.* Oakland, CA: New Harbinger Publications.

Halley, F. M. (1991). Self-regulation of the immune system through biobehavioral strategies. *Biofeedback and Self-Regulation, 16*(1), 55–73.

Herbert, T. B., & Cohen, S. (1993). Depression and immunity: A meta-analytic review. *Psychological Bulletin, 113,* 472–486.

Houldin, A. D., McCorkle, R., & Lowery, B. J. (1993). Relaxation training and psychoimmunological status of bereaved spouses. *Cancer Nursing, 16*(2), 47–52.

Jacobson, E. (1938). *Progressive relaxation.* Chicago: University of Chicago Press.

Johnson, N. L. (1991). Physiological and emotional responses to taped music programs in intensive care units. *Masters Abstracts International,* 31–02, 0758 # 71762.

Kiecolt-Glaser, J. K., Pennebaker, J. W., & Glaser, R. (1988). Disclosure of traumas and immune function: Health implications for psychotherapy. *Journal of Consulting and Clinical Psychology, 56*(2), 239–245.

Kobasa, S. (1984). How much stress can you survive? *American Health, 3*(7), 64–77.

LeCron, L. (1964). *Self-hypnosis* (pp. 78–92). New York: Signet.

Levy, S. M., Huberman, R. B., Whiteside, T. J., Sanzo, K., Lee, J., & Kirkwood, J. (1990).

Perceived social support and tumor estrogen/progesterone receptor status as predictors of natural killer cell activity in breast cancer patients. *Psychosomatic Medicine, 52*(1), 73–85.

Meichenbaum, D., & Cameron, R. (1974). Modifying what clients say to themselves. In M. Mahoney & R. Cameron (Eds.), *Self-control: power to the person.* Monterey, CA: Brooks/ Cole.

Post-White, J., & Johnson, M. (1991). Complementary nursing therapies in clinical oncology practice: Relaxation and imagery. *Dimensions in Oncology Nursing, 5*(2), 15–20.

Quinn, J. F., & Strelkaukas, A. J. (1993). Psychoimmunology effects of therapeutic touch on practitioners and recently bereaved recipients: A pilot study. *Advanced Nursing Science, 15*(4), 13–26.

Scandrett, S., & Uecker, S. (1985). Relaxation training. In G. Bulecheck & J. McCloskey (Eds.), *Nursing interventions: Treatments for nursing diagnoses* (pp. 22–48). Philadelphia: W. B. Saunders.

Selye, H. (1956). *The stress of life.* New York: McGraw-Hill.

Slyfield, C. M. (1992). The effect of music therapy on patient's pain, blood pressure, and heart rate after coronary artery bypass graft surgery. *Masters Abstracts International,* 31-03, 76, #11351497.

Snyder, M. (1984). Progressive relaxation as a nursing intervention: An analysis. *Advances in Nursing Science, 6*(3), 47–58.

Zahourek, R. (1978). *Use of relaxation and hypnotic techniques in the care of the difficult patient.* Workshop for nurses at Downstate Medical Center, Brooklyn, NY, November 1, 1978.

Zeagans, L. (1982). Stress and the development of somatic disorders. In L. Goldberger & S. Brezwitz (Eds.), *Handbook of stress: Theoretical and clinical aspects.* New York: Free Press.

CHAPTER 14

Smoking Cessation

Charlene Long

According to the Centers for Disease Control (CDC), cigarette smoking is the chief avoidable cause of illness and death in the United States (U.S. Department of Health and Human Services [DHHS], 1999a). Certainly prevention is the ideal way to control this problem. This is something that should be considered early in everyone's life. However, a large number of Americans still smoke, and it has been found that if both parents smoke there is a 90% chance that a child will smoke. If only one parent smokes, there is a 45% chance that a child will smoke (Lynch & Bonnie, 1994).

In 1964, the U.S. Public Health Service issued its first report on smoking and health, and America's smoking epidemic began to decline. At that time, approximately 40% of all Americans smoked (Ray & Ksir, 1993). Although there has been a decline in smoking among American adults since the 1960s, according to *Healthy People 2010,* (USDHHS, 1999a) approximately 24% of Americans over the age of 18 years continue to smoke. Forty-eight million Americans smoked in 1997, the same rate as in 1995. Data from U.S. agen-

cies show that tobacco kills more Americans each year than alcohol, cocaine, crack, heroin, homicide, suicide, car accidents, fires, and AIDS *combined.*

Studies have shown that tobacco is more addictive and difficult to give up than most other substances (Battijes, 1988; Bobo, 1989; Bobo & Davis, 1993). There are more than 4,000 known chemicals in tobacco (Sims, 1994), and dozens of these chemicals are known to be toxic to the body. Nicotine is one of the most toxic chemicals in tobacco and is, in fact, used in many insect sprays. For nicotine to be released from the tobacco, it must be burned; it is released along with many other toxic compounds including carbon monoxide and tar when the tobacco is burned during cigarette smoking (Bennett & Woolf, 1991).

Tobacco affects all organ systems of the body. The mechanisms of tobacco effects have been studied primarily in relation to nicotine, carbon monoxide, catecholamines, and nicotine metabolites (Sullivan, 1995). Nicotine is believed by most investigators to be the compound primarily responsible for the pharmacological effects of smoking. The lungs readily absorb nicotine, and after one puff, nicotine reaches the brain in about two seconds (Sims, 1994).

CONSEQUENCES OF TOBACCO USE

The American Lung Association (1999) reports that smoking-related diseases claim an estimated 430,000 American lives each year. The U.S. Department of Health and Human Services (1999b) reports that one in every six deaths in the nation is linked to smoking (approximately 1,200 per day). The health risks of smoking such as heart and vascular disease and stroke; cancer of the lung, pharynx, larynx, esophagus, liver, pancreas, and bladder, emphysema and other respiratory diseases, slowed wound healing, and stomach ulcers are well known (Hays, Dale, Hurt, & Croghan, 1998; USDHHS, 1999b).

According to the American Lung Association (1999), approximately 22.5 million American women are smokers. Although the American public is concerned about breast cancer, more American women die annually from lung cancer than from any other type of cancer: There were 68,000 female deaths from lung cancer in 1999 compared to 43,400 female deaths from beast cancer (USDHHS, 1999b).

The most distressing statistic is that one third of all women of childbearing age in the United States are smokers. Even more alarming is the fact that 20% to 25% of them continue to smoke during their pregnancies even with evidence of potential damage to the fetus. The rate among adult men is declining while there is an increasing number of female teenage smokers.

Maternal tobacco use is associated with mental retardation, spontaneous abortions, low birth weight, birth defects such as cleft lip and palate, and respiratory prob-

lems such as bronchitis, asthma, and sudden infant death syndrome (Sullivan, 1995). Passive smoking also contributed to an increased need for emergency room visits. Children living with smokers visited emergency rooms 63% more often than children from nonsmoking households (Evans et al., 1987).

If current patterns persist, an estimated five million persons under the age of 18 years will die prematurely from a smoking-related disease (USDHHS, 1999a). In addition, smoking costs the United States approximately $97.2 billion each year in health care costs and lost productivity. For this reason, it is vital to assist those who desire to quit smoking and to help keep young people from starting.

Tobacco dependence has been compared to other forms of drug dependence and found to be very similar. They are all complex processes. Users report that the effect of smoking is both euphoric and tranquilizing (Sullivan, 1995). The effects are not as dramatic as the emotional and behavioral changes with other abusive substances; however, after repeated use, the pleasurable effects do occur. The pleasurable effects are a part of the addiction process of tobacco. Tolerance to the substance develops, withdrawal symptoms occur upon cessation, and the user believes that the drug reduces anxiety or stress (Bennett & Woolf, 1991).

A smoker who is age 35 or older has twice the risk of stroke than the nonsmoker. In addition, the smoker has 6 times the risk of mouth cancer, 10 times the risk of laryngeal cancer and chronic obstructive pulmonary disease (emphysema and bronchitis), and 12 times the risk of lung cancer. The risk for coronary heart disease and heart attack is twice as high among smokers than among nonsmokers (National Institutes of Health [NIH], 1993).

Smoking is associated with heart and blood vessel disease, chronic bronchitis and emphysema, gastritis and ulcers, and cancer of the lungs larynx, pharynx, oral cavity, esophagus, pancreas, and urinary bladder. Young women who smoke and take birth-control pills are 17% more likely to have a stroke. Many physicians refuse to prescribe birth-control pills for smokers.

There is controversy about whether exposure to secondhand smoke leads to increased health risks, and further research is needed in this area. However, the U.S. Surgeon General's Report in 1986 reported that: (a) secondhand smoke is a cause of disease including lung cancer in healthy nonsmokers; (b) children of parents who smoke compared with children of non-smoking parents have an increased frequency of respiratory diseases, sudden infant death syndrome (SIDS), and inner ear infections; and (c) simply separating smokers and nonsmokers within the same air space (such as restaurants, airplanes, etc.) may reduce but does not eliminate tobacco smoke exposure. Nicotine is found in the blood of nonsmokers exposed to secondhand smoke. Secondhand smoke exposure also has serious health effects. Studies have found that among nonusers of tobacco 88% had detectable levels of serum cotinine, a biological marker for exposure to secondhand smoke (Pirkle et al., 1996). The results of most studies indicate that there is no safe threshold of exposure to cigarette smoke (USDHHS, 1999b).

Chewing tobacco is a potent cause of mouth cancer and other oral diseases. A national survey of household residents 12 years of age and older found that 11% had tried chewing tobacco, snuff, and other smokeless tobacco and that 3% used chewing tobacco almost daily. Young boys are at major risk since many sports heroes use smokeless tobacco, and smokeless tobacco users are also more likely to use alcohol, cigarettes, and marijuana. They are more likely to report poor health and hospitalization and to report symptoms of depression than nonusers. A number of retired major league baseball players are telling kids, "Don't start" (AARP, p. 6).

In addition to real and potential health risks, tobacco consumption and exposure to smoke impose an enormous economic burden on society. An estimated $23 billion dollars in medical costs can be attributed to tobacco use or exposure. Another $43 billion is lost to society because of illness or premature death.

Nicotine is also a gateway drug. Two thirds of those who smoke one pack a day also use illicit drugs, while only 10% of those who have never smoked do so. The initiation of daily smoking is highest in junior high school, that is, at 12 to 14 years. The smoking rate among 18- to 24-year-olds rose from 24.8% in 1995 to 28.7% in 1997 (USDHHS, 1999a). The decrease has been greatest among college graduates, dropping by half while hardly changing among those with less than a high school education. In addition, cigarettes will kill one in five people in industrialized countries or at least 250 million people. This is more than the entire population of the United States.

Healthy People 2010, a report from the U.S. Department of Health and Human Services (1999a), has targeted the reduction of cigarette smoking to 12% of adult smokers (18 years and older) by the year 2010. The baseline data for this projected goal are from 1997, which showed that 24% of the adult population were cigarette smokers (USDHHS, 1999a). The report also recommended a reduction in tobacco product use among students in grades nine through 12 from 43% in 1997 to a target of 21% in 2010. Research has found that the beginning cigarette smoker tends to be an adolescent between the ages of 12 and 18 who is from a lower socioeconomic group and is likely to be a high school drop-out (Dappen, Schwartz, & O'Donnell, 1996; Lamkin, Davis, & Kamen, 1998). Having a friend who smokes has been consistently identified as the primary factor influencing smoking behavior (Ary & Biglan, 1988). This has major implications for prevention of smoking among young people.

BENEFITS OF SMOKING CESSATION

The U.S. Department of Health and Human Services National Institutes of Health (1999b) indicates that good reasons to stop smoking for teenagers include bad breath, stained teeth, cost, lack of independence (controlled by cigarettes), sore throats, coughing, difficulty breathing (may affect sports, and frequent respiratory infections). Good reasons to stop smoking for pregnant women include the increased risk of spontaneous abortion and fetal death and increased risk of low birth weight babies. Parents should stoop smoking because of increased coughing and respiratory infections among their children and because they are poor role models. New smokers will find it easier to smoke now rather than later, and long-term smokers will have a decreased risk of heart disease and cancer if they stop now. Those with a family history of heart disease or cancer are at a higher risk if they smoke.

Asymptomatic adults who smoke are at twice the risk of heart disease, six times the risk of emphysema, ten times the risk of lung cancer, and have five to eight years shorter lifespans than those who do not smoke. In addition, the cost of cigarettes, increased sick time, bad breath, inconvenience and social unacceptability, and more wrinkles make smoking less satisfac-tory. For symptomatic adults, smoking is correlated with more upper respiratory infections and coughs, sore throats, dyspnea (difficulty breathing), ulcers, angina, claudication, osteoporosis, esophagitis, and gum disease. All smokers will save money by stopping smoking, feel better, improve their ability to exercise, may be able to work more with less illnesses, live longer and enjoy life, grandchildren, and retirement (USDHHS, 1991).

U.S. Department of Health and Human Services Clinical Practice Guideline Number 18 on Smoking Cessation (April, 1996) indicates that the components of clinical interventions designed to enhance motivation are the "4 Rs" (p. 64): relevance, risks, rewards, and repetition. Relevance includes motivational information relevant to patient's disease status, family or social situation, health concerns, age, and other important patient characteristics.

Tips for using this model include:

1. Ask the individual to identify potential risks or negative consequences of smoking.
2. Emphasize those most relevant to the client.
3. Identify the rewards or the potential benefits of quitting smoking. (Those most relevant to the individual should be highlighted. Examples would include improved health, enhanced taste, improved sense of smell, monetary savings, setting a good example for kids, and performing better in sports.)
4. Use repetition. Provide motivational information every time you see an unmotivated client.

Benefits from stopping smoking begin almost immediately according to Andrews (1998); see Table 14.1. Twenty minutes after the last cigarette, the blood pressure,

TABLE 14.1   Benefits from Stopping Smoking

After Last Cigarette	Benefits
Within 20 minutes of last cigarette	• Blood pressure drops to normal • Pulse rate drops to normal rate • Body temperature of hands, feet increases to normal
8 hours:	• Carbon monoxide level in blood drops to normal • Oxygen level in blood increases to normal
24 hours:	• Risk of heart attack decreases
48 hours:	• Nerve endings start regrowing • Ability to smell and to taste things is enhanced
72 hours:	• Bronchial tubes relax, making breathing easier • Lung capacity increases
2 weeks to 3 months:	• Circulation improves • Walking becomes easier • Lung function increase up to 30%
1 to 9 months:	• Coughing, sinus congestion, fatigue, shortness of breath decreases • Cilia regrow in lungs, increasing ability to handle mucus, clean the lungs, reduce infection • Body's overall energy level increases
5 years:	• Low birth weight: Baby's risk lowered if mother quits before pregnancy or during first trimester • Lung cancer death rate for average smoker (one pack a day) decreases from 137 per 100,000 people to 72 per 100,000 • Stroke risk reduced to level of nonsmoker within 5 to 15 years
10 years:	• Lung cancer death rate for average smoker drops to 12 death per 100,000—almost the rate of non-smokers • Precancerous cells are replaced • Other cancers decrease such as those of the mouth, larynx, esophagus, bladder, cervix, kidney and pancreas. (There are 30 chemicals in tobacco smoke that cause cancer.)
15 years:	• Coronary heart disease down to level of nonsmoker classification

pulse, and temperature of hands and feet return to normal. After 8 hours, carbon monoxide levels drop and oxygen levels in the blood increase to normal. Within 24 hours, the chances of heart attack begin to decrease. After 48 hours, nerve endings start regrowing and the ability to smell and taste is enhanced. Seventy-two hours after quitting smoking bronchial tubes relax, making breathing easier, and lung capacity increases. Circulation improves, walking becomes easier, and lung function increases up to 30% within 2 weeks to 3 months after quitting smoking. Between 1 and 9 months after quitting smoking,

coughing, sinus congestion, fatigue, and shortness of breath decreases. Cilia regrow in lungs, increasing the ability to handle mucus, clean the lungs, and reduce infection. In addition, the body's overall energy level increases. After 5 years, the lung cancer death rate for the average smoker (one pack a day) decreases from 137 per 100,000 people to 72 per 100,000. After 10 years, lung cancer death rate corresponds to that of nonsmokers, and after 15 years the risk of coronary heart disease equals that of a nonsmoker. In addition, other cancers such as those of the mouth, larynx, esophagus, bladder, kidney, and pancreas decrease (Andrews, 1998). Your teeth are also whiter, your breath fresher, you enjoy the flavor of food more, your clothes and car no longer smell of stale smoke, and you generally feel better.

RESEARCH ON SMOKING CESSATION

Support from family and friends and positive messages from community practitioners may be the most important factors in helping people quit smoking for good. The American Lung Association is involved in research efforts to understand how the practitioner can help people stop using tobacco. It is important to be aware of current research on smoking cessation in order to offer the client the best assistance possible.

A study reported in the British Medical Journal (Davidsson, Rossner, & Westin, 1999) indicated that women who were concerned about weight gain were more likely to quit if their smoking cessation program combined nicotine gum with a special low-calorie diet. Fifty percent of those individuals studied quit smoking after a 16-week cessation program that included nicotine gum and a commercial, very low-calorie diet. In contrast, only 35% of nondieting women were able to quit smoking after 16 weeks. A year later, 28% of the diet group were still not smoking, compared with just 16% percent of the other group.

Results of a national study conducted in July 1999 by the American Lung Association (ALA, 1999) indicated that nearly 70% of smokers want to stop smoking and have tried to do so an average of 5.3 times each. This study included interviews of 1,001 cigarette smokers aged 18 and over who had tried to quit at least once but were unsuccessful. The average smoker in the group had been smoking 19 years and was smok-

ing about one pack per day. Younger smokers (18–34 years old) smoked 3 to 4 fewer cigarettes per day than smokers over the age of 35 years. Men had attempted to stop 1.4 times more than women. Smokers over 50 years of age had tried twice as many times as those under 50 (8.0 vs. 4.4), and 7 out of 10 (69%) of those interviewed were planning to quit again in the next six months (ALA, 1998).

Addiction was the reason cited most often for smokers' decisions to smoke (82% rated this a 4 or 5 on a 5-point importance scale). Women were more likely to say that they smoked to relieve stress or to have something to do with their hands.

Several studies have shown that structured smoking cessation interventions do affect smoking abstinence (Stanislaw & Wewers, 1994; Padula & Willey, 1993; Resnicow et al.; McDonald, 1999; Osler et al., 1999; Hudmon et al., 1999; Allen et al., 1999; Perkins et al., 2000). Further study is needed in this area. The implication for health care practitioners would be that paying attention to smoker's smoking behavior can affect cessation.

Osler et al. (1999) found that quitting smoking was positively associated with male gender and cigar smoking and negatively associated with the amount of tobacco smoked, inhalation, and alcohol consumption. Smoking cessation among women was positively associated with level of education and lower body mass index. Cohabitation status, leisure activity, or bronchitis symptoms did not affect smoking cessation. Implications for the health care practitioner would be to target persons who smoke more heavily and lean, poorly educated women.

The majority of the smokers interviewed had tried to quit without the benefit of nicotine therapy: Three out of four (73%) had tried "cold turkey," and two out of five (44%) had gradually reduced their cigarette consumption (ALA, 1998).

The reasons smokers gave for returning to smoking included missing the comfortable feeling that smoking gave them (42%), needing something to do with their hands (41%), and stress or nerves. A majority of those interviewed indicated that they did not understand how nicotine affected them. Seventy-two percent believed that nicotine causes cancer while 62% believed that products containing nicotine might help smokers stop smoking. Four out of ten of those interviewed (39%) indicated that they were confused about products available to assist with stopping smoking.

The results of the ALA study indicated that smokers needed support when attempting to quit (ALA, 1998). In response, the American Lung Association developed its Quit Smoking Action Plan. This plan outlines in very simple terms the steps a smoker can take to enhance the likelihood of success in smoking cessation. The three key elements of the plan include preparation to quit smoking, medications, and how to remain smoke-free. Since smokers smoke for a variety of reasons, there needs to be a wide array of tools available to suit their personalities.

The American Lung Association's smoking cessation programs found that quit rates varied. The Freedom from Smoking Group Clinic showed a 51% quit rate at the end of the clinic with a continuous quit rate of 27% at the end of one year (ALA, 1986). Other programs varied, but all results were positive.

WAYS TO ENCOURAGE SMOKING CESSATION

There are a variety of methods for assisting clients in kicking the smoking habit. First, you may have to prove to clients that they are truly addicted to cigarettes. The following quiz can be used to identify whether a client is addicted:

1. Do you smoke your first cigarette within 30 minutes of waking up in the morning?
   Yes   No

2. Do you smoke 20 cigarettes (one pack) or more each day?
   Yes   No

3. At times when you can't smoke or don't have any cigarettes, do you feel a craving for one?
   Yes   No

4. Is it tough to keep from smoking for more than a few hours?
   Yes   No

5. When you are sick enough to stay in bed, do you still smoke?
   Yes   No

   If you answered yes to two or more questions, you may be addicted to cigarettes. The more yes answers you gave, the more likely that you are addicted to the nicotine in cigarettes (ALA, 1999).

Smokers must decide if they really want to quit. Quitting can be beneficial not only to the individual, but also to the persons around them because health risks are reduced for both. Encourage smokers to determine why they want to quit smoking. Use the "Reasons for Quitting Smoking" in Box 14.1 to help smokers quit smoking.

Give smokers a list of resources in the community to assist in smoking cessation. Ask clients frequently about smoking cessation and offer frequent encouragement. If a client slips and smokes a cigarette or two, ask them to give themselves forgiveness.

Box 14.1   Reasons for Quitting Smoking

"For my health—to lower my chances of lung cancer, heart disease, and other serious illnesses."

"So my family will be healthier."

"I want to be in control of my life."

"So I won't smell of cigarettes and my teeth won't be yellow."

"To set a good example for my family."

"Out of respect for my body."

"So I'll feel better—I won't cough so much and I'll have more energy."

"Smoking is a waste of money."

"My other reasons to quit:"

(ALA, 1993)

Tell them that millions of people who have quit smoking slip, but that many of these smokers end up quitting for good. Ask clients why they slipped up and help them draw up a plan listing specific measures to take if the situation comes up again.

There are a variety of reasons that someone smokes (ALA, 1991). These include stimulation, handling (which includes holding the cigarette, lighting up, etc.), pleasure, relaxation, tension reduction, craving, and habit. If a client identifies one or more of these reasons as the most important, strategies can be planned to control them. You can also help identify what triggers the urge to smoke. Some typical triggers are playing cards, drinking coffee, watching TV, finishing a meal, being on a work break, and having a drink.

Other roadblocks to quitting can be identified and dealt with. Clients who express concern that they will gain too much weight need to be encouraged to eat healthful snacks and to exercise. Box 14.2 provides examples of healthy snacks.

Box 14.2   Healthy Snacks

Berries
Peaches
Cantaloupe
Plums
Pears
Fresh or canned pineapple
Apples
Carrots
Celery
Broccoli
Raisins
Air-popped popcorn
Banana
Small bran muffin
Cereal without sugar and milk
Frozen grapes
Sugarless gum and candy
Tomato Juice
Diet soda
Fruit juice
Water

The reason many people gain weight after giving up smoking is that they start to burn calories a little more slowly (ALA, 1993) and because food tastes better. Some people turn to food instead of cigarettes when they want to do something with their hands. Some comments to make to smokers are: "You may not gain any weight if you stop smoking. The general rule is that a person may gain between 5 and 8 pounds after stopping smoking" (Sullivan, 1995). "A few extra pounds are not nearly as bad for your health as smoking." "Let's find some ways for you that will reduce possible weight gain." "Exercise will help you burn calories faster and avoid gaining weight."

Some other ways for clients to control their hunger include:

Drinking a large glass of a low-calorie beverage.

Keeping your hands busy by sewing, working on a puzzle, writing a letter, or washing your hair.

Eating slowly. Don't eat on the run.

Making a list of five things you'll do before eating anything such as stretching for 2 minutes, trimming or filing your nails, or washing your face.

Making a phone call to a friend.

The following are additional ways to adjust eating habits to control weight:

1. Eat meats that are low in fat and calories such as veal, chicken, turkey, and fish; green leafy vegetables which are low in fat and calories and high in vitamins and minerals; fresh fruits, vegetables, and fish (low in fat and calories but filling and high in vitamins and minerals).

2. Control your sugar intake; sugar is high in most diets and turns into body fat.

3. Eat three meals a day to keep blood sugar levels at an even keel and prevent headaches and nervousness. (This also prevents eating large amounts at a time if you are desperately hungry.)

4. Bake foods rather than frying; watch intake of starchy foods such as potatoes, pasta, noodles, rolls, breads, croutons, and crackers; and keep alcohol intake low. Alcohol is very high in calories and doesn't provide nutrients. Alcohol may also be a trigger to smoking.

5. The American Lung Association (1986) recommends these four tips:
   (a) Using milk, preferably skim milk, in coffee and tea.
   (b) Cooking with herbs and spices, rather than butter or margarine, and avoiding gravies and creamy sauces.
   (c) Eating lots of salads with light dressings such as light oil and vinegar.
   (d) Starting meals with clear soups or broth, carrot sticks and celery stalks, or a small salad.

6. Exercise helps many people control their weight while quitting smoking and reduces the tension connected with smoking cessation. It may be as simple as choosing to climb the stairs instead of using the elevator or getting off the bus a stop or two early. Walking is a way of keeping your mind off smoking as well as making you feel better keeping the weight off. Walking for 20 minutes at a steady pace three or four times a week is good for your body. If you're over the age of 40 years and have physical problems, check with your doctor before starting any exercise plan.

7. A partner who smokes can be very distressing when you're trying to quit. Ask your partner not to smoke around you and not offer you cigarettes. If you plan to buy your own cigarettes, the urge may pass before you arrive at the store.

8. Keep trying to quit. Most smokers try and fail several times before succeeding. It has been found that the more times a smoker has tried and failed to quit, the better the chance of success the next time (ALA, 1998).

9. There are a variety of ways to stop smoking. Most ex-smokers stop smoking "cold turkey" (immediate stoppage). Cutting back gradually doesn't seem to work as well as stopping abruptly, possibly because the smokers end up inhaling more deeply on the cigarettes they do smoke in order to keep their nicotine levels up.

10. If you're highly addicted, seek support programs. The American Lung Association and the American Cancer Society have support programs available.

11. Ask your non-smoking friends to give you positive support and praise for attempting to stop. If you fail, ask them to try giving you support again later.

12. All reminders of smoking such as lighters or ashtrays should be thrown out.

13. If you smoke at certain times, plan other activities during those times.

14. Try hypnotherapy.

Some additional tips for quitting are shown in Box 14.3, "Tips for Quitting."

The practitioner can use the following steps to encourage smoking cessation (Andrews, 1998; Lindell & Reinke, 1999).

1. *Ask.* The first step is to identify smokers. A routine question at each visit should address smoking behavior. The answer should be recorded along with the rest of the vital signs and should be easy to note by anyone looking at the chart. There are several tests that can be used to determine the degree of dependence. Interest in quitting should also be determined at each visit and assistance offered depending on responses.

2. *Advise.* Give straightforward information about the health risks, which can be personalized using information from the history and review of symptoms. Rewards of cessation, both physical and financial, can be mentioned. The importance of stopping can be related to the person's current state of health or illness. This information should be repeated as needed.

3. *Assist.* When the smoker is ready to quit, behavioral modification and an agreed-upon stop date should be discussed. Referrals to smoking cessation programs can also be made at this point. At all stages, support and encouragement is appropriate and necessary.

4. *Arrange follow-up.* This is a crucial aspect of care especially during the first 2 weeks of cessation due to the high relapse rates during this time.

The health care provider can also provide a list of suggestions for controlling cravings during the cessation process. An example would be to snack on carrot sticks, drink lots of cold water, go for long walks, dispose of all smoking equipment, and stay away from places where smoking is common.

CASE STUDY

Mary P., a practitioner in a community-based wellness program, plans to open a smoking cessation class to the public. She has completed the Freedom from Smoking course at the American Lung Association and studied hypnosis and behavior modification during her master's program.

Mary's first project would be a needs assessment of the patients attending her program and in the surrounding community and determine an ideal time for the classes.

1. In order to get the most students, what times might be good to offer the classes?

Box 14.3   Tips for Quitting

- Plan a quitting date that may have significance to you or that may just be a good time in your mind to quit.
- Take up knitting or fool with a coin or bead when your hands want to play.
- Change your routine. If you love an after-lunch cigarette, get right up from the table after eating instead of lingering.
- If you fear gaining weight, stock up on sugarless gum, mints, celery sticks, carrots, grapes, popcorn, and other low-calorie foods.
- Exercise instead of smoking and get more sleep so you won't feel tired when you quit smoking.
- Reward yourself by stashing away your cigarette money, and at the end of a week or two treat yourself to a little luxury. Think of what you want in terms of the cost in cigarettes.
- Request no-smoking sections in planes, restaurants, and trains.

---

2. How would Mary publicize the classes?

3. What questions would Mary ask the class about past attempts at smoking cessation? Would Mary expect that the class members were making their first attempts at smoking cessation?

4. What would Mary ask the class members about how smoking makes them feel?

5. What suggestions would Mary give about how to stop smoking?

6. What would be some of the concerns expressed by the class members that might affect their ability to stop smoking?

7. Discuss funding for the program. How would supplies be obtained and how could medications be obtained for support?

SUMMARY

Smoking is an addiction that causes short-term and long-term physical and psychological effects to the smoker. Cigarettes are costly to the individual and the country in terms of lost productivity and loss of life. Smoking-related diseases such as heart and vascular disease, lung disease, and cancer claim an estimated 430,000 American lives each year. Nicotine, the primary toxin in cigarettes, is a gateway drug to other drug use. In spite of these facts, approximately 3,000 young people begin using cigarettes every day.

There are several ways to assist the smoker to stop smoking. First, and foremost, the person must want to quit. If a person doesn't want to quit, another person cannot make the first person quit. The health care provider should give reasons why quitting is beneficial for the health of the person. The health care provider needs to be knowledgeable about the addictive qualities of tobacco/nicotine. By assisting the smoker with direct pharmacological as well as psychological support, the health care provider can provide appropriate care.

SMOKING CESSATION RESOURCES

The National Cancer Institute
9000 Rockville Pike, Building 31, 10A-24

Bethesda, MD 20892
(800) CANCER

National Health, Lung, and Blood Institute
Information Center
P.O. Box 30103
Bethesda, MD 20824-0105
(301) 251-1222

American Cancer Society
1599 Clifton Road
Atlanta, GA 30329
(800) ACS-2345

American Health Association National
Center
7272 Greenville Avenue
Dallas, TX 75321
(800) AHA-USA1

American Lung Association
1740 Broadway
New York, NY 10019-4272
(212) 315-8700; (800) LUNG-USA

Office on Smoking and Health Centers for
Disease Control and Prevention
Mail Stop K-50, 4770 Buford Hwy., N.E.
Atlanta, GA 30341-3724
(770) 448-5705; (800) CDC-1311; FAX
(770) 332-2552
Database on CD-ROM: (202) 783-3238

The American Lung Association (1991)
offers a variety of smoking cessation programs. These programs include smoking
cessation classes in the community and at
many area hospitals, hypnotherapy at variety of sites, Freedom from Smoking classes,
and smokers anonymous and nicotine
anonymous groups. Hospital-based support programs are often available through
the rehabilitation or wellness departments.

REFERENCES

Albanese, J. (2000). How can we reach teenage smokers? *Nursing Spectrum, 10*(11), 12–14.

Allen, S. S., Hats Kami, D. K., Christianson, D., & Nelson, D. (1999). Withdrawal and premenstrual symptomatology during the menstrual cycle in short-term smoking ab-stinence. *Nicotine and Tobacco Research, 1*(2), 129–142.

AMA News (Oct. 23, 2000). Articles question Joe Camel's success, influence on teen smoking. *Marketing News.*

American Association of Retired Persons. (1996). Smokeless tobacco under fire. *AARP Bulletin, 37*(6), 6–7.

American Lung Association. (1986). *Freedom from smoking.* American Lung Association.

American Lung Association. (1991). *Stop smok-ing: A guide to your options.* West Palm Beach, FL: American Lung Association.

American Lung Association. (1999). *Nicotine ad-diction and cigarettes.* West Palm Beach, FL: American Lung Association.

American Lung Association. (2000). *Tobacco fac-toids.* West Palm Beach, FL: American Lung Association.

Andrews, J. (1998). Optimizing smoking cessa-tion strategies. *The Nurse Practitioner, 23*(8), 47–67.

Ary, D. V., & Biglan, A. (1988). Longitudinal changes in adolescent cigarette smoking behavior onset and cessation. *Journal of Be-havioral Medicine, 11*(4), 361–382.

Battjes, R. J. (1988). Smoking as an issue in alcohol and drug abuse treatment. *Addictive Behaviors, 13,* 225–230.

Bennett, E. G., & Woolf, D. S. (Eds.). (1991). *Substance abuse: Pharmacologic, developmental, and clinical perspectives.* Albany, NY: Delmar.

Bobo, J. K. (1989). Nicotine dependence and alcoholism epidemiology and treatment. *Journal of Psychoactive Drugs, 21*(3), 323–329.

Bobo, J. K., & Davis, C. M. (1993). Cigarette smoking cessation and alcohol treatment. *Addiction, 88,* 405–412.

Dappen, A., Schwartz, R. H., & O'Donnell, R. (1996). A survey of adolescent smoking pat-terns. *Journal of the American Board of Family Practice, 9*(1), 7–13.

Evans, D., Levison, M. J., Feldman, C. H., Clark, N. M., Wasilewski, Y., Levin, B., & Mellins, R. B. (1987). The impact of passive smoking on emergency room visits of urban children with asthma. *American Review of Respiratory Diseases, 135*(3), 567–572.

Hays, J. T., Dale, L. C., Hurt, R. D., & Croghan, J. T. (1998). Trends in smoking related diseases. *Postgraduate Medicine, 104*(6), 56–66.

Hudmon, K. S., Gritz, E. R., Clayton, S., & Nisenbaum, R. (1999). Eating orientation, postcessation weight gain, and continued abstinence among female smokers receiving an unsolicited smoking cessation intervention. *Health Psychology, 18*(1), 29–36.

Lamkin, L., Davis, B., & Kamen, A. (1998). Rationale for tobacco cessation interventions for youth. *Preventive Medicine, 27*(5), P43, A3–8.

Leon, L., & Rosen, D. C. (1999). Smoking cessation—Developing a workable program. *Nursing Spectrum, 9*(7), 12–14.

Lindell, K. O., & Reinke, L. F. (1999). Nursing strategies for smoking cessation. *The American Nurse, 31*(2), A1–A8, 249–256.

Lynch, B. S., & Bonnie, R. J. (Eds.). (1994). *Growing up tobacco free.* Washington, DC: National Academy Press.

National Cancer Institute. (1993). *Cancer facts.* Washington, DC: Author. National Institutes of Health.

Osler, M., Prescott, E., Godtfredsen, N., Hein, H. O., & Schnohr, P. (1999). Gender and determinants of smoking cessation: A longitudinal study. *Preventive Medicine, 29,* 57–62.

Padula, C., & Willey, C. (1993). Tobacco withdrawal in CCU patients. *Applied Nursing Research, 12*(6), 305–312.

Perkins, K. A., Levine, M., Marcus, M., Shiffman, S., D'Amico, D., Miller, A., Kevins, A., Ashcom, J., & Broge, M. (2000). Tobacco withdrawal in women and menstrual cycle phase. *Journal of Consulting and Clinical Psychology, 68*(1), 176–180.

Pirkle, I. L., Flegal, K. M., Bernet, I. T., Brody, D. J., Etzel, R. A., & Maurer, K. R. (1996). Exposure of the U.S. population to environmental tobacco smoke: The third National Health and Nutrition Examination Survey, 1988 to 1991. *Journal of the American Medical Association, 275*(16), 1233–1240.

Ray, O., & Ksir, C. (1993). *Drugs, society, and human behavior* (6th ed.). St. Louis, MO: Mosby-Yearbook.

Rigotti, N. A. (1993). Why we must help parents stop smoking. *Respiratory Care, 38*(9), 982–984.

Stanislaw, A. E., & Wewers, M. E. ((1994). A smoking cessation intervention with hospitalized surgical cancer patients: A pilot study. *Cancer Nursing, 17*(2), 81–86.

Sullivan, E. J. (1995). *Nursing care of clients with substance use.* St. Louis, MO: Mosby.

U.S. Department of Health and Human Services. (1999a). *Healthy People 2010: National health promotion and disease prevention objectives* (Conference Ed.). Washington, DC: Author.

U.S. Department of Health and Human Services. (1999b). A report of the Surgeon General. Centers for Disease Control. Atlanta, GA: Author.

CHAPTER 15

Violence-Prevention Skills

Carolyn Chambers Clark

THE CAUSES AND EFFECTS OF VIOLENCE

The causes and nature of violence are complex, but social and environmental factors clearly play a major role. Every day in the United States, three children die of abuse and neglect. An estimated 3 to 4 million women are abused by their partners annually (Capaldo & Lindner, 1999), and 25% to 40% of all women in the United States have been physically assaulted by a spouse or male partner (Abner, 1995), and battering or abuse during pregnancy is a widespread problem (Campbell, 1998, 1999). For a free kit on domestic violence and child custody, visit the Website www.nowldef.org.

Two out of every five American households with children contain guns, and 25% of those guns are either loaded or unlocked. It's not surprising that 15 children are killed with guns in this country every day. Only 29% of parents with guns in their home believe that the most important message about gun safety is that "guns kept in the home kill family members more often than they kill in self-defense" (Sutherland,

1999). Violent crime has fallen faster in states where carrying concealed weapons (CCW) is strictly regulated or prohibited than in states with lax CCW laws (Handgun Progress Report, 1999).

Being a witness to a violent event can lead to trauma. Witnessing violence can create aggression, anxiety disorders such as acute and posttraumatic stress, relationship problems, and a disruption in the development of empathy (Osofsky, 1995). In one study of a major city, up to 90% of elementary school children witnessed violence and 33% witnessed a homicide (Groves, Zuckerman, Maran, & Cohen, 1993).

Violence is perpetuated when the victim identifies with the abuser and becomes violent. There may also be important connections between violence toward animals and violence toward humans. Violence toward animals is often predictive of violence toward humans. Companion animals, as well children and relatives, are often victims in battering situations (Ascion, 1996). You will need to work more closely with humane officers and animal cruelty personnel to report animal cruelty as a first step toward preventing battering (Capaldo & Lindner, 1999).

Physical violence often starts when individuals do not have the words to express their negative emotions. They must learn how to identify and give name to their feelings, and learn to listen. You can be instrumental in teaching communication skills that can defuse physical violence.

EMOTIONAL INTELLIGENCE PREVENTS VIOLENCE

Emotional intelligence is the ability to understand, manage, and express feelings to enhance learning, relationships, problem-solving, and adaptation to the demands of growth and development. Emotional intelligence includes self-awareness, control of impulsivity, cooperation with and caring for self and others. Behaviors that can enhance emotional intelligence, thereby reducing violence, are shown in Table 15.1.

COMMUNITY SERVICE PARTICIPATION

Recent research has demonstrated that participation in community youth service can reduce violence in the community (O'Donnell et al., 1999). The purpose of the study was to examine whether participation in a school-sponsored program could reduce self-reported violent behaviors among young urban adolescents. A total of 972 seventh- and eighth-grade students at two public middle schools were surveyed at baseline and 6 months later. The intervention school received the Reach for Health classroom curriculum, which includes a 10-lesson unit focused on violence prevention. Half of the students in the intervention school were also assigned by classroom to participate in analyses showed that eighth graders who participated in the Community Youth Service program had a statisti-

cally significant decrease in violent behavior. The eighth graders reported less violence at follow-up than their curriculum-only counterparts or students in the control school. Teaching young adolescents to become involved in community service can prevent their future violent acts.

COACHING YOUNG WOMEN TO SPOT AN ABUSIVE RELATIONSHIP

Thirty-three percent of teenagers experience physical violence in dating relationships, and 30% of young women who are murdered are killed by their husband or boyfriend. You can help prevent the violence faced by young women by coaching them on the 10 signs to watch for, listed in Box 15.1 (Spitzer, 1999).

HELPING SEXUAL ABUSERS REDUCE THEIR VIOLENT BEHAVIOR

Sex offenders are represented at every social, educational, occupational, and economic level. Only a small percentage are strangers; most are parents, grandparents, stepparents, siblings, relatives, friends and neighbors, and most are men. They are often considered untreatable.

Scheela (1999) described a program to help sex offenders stop their violent behavior. Steps in treatment included:

1. *Disclosure.* The offender states and writes down all the details of his abuse.
2. *Empathy document.* The offender writes about specific abuse episodes as if he were the victim, detailing the thoughts and feelings of his victim before, during, and right after, and possible lifelong effects.
3. *Apology letter.* The offender writes an apology to his victim(s) and decides whether to send the message or not.

TABLE 15.1   Emotional Intelligence

Behavior	Example Behavior
Validate infant's empathic response to another infant's cries.	"You're upset that Danny is crying."
Help children acknowledge their feelings.	"You're angry because the teacher scolded you."
(Grades 1–3)	Draw simple faces on paper that depict various emotions and write "I feel _____" under each face. Ask the children to fill in the blanks; then role-play situations that might evoke these emotions. Point to the face that describes how they feel and then say the words aloud.
(Grades 4–6)	Choose a feeling (e.g., pride) and talk about a time in your life when you felt proud and what made you feel that way. Encourage the children to share a time with a partner or you when they felt pride; then listener paraphrases the story; then roles are reversed.
(Grades 7–9)	Teach the children seven questions to ask to help others resolve conflicts: What is it you need? What do you think the problem is? Can you think of a way that we might solve this problem? Would you be happy with this solution? Do you both agree to this solution? Can we talk again to make sure the problem is really solved?
Enhance self-esteem and pride (Grades 1–3)	Write down all the child's good qualities; ask the child to make a similar list and choose a quality from the lists of which she/he is most proud; create a special name tag for the child to wear
(Grades 4–6)	Ask children to write their life stories, including doing research on the day they were born by interviewing family members
(Grades 7–9)	Ask each child to create a family tree by writing on the branches the names of people who have influenced his/her life in a positive way and their most admirable quality; have the child discuss how they have developed or can develop these qualities in himself/herself.
Teach children to respect differences.	
(Grades 1–3)	Start a pen-pal program with children different cultural, religious or political beliefs.
(Grades 4–6)	Ask students to search newspapers and magazines for images that challenge preconceived ideas about roles (nurse, doctor, car mechanic, model, police officer, dancer, criminal).
(Grades 7–9)	Ask students to (a) point out any stereotypes they see in the media; (b) write letters to companies that create ads using negative stereotypes; (c) create positive images to include in the letters.

(continued)

TABLE 15.1   *(continued)*

Behavior	Example Behavior
Teach children to care.	Help them start a garden.
	Teach children to respect all creatures by adopting an animal from a local shelter or by making a bird feeder.
	Teach children to respect the environment by visiting a national park, botanical garden, or nature park.
	Support their participation in a charitable event (walkathon or dance-athon) or in tutoring another child.
	Bring them to a local shelter or soup kitchen to volunteer.
	Help a child write a letter to protest unkind treatment or to voice support.
	Make a pact with a child to always say please and thank you.
Organize a "Kids Peace Day" to empower children. Teach them to work with others and to share what they've learned about peace and violence prevention.	Children become the teachers and providers of goods and the adults learn about peace from them.

Box 15.1   Spotting an Abusive Relationship

1. Your partner is jealous and possessive toward you.
2. Your partner tries to control you by being bossy and never considers your opinions.
3. Your partner scares you, making you afraid of how he will react to things you do or say.
4. Your partner has a quick temper and a history of violence toward others.
5. Your partner pressures you into doing things you do not want to do such as having sex or breaking the law.
6. Your partner abuses illegal drugs and alcohol.
7. Your partner blames you for his problems, including those he brings on himself.
8. Your partner has a history of bad relationships.
9. Your partner believes that men should take the lead in relationships and women should follow.
10. Your family and friends have warned you about your partner or have told you they are worried for your safety.

4. *Autobiography.* The man writes about his past including family of origin, education, occupation, military, marital, health, crimes, social and sexual development, and is encouraged to find patterns that contributed to his abuse.

5. *Abuse cycle.* The offender identifies how his thoughts and feelings led to abuse and kept it going. He pinpoints thought distortions, dysfunctional coping patterns, fantasies, control and abuse behaviors.

6. *Safety plan.* The man synthesizes what he has learned and develops a plan to prevent future abuse behaviors.

HELPING PARENTS REDUCE MALTREATMENT OF THEIR CHILDREN

There are few well-conducted and adequately controlled studies showing that abusive parenting can be changed by training (Stevenson, 1999). According to Wolfe and Wekerle (1993) parents who abuse their children have learning needs that, if met, can result in a reduction of violent behavior. These parents have learning needs in the following areas:

1. Reducing their distress and enhancing general coping behaviors.
2. Controlling anger and reactivity so they can stop reacting to child provocation.
3. Teaching, disciplining and appropriately stimulating their children.
4. Expanding their expectations of child behavior.
5. Reducing their dependence on alcohol, drugs, prostitution, and subcultural peer groups.
6. Increasing their social supports.

Several studies have demonstrated that when parents learn how to meet these needs, they are less abusive with their children (Gaudin, Wodarski, Arkinson, &

Avery, 1990; Irueste-Montes & Montes, 1988; Wolfe & Wekerle, 1981; Lutzker & Rice, 1984). Teaching parents these skills can be an important step toward reducing their violence.

GANG SUPPRESSION AND INTERVENTION

The National Youth Gang Suppression and Intervention Program developed policies and procedures to mobilize community efforts by police, prosecutors, judges, probation and parole officers, corrections officers, schools, employers, community-based agencies, and a wide range of grassroots organizations to stop violent gangs. Social disorganization and a lack of social opportunities largely account for gangs; and racism and deficiencies in social policy are also contributing factors (Spergel et al., 1996).

The first step in intervening in gang violence is to assess the problem. Representatives of criminal justice and community agencies, grassroots organizations, schools, churches, local businesses, and gangs should participate in describing the nature of violence and recommend appropriate solutions. A consensus must be developed.

Local councils or statutory commissions need to be established to set policy and coordinate programs. The community process goes through several stages before a program with positive impact can be developed. The list below shows the stages of community process and their identifying characteristics. Use it when participating in or leading a community process to reduce gang violence.

Stage	Indicants
Initial organizing	• Denial, initial organizing, and policymaking

Middle	• Goal and problem displacement
	• Community conflict
Third stage	• Charges of ineffective programs, institutional racisms, and corruptions
Moral leadership development	• Develop accountability to make sure the right programs are launched and the right youth are targeted for services

Local citizen leadership should be developed. A variety of organizing and management skills can be taught to this cadre of community members, including how to efficiently marshal pickets or persuade local legislators to vote for or against a particular gang-related measure; conduct meetings or interagency negotiations; and develop cooperative community group and agency agreements regarding gang programs.

When establishing goals and objectives for a program, make sure comprehensive strategies—remedial education, training, jobs, outreach services—are provided. Ensure that a balance is created between strategies focusing on individual or family change and those demanding system change such as the development of a local youth conservation corps. Long-term sustained efforts may be needed when vulnerable and hardcore youths are involved.

Some interventions that show promise include:

• Close supervision and possible incarceration of gang leaders and repeat offenders
• Remedial education for targeted youth gang members in middle school and job orientation, training, place-ment, and mentoring for older gang members
• Referring fringe members and their parents to youth services for counseling and guidance
• Using crisis intervention techniques to mediate gang fights
• Providing preventive services for youths who are at risk for joining gangs
• Patrolling community "hot spots"
• Safe zones around schools (Spergel et al., 1996).

A mobilized community is the best approach to gang problems. Consistent policies and communication result in greater social control and support and more effective targeting of the problem. Local leaders must be recruited and encouraged to participate so that racial and class conflicts are avoided or at least kept to a minimum.

Gang members must be held accountable for their criminal acts but also have opportunities to change or control violent behavior. Youth must also be taught the consequences of their actions.

Mobilizing a community to action requires cooperation and collaboration of key groups and activists. Care must be taken not to let community organizations focus on protecting their turf, rivalry, and conflict. Failure in community mobilization can occur due to insensitivity to community racial, ethnic, or class interests.

A community plan to reduce gang violence can only proceed when leaders are committed to the resolution of problem. The plan must be supported by key political and economic forces in the community and the developmental needs of local agency and community groups.

The police department may establish a gang detail or designate one or more officers as gang specialists. When working in the community, you must be able to network effectively with key political, economic, agency, and police leaders. A good start would be to meet with leaders in these organizations and let them know your violence prevention goals after learning theirs.

Gang members often bring their violence to schools. Many are bored with class and feel inadequate there and drop out of school as soon as they can. They never developed good learning skills and have experienced academic and social failure in school from an early age. They do not identify with teachers and staff and may distrust and dislike them intensely.

Schools can effectively control or suppress gang violence by developing a gang code with guidelines specifying appropriate response by teachers and staff to different kinds of gang behavior; keeping communication open between school personnel, parents, community agencies, and students; distinguishing between gang- and non-gang activity so as not to exaggerate the scope of the problem (Spergel et al., 1996).

One view of gang activity is that it fills the vacuum for youth who have been undertrained and underrehabilitated and systematically ignored or excluded from special education or work programs. Violence prevention activities must be forged in close cooperation with local businesses and must focus on school dropouts aged 16 to 24 to include remedial education, training, job placement, or employment and career development. A job bank should be created with the expectation of testing the hypothesis that young gang members can relinquish their roles in gangs and become hard-working, loyal, and productive members of the community.

To determine the effectiveness of grassroots projects dealing with gangs, use the following indicants: (a) the number of people who participate in projects; and (b)

whether community actions are associated with a decline or change in the character of the problem (Spergel et al., 1996).

HELPING PARENTS DEAL WITH THE EFFECTS OF TELEVISION VIOLENCE

Most American children spend more time watching television (21 to 30 hours a week) than participating in any other activity except sleeping (American Academy of Pediatricians, 1995). American television is the most violent in the world with 3 to 5 acts of violence per hour during primetime and 20 to 25 acts per hour during Saturday morning so-called children's programming. By age 18, most individuals have viewed 200,000 acts of violence on television (Dowell, 1998).

Although each child has a unique reaction to television programs, it is recommended that families do the following:

1. Limit television viewing to 2 hours per day.
2. Develop alternative activities with and for their children including reading, athletics, hobbies, art or other imaginative play.
3. Use a blocking device to block violent programs.
4. Explain and discuss the meaning of programs and commercials with children.
5. Encourage informed decision-making about violent programs.
6. Discuss television characters' motivation, making value judgements pointing out good and bad behavior.
7. Ask, "Is this real?" or "How is this different from what we do at home?" and "What would happen if you did that?"

CONFRONTING SCHOOL VIOLENCE

Children who are violent share a common profile (Tolnai, 1998; National School Safety Center, 1999; Skloot, 1998).

- They are male;
- have a troubled family environment, including their parents or other adults who help them acquire weapons;
- have witnessed or have been a victim of abuse or neglect;
- have had erratic harsh discipline, no reward for socially acceptable behavior, and a coercive style of parenting where they have learned that aggression pays off;
- have a history of tantrums and uncontrollable angry outbursts;
- habitually make violent threats when angry;
- have a background of drug, alcohol or other substance abuse or dependency;
- are preoccupied with weapons, explosives, or other incendiary devices;
- have previously been expelled from school;
- display cruelty to animals;
- have a poor relationship with peers, often feeling picked on or inferior, but a strong need to belong;
- strongly identify with violence: TV shows, movies, or music expressing violent themes and acts;
- tend to blame others for difficulties and problems;
- reflect anger, frustration, and the dark side of life in school essays or writing projects;
- are involved with a gang or antisocial group on the fringe of peer acceptance;
- are often depressed or have significant mood swings;
- have threatened or attempted suicide;
- have little or no support or supervision from parents or a caring adult;
- have been bullied or bully peers or younger children.

According to the National School Safety Center's Web site (http://www.nssc.org) these characteristics should serve to alert school administrators, teachers, and support staff to address the needs of troubled students through meetings with parents, school counseling, guidance and mentoring services, and referrals to appropriate health and social services and law enforcement personnel. Such behavior should also be an early warning signal for schools to plan crisis prevention and intervention procedures to protect the health and safety of other students and staff (Stewart, 1998; Skloot, 1998).

Culture may play a role in violence. For example, Hispanic students have a strong sense of group through their family ties and tend to express their violence in groups. Anglo children are more to be brought up with an emphasis on the individual. Their violence is more apt to manifest as individual versus individual or individual versus a group (Stewart, 1998).

Other factors contribute to violence in schools. The availability of guns, especially multiple-round arms, has increased. There has also been an increase in drug trafficking in the school setting (Stewart, 1998).

The following interventions may be helpful in addressing school violence:

1. Use parents as monitors and teacher's aides.
2. Hold regular meetings about violence issues.
3. Train staff in violence prevention, including identifying at-risk students and what to do during a crisis.

4. Offer extra help with schoolwork, providing referrals and listening to at-risk students.
5. Teach anger-management, appreciation of diversity, and mediation.
6. Share information with school personnel about children who fly off the handle easily, who have broken their wrists by striking walls, or who have unaddressed emotional or medical conditions (increasing frustration).
7. Train "security dads" to patrol, befriend students, and attend games or activities for kids who have no one to cheer them on.
8. Establish a culture that says, "Fighting and violence are not accepted here."
9. Teach age-appropriate skills in self-esteem development, stress management and reduction, and refusal skills to help youth resist drugs or alcohol.
10. Establish ongoing reward systems for good school citizenship and other incentives for good behavior.
11. Use a dress code and prohibit gang signs, shouting gang slogans, and writing gang slogans.
12. Consistently discipline students with punishment that escalates with the number or severity of infractions to demonstrate the school's seriousness.
13. Create a climate of ownership and school pride in students.
14. Establish a parents' center.
15. Make sure there is an active student component in all programs, including making the school welcoming and safe.
16. Establish collaborative partnerships and a school communication network (Schwartz, 1999; Stephens, 1994).

Parents can be taught the following violence prevention skills:

1. Enhance their child's frustration tolerance by saying no to their children and then serving as a role model by dealing calmly with the anger that might arise.
2. Encourage their children's participation in activities that provide adult supervision and focus on process not outcome, including choir, band, debate team, drama club, and sports.
3. Discuss television violence with their children, including pointing out that the long-term effects of violence are not shown.
4. Help their children identify the danger zones in schools and find ways to stay away from them.
5. Identify significant or sudden changes in their children's mood (irritability, anger), appearance (tattoos, body piercing, black lipstick, heavy makeup), or behavior (withdrawal, secretiveness, outbursts of violence, or involvement with the occult or hate groups).
6. Trust their evaluation: If they think something is wrong, seek help from a mental health professional and be persistent in finding someone who can teach the child new behaviors, not just medicate them.

PREVENTING WORKPLACE VIOLENCE

It is important to remember that the workplace is a microcosm of society, and violent behavior does not operate in a vacuum. A careful analysis of violent incidents reveals that they are often the culmination of long-standing, identifiable problems, conflicts, disputes, and failures. When materialism reigns, product is more important than people. This poisonous influence distances individuals from their feelings. To reduce workplace violence, policies must be the result of employee and employer collaboration and communication or they will result in scapegoating, denial and even violence (Braverman, 1999).

Sources of Organizational Stress

To prevent violence in the workplace, the sources of stress and strain must be identified first. Causes of workplace violence range from an accident that kills or maims to an episode or pattern of abuse or harassment to continuing stress from organizational restructuring. Organizational leaders who are prepared for crisis know that stress directly affects their employees and will be alert to the following danger signals:

- Conflicts occur between employees, including fights, threats, harassment, or breakdown in work group functioning
- An increasing diversity in the workforce that results in discrimination and sexual harassment claims
- Downsizing and restructuring occurs in a climate of disrespect without expressions of positive gratefulness for employee contributions
- Drug and alcohol abuse and even domestic violence occurs in the workplace
- Unstable and problematic employee and employer behavior is on the increase
- The workplace is a high-risk industry, including retail, transportation, and health care (Braverman, 1999).

Violence Prevention Plans

Once signs of a violence-prone organization are noted, and preferably before they are identified, the following steps need to be taken:

1. Support from the top must be enlisted.
2. Form a violence prevention team.
3. Perform a workplace violence-risk audit.
4. Develop policies and procedures for employees in collaboration with labor that are within the law on: what to report, to whom, and how to investigate reports of violence or threatened violence system-wide. (A referral through an established health care delivery network will not provide a system-level assessment and to provide medical, legal, security, and mental health information after a report has been made. If violence is imminent, take team action to contact law enforcement, secure the facility, notify potential targets, and arrange for surveillance of the threatening employee. may carry a threat of punishment.) Also have a commonsense procedure and policy for terminations and layoffs that respect the employee.
5. Conduct training in the policy and procedures, including how to approach an employee suspected of violent or self-destructive behavior. Conduct a face-to-face investigation, gathering all related information (including asking the employee for permission to talk to past treatment sources), informing the employee that company policy requires a danger-of-violence assessment and that information about that topic only will be shared with the employee and appropriate human resources, medical, and mental health representatives.

6. Establish violence education, assessment, and counseling that is employer managed and financed and nonpunitive.

Threat-of-Violence Assessment

The threat-of-violence assessment includes a process of gathering information and making appropriate decisions. An assessment proceeds step-by-step and involves (a) determining the risk, (b) establishing a "time-out" period, and (c) engaging the at-risk employee as an active willing participant in the process.

The information in Box 15.2 can be used to complete the assessment and decision-

making process once an at-risk individual has been identified.

TEACHING ANGER-CONTROL SKILLS

Violence is the acting out of anger. Learning communication skills can help reduce the tendency to act out anger. Rules that need to be learned and practiced include the following:

1. I can take a time-out when I feel myself getting angry. I can make a contract with myself to take a time-out. Simply

---

Box 15.2 Threat-of-Violence Assessment and Decision-Making Process

Determination of risk

Has a weapon been displayed?
Has clear intent or a plan been expressed?
Does the individual have the means to carry out the plan?
How imminent is the threat?

Involvement of employee in assessment phase

Defer decisions; put employee on leave with pay.
Ask the individual to be an active, willing participant, and to meet with a manager and a middle manager or human resource representative.
Explain that no decision will be made until the conclusion of fact findings and that he/she is innocent until proven guilty.
Explain the assessment process and demystify and explain any contact with professionals.
Any mental health professional must understand workplace issues and be willing to deal with employees in the context of their work environment.
Examine multiple sources of information: the employee's words, other employees with relevant information, medical and personnel records (obtain employee's informed consent).
Questions to be answered include:
Where is the record of discipline for past problems?
Where is the documentation of performance or claims for medical disability?
What is the history of changes, morale issues, or complaints in the work unit?
What is known about what else may be going on in the employee's life?

walking away when I'm angry will not work unless there is a clear communication to the other person: "I'm upset. I'm going to leave before I hurt someone or break something. I will return when I can talk without losing my temper." The angry person should go to a safe place to calm down. Taking a brisk walk, drinking a cup of chamomile tea, reading an interesting book, or listening to a relaxation tape can help.

2. I can practice prevention by learning to relax. Listening to relaxation tapes and learning relaxation skills will help reduce body tension and the tendency to get angry. Some quick relaxers include softening my eyes, breathing abdominally, tightening a few muscles then relaxing them, thinking relaxing thoughts ("I am not going to let this upset me," and "I can stay in control and keep relaxed").

3. I can quit trying to control other people. I can let go of an idea and not argue. Some ideas for loosening control that I will use include: Forget about trying to make everyone agree with me; learn to say what I have to say once and only once. Realize that difference is good; accept it. Make requests, not demands and threats. Never ask a yes-no question unless I can accept the answer. Learn to live with other people's choices. Be grateful if I get what I want by asking for it; be polite even if I don't get what I want.

4. I can reward people when they do what I want. I can reward people when they do what I want by praising them, giving monetary rewards or food, letting them use something I have, doing something for them in return for their doing what I want; by being understanding and just simply listening to what someone else has to say.

5. I can speak softly and not curse. I don't have to shout or swear to get what I want.

6. I can take responsibility for everything I say or do. I can stop saying, "You make me angry," and start saying, "I'm making myself angry." I can begin every day by vowing to respect other people. I can pay attention to others and begin to praise out loud whatever I like. I can avoid calling people names and let others take the responsibility for their own choices. I can stop giving others the silent treatment and speak up about my anger and find solution to the problem.

7. I can tell others what bothers me in a direct, specific, and polite manner.
   (a) I can be direct: "I'm angry because we agreed you'd do the dishes and they're still in the sink." (I can avoid lectures, angry silence, and guilt: "If you loved me you would . . . ").
   (b) I can be specific. "Please close the door when you're playing CDs."
   (c) I can be polite and avoid being rude or crude. I can respect other people even when angry.

8. I can use *I* Statements. An *I* statement has three parts: Voicing a specific behavior that bothers me ("You spent the car payment money on clothes"); reporting the feeling experienced ("I feel angry and afraid"); requesting a change in behavior ("I want you take the clothes back right now").

9. I can challenge irrational thoughts that keep me angry.
   (a) I can avoid "awfulizing" by refusing to turn disappointments into disasters. I can ask: "If this were the last day of my life, would this really matter?" Or "Compared to the worst thing that's ever happened to me, how does this rate?"
   (b) I can avoid demonizing by refusing to blame other people just because they disagree with me.

(c) I can realize the world is neither good nor bad, it just is.
(d) No matter what my background, I'm responsible for how I behave.
(e) I will refuse to make excuses and realize I can and will control my anger.
(f) I can avoid blaming past experiences for current anger.
(g) Just because someone asks me to do something doesn't mean they're bossing me; I can say no if I want to.
(h) I can challenge my own ideas that make me angry because I'm in charge of what I think.

10. I can prevent resentment.
(a) I can stick to the issue and not bring in old hurts.
(b) I can ask myself what the problem is and figure out what to do to fix it.
(c) I can get help if I need it.
(d) I am responsible for my own happiness.

11. I can quit raging by learning to forgive.
(a) I realize that forgiving is choice.
(b) I forgive for the sake of my own health, not for the other person.
(c) I can decide to forgive somebody, realizing it takes time.
(d) I can forgive myself for all the hate I've been carrying around, for wasting years of my life resenting others, and for the stupid things I've done in the name of hate.
(e) I can make a list of people I need to forgive, including myself.
(f) I can write down the reasons I need to forgive people, how forgiving them will help me, how my hatred is hurting me, and what the result of all this hate has been.
(g) I can list the angry thoughts I have most often.
(h) I can list the things I do because of my hate (make late night calls and hang up, start rumors, put sugar in their gas tank, avoid them, etc.).
(i) I can make a promise to stop hateful thoughts and actions, and begin with one or two people on my list.
(j) I can write down two or three good things about each person I resent.
(k) I can pray for them, send angels to help them, or think of one nice thing that could happen to them (Potter-Efron, 1994).

Three UNICEF Websites that may be of use to you or your clients are:

UNICEF. Respect differences. [On-line]. Accessed 8/8/99. Available: http://www.unicefusa.org/issues96/sep96/guide/talking.html.

UNICEF. Try talking it out. [On-line]. Accessed 8/8/99. Available: http://www.unicefusa.org/issues96/sep96/guide/friend.html.

UNICEF. Love yourself. [On-line]. Accessed 8/8/99. Available: http://www.unicefusa.org/issues96/sep96/guide/build.html

REFERENCES

Abner, C. (1995). Battering in the womb. *Massachusetts Psychological Association Quarterly, 38*(4), 8.

American Academy of Pediatricians. Committee on communications, children, adolescents and television. *Pediatrics, 96*, 786–787.

Ascione, F. T. (1993). Children who are cruel to animals: A review of research and implications for developmental psychopathology. *Anthrozoos, 1*(4), 226–247.

Braverman, M. (1999). *Preventing workplace violence: A guide for employers and practitioners.* Thousand Oaks, CA: Sage.

Call, L. (1999). Emotional intelligence in children. *Prevention Forum, 19*(3), 16–17.

Campbell, J. C. (1998). *Empowering survivors of abuse: Health care, battered women and their children.* Thousand Oaks, CA: Sage.

Campbell, J. C. (1999). If I can't have you no one can: Murder linked to battery during pregnancy. *Reflections, 25*(3), 8–12.

Capaldo, T., & Lindner, L. (1999). Resensitizing society: Understanding the connection between violence toward human and non-human animals. *The Forensic Examiner, 8*(7, 8), 28–30.

DeAngelis, T. (1995). Research documents trauma of abuse. *Monitor: Journal of the American Psychological Association, 26*(4), 34.

Dowell, D. L. (1998). Effects of television on children: A review of the literature and recommendations for nurse practitioners. *The American Journal for Nurse Practitioners, 2*(1), 31–37.

Gaudin, J. M., Wodarski, J. S., Arkinson, M. K., & Avery, L. S. (1990). Remedying child neglect: Effectiveness of social network interventions. *Journal of Applied Social Sciences, 15,* 97–123.

Groves, B. M., Zuckerman, B., Maran, S., & Cohen, D. (1993). Silent victims: Children who witness violence. *Journal of the American Medical Association, 269*(2), 262–263.

Gun Control Progress Report. (1999). A look at the states. p. 2. Author.

Irueste-Montes, A. M., & Montes, F. (1988). Court-ordered vs. voluntary treatment of abusive and neglectful parents. *Child Abuse and Neglect, 12,* 33–39.

Lutzker, J. R., & Rice, J. M. (1984). Project 12-ways: Measuring outcome of a large in-home service for treatment and prevention of child abuse and neglect. *Child Abuse and Neglect, 8,* 519–524.

National School Safety Center. [On-line]. Accessed 1999, August. Available: http://www.nss1.org/reporter/checklist.htm.

O'Donnell, L., Stueve, A., Doval, A. S., Duran, R., Atnafou, R., Haber, D., Johnson, N., Murray, H., Grant, U., John, G., Tang, J., Bass, J., & Piessens, P. (1999). Violence prevention and young adolescents' participation in community youth service. *Journal of Adolescent Health, 24*(1), 28–37.

Osofsky, J. (1995). The effects of exposure to violence on young children. *American Psychologist, 50*(9), 786.

Potter-Efron, R. (1994). *Angry all the time: An emergency guide to anger control.* Oakland, CA: New Harbinger.

Scheela, R. (1999). Sex offenders with guts to change. *Reflections, 25*(3), 13–15.

Schwartz, W. An overview of strategies to reduce school violence. [On-line]. Accessed 1999, August. Available: http://eric-eb.tc.columbia.edu/digests/dig115.htm

Skloot, R. (1998). Violence in the schools: History, evolution and prevention. *Prevention Forum, 19*(1), 6–8.

Spergel, I., Chance, R., Ehrensaft, K., Regulus, T., Kane, C., Laseter, R., Alexander, A., & Oh, S. (1996). *Gang suppression and intervention: Community models.* Washington, DC: U.S. Department of Justice.

Spitzer, E. (1999). Spotting an abusive relationship. [On-line]. Accessed 1999, August. Available: http://www.oag.state.ny/us/family/warnings.

Stephens, R. D. (1994). Planning for safer and better schools. *School Violence Prevention, 23*(2), 204–215.

Stevenson, J. (1999). The treatment of the long-term sequelae of child abuse. *Journal of Child Psychology and Psychiatry, 40*(1), 89–111.

Stewart, M. (1998, September/October). RNs confront causes, consequences of school violence. *The American Nurse,* 16–17.

Sutherland, M. W. (1999, February 22). The killing fields: Our schools, small towns and the suburbs. *The Nursing Spectrum,* 16–17.

Tolnai, E. (1998). Research update: Childhood aggression. *Prevention Forum, 19*(1), 17–18.

Wolfe, D. A., Kaufman, K., Aragona, J., & Sandler, J. (1981). *The child management program for abusive parents: Procedures for developing a child abuse intervention program.* Winter Park, FL: Anna Publishing.

Wolfe, D. A., & Wekerle, C. (1993). Treatment strategies for child physical abuse and neglect—a critical progress report. *Clinical Psychology Review, 13,* 473–500.

CHAPTER 16

Environmental Wellness

Carolyn Chambers Clark

ENVIRONMENTAL WELLNESS: A HOLISTIC PERSPECTIVE

When a part of the world is harmed, everything within the whole is affected. Operating from this view means you include the broader environment as client. It is insufficient to suggest health care treatment after exposure to hazardous materials. The issue of a nearby toxic dump, unsafe water, and other environmental problems must also be addressed.

Being a holistic practitioner in this broader view includes:

- learning everything you can about community environmental problems, including who knows about the problem, its history, level of threat, research outcomes, popular literature, expert opinion, stories of those being affected, regulatory guidelines, jurisdiction, and what has already been tried
- helping to ensure that the by-products of your processes and services do not adversely affect environmental quality
- assisting regulatory agencies in assessing the effect of all synthetically

produced chemicals on overall health and wellness

- influencing the systematic management of waste so the quality of life is enhanced
- taking a stand against the disturbance of natural ecosystems that keep infectious organisms and disease vectors in check
- taking action to enhance sustainable economic development (as opposed to unbridled growth) including: stabilizing world population, reversing deforestation, cleaning up the world's water supply, and reducing the billions of tons of toxic wastes added to the atmosphere yearly
- undertaking research or political efforts to ensure more money is spent on the study of chemical interactions with living things and the environment (Schuster, 1997).

MAJOR ENVIRONMENTAL ISSUES

The environment is pivotal to health and wellness. Twenty-five to 33% of the global burden of ill health can be attributed to environmental factors. Environmental health and wellness actions include promoting safe conditions that enhance well-being and protect individuals from environmental factors that may adversely affect their level of wellness.

Children under 5 years of age bear the largest burden of environmental threats (Smith, Corvalan, & Kjellstrom, 1999). Fourteen million American children between the ages of 7 and 17 live in poverty, with no electricity, no toilets, and in unsafe environments (Free, 1999). According to Theresa Kilbane of UNICEF (1999) improving the environment of these children includes:

- Security of tenure. Many children and their families live under the threat of eviction or forced removal because title to the land they live on is illegal.
- Safe location. Children should live away from open sewers, mudslides, and other dangerous hazards. Access to health centers, schools and safe play places must be found.
- Safe and sufficient water and sanitary removal of waste.
- Food storage and cooking facilities that keep food safe from spoilage and infestation by animals or insects and are properly ventilated.
- Houses built with safe construction materials that are moisture-proof, well-ventilated, and easy to clean and that will not harbor rodents and insects.
- A living environment that meets everyone's needs for privacy, reachability, and observability (of young ones by their parents).

Environmental safety is an important issue for children. Because of their patterns of exposure and their biological vulnerability, children are highly susceptible to injury from these exposures. As a health and wellness promotion professional, you are in a unique position to help:

- assess patterns of children's exposure to hazardous chemicals from hazardous waste disposal sites
- quantify children's vulnerability to environmental toxicants
- assess causal associations between environmental exposures and disease
- empower community members to protect their children from potential injury

Three to 4 million children and adolescents in the United States live within 1 mile of a designated Superfund hazardous waste disposal site and are at risk of exposure to toxic chemicals released from these sites into air, groundwater, surface water, and surrounding communities (Smith et al., 1999).

Adults are also at risk. More than 19 million individuals, 44% of whom are 50 or older, live in manufactured housing or mobile homes. Yet the current legislation fails to address safety, quality, and warranty protections. Current federal standards for the manufacture of mobile homes are not adequately enforced nationwide, yet three fourths of owners have had significant problems with their mobile home (Mobile-home bills need more teeth, 1999).

As a wellness facilitator, you can help these individuals obtain healthier living facilities. Provide the following toll-free numbers to call:

- The U.S. Department of Housing and Urban Development (800) 927-2891
- The Federal Trade Commission (877) 382-4357.

Air Pollutants

Air quality is a major factor in environmental wellness. Air pollution is correlated with a rise in the overall death rate from respiratory and cardiovascular diseases. Worsening of lung function and other symptoms occur when air quality falls, and this leads to an increase in the number of health care visits and hospitalizations (Ballester, Tenias, & Perez-Hoyos, 1999).

The burning of hospital wastes is a major source of air pollution near medical centers. The technology for clean disposal of hazardous wastes has existed for years, including the conversion of the remains to recycled products. For more information on one type of environmentally sound technology visit the Web site *http://www.star-tech.net.*

With the increased use of air-conditioning, potentially severe airborne diseases have emerged. One way to counteract this danger is to use high-efficiency filters and low-risk components in air-conditioning systems (Parat, Perdrix, & Baconnier, 1999).

A common danger in home and in many other settings is secondhand tobacco smoke. Use the following facts to inform clients and to work for smoke-free policies in your community:

- Secondhand smoke causes lung cancer and an estimated 3,000 deaths a year in healthy nonsmokers (30 times as many lung cancer deaths as all regulated air pollutants combined).
- Secondhand smoke is responsible for other respiratory problems in non-smokers including coughing, phlegm, chest discomfort, reduced lung function, and reddened, itching, watering eyes.

- More than 4,000 chemical compounds have been identified in tobacco smoke with at least 43 that are known to cause cancer in humans or animals.
- At high exposure levels, nicotine is a potent and potentially lethal poison; secondhand smoke is the only source of nicotine in the air.
- More than 90% of Americans favor restricting or banning smoking in public places.
- Forty-six states and the District of Columbia in some manner restrict smoking in public places (Centers for Disease Control and Prevention [CDC], 1993).

Food Toxins

During the 21st century, foodborne diseases can be expected to increase, especially in developing countries, due to environmental and demographic changes, climatic changes, changes in microbial and other ecological systems, and decreasing freshwater supplies. The increasing age of human populations, unplanned urbanization, and migration and mass production of food due to population growth and changed food borne habits will also result in the degradation of sanitation and the immediate human environment. Mass tourism and international trade is causing foodborne and feedborne pathogens to spread transnationally. As new toxic agents are identified and new toxic effects recognized, the health and trade consequences of toxic chemicals in food will also have global implications (Kaferstein & Abdussalam, 1999).

In August 1999, the U.S. Environmental Protection Agency announced a partial ban on the use of the broad-spectrum insecticide methyl parathion, targeting foods commonly eaten by children, including all fruits, carrots, fresh peas and beans, and tomatoes. This insecticide is neurotoxic to humans and kills birds, aquatic life, and honey bees.

The action was the EPA's first major step under the Food Quality Protection Act of 1996. Methyl parathion will continue to be allowed on corn, oats, rice, soybeans, sugar beets, wheat, potatoes, and other foods (EPA Fact Sheet, 1999).

Some of the steps to take personally and with clients include:

- Growing at least some portion of your own food
- Choosing organically grown local foods whenever possible
- Asking the EPA to prohibit the use of dangerous pesticides on all foods

Soil and Water Contaminants

Copper in tap water has caused numerous gastrointestinal symptoms and a series of severe systemic diseases including liver cirrhosis. All symptoms were correlated with copper plumbing in the home. Pathologically high concentrations of non-ceruloplasmin-bound copper in serum or elevated copper levels were found in the urine. The researchers concluded that copper poisoning must be considered as a possible cause of chronic gastrointestinal diseases in communities in which copper plumbing is common (Eife et al., 1999; Stenhammar, 1999).

Heavy metal and parasite contamination of drinking water is a major concern. Bringing drinking water to a rolling boil for 1 minute will kill most harmful bacteria and parasites. Another method is to install a counter-top distiller that boils water and then condenses the vapor. A distiller will eliminate most minerals, including arsenic, but may not eliminate some other chemicals. An under-the-sink system that uses reverse osmosis can remove many contaminants, including industrial chemicals, nitrates, toxic metals (e.g., barium and chromium), and lead. Faucet-mounted water filters can eliminate lead and chlorine byproducts (e.g., chloroform) and improve the taste of drinking water, but will not all remove parasites. In either case, it is important to change filters as advised by the manufacturer.

The government has long required public water utilities to test for a long list of natural and human-made pollutants. As of 1999, a new federal law requires water utilities serving more than 10,000 people to send an annual report directly to their customers that includes exactly what is in drinking water when it leaves a treatment plant and whether it approaches government safety levels. If a water utility serves fewer than 10,000 people, this information will be available at a public library or in a local newspaper. Pollutants of special concern include:

- **Arsenic:** At its current level of 50 mcg per liter, it carries a lifetime cancer risk from 1 in 1,000 to as high as in 100, according to the National Research Council. If water has an arsenic level higher than 10 mcg/l, use a water distiller, the only product currently certified to remove this pollutant.
- **Chlorination by-products:** Chlorination reacts with organic matter to produce chloroform and triholmethanes, suspected carcinogens. The current government safety limit is 80 mcg/l. Pregnant women or those planning a pregnancy should drink filtered water to reduce the risk of miscarriage and install a water filter on showers to re-

duce the amount of chlorine absorbed through the skin.

- **Cryptosporidium:** This parasite was responsible for the largest outbreak of disease from a contaminated water supply. Although healthy adults recover, this parasite can be fatal to 50% of those diagnosed with cancer or HIV/AIDS.
- **Lead:** Lead, lead-soldered pipes, and some brass faucets can add lead to water supply that left the treatment plant lead-free, and fluoride added to drinking water may increase the absorption of lead (Masters, 1999; Frazer, 1999).

To find a certified testing laboratory near you, call the Environmental Protection Agency's Safe Drinking Water Hotline at (800) 426-4791 or visit the EPIA Web site at *www.epa.gov/safewater*. If the lead level is more than 15 parts/billion, filter drinking water ("Fit to drink," 1999).

The chlorine added to drinking water in the United Stated has produced dramatic reductions in waterborne diseases such as typhoid fever. But other dangers may be lurking. Statistical analysis and metanalysis of well-designed studies indicate that drinking chlorinated water is correlated with a 21% greater risk of bladder cancer and a 38% greater risk of rectal cancer than drinking nonchlorinated water (Fackelmann, 1992).

Spread of Infectious Disease

Infectious diseases are the third leading cause of death in the United States, and the leading cause worldwide (Binder et al., 1999). A major source of infectious disease spread is human feces. One of the most common parasites spread in this manner is the roundworm. The common cold can be spread by touching the hand of an in-

fected person and then touching the face or eyes, letting the organisms gain entrance into the body. The spread of both organisms can be better controlled by:

- washing the hands after exposure to organisms
- using only safe drinking water,
- excluding or segregating ill individuals,
- routine cleaning of work or play objects,
- separation of food-handling from bathrooms or diaper-changing areas,
- cleaning all exposed surfaces (e.g., bathrooms, diaper-changing kitchens) after each use.

Changes in animal production practices (increasing the number of animals raised per unit area, automated animal feeding, and the use of antibiotics to increase animal growth rates have introduced new risks to animal handlers. Risks to the meat-eating population have also increased as bacteria become more resistant to antibiotics.

Bacteria live on and in the human body in astonishing numbers. Most are harmless, some even help digest food. Use of broad-spectrum antibiotics can wipe out microbial competition, leaving the strong, resistant bacteria behind to multiply unchecked. Modern travel and trade mean contact with resistant pathogens are a handshake, hospital visit or airplane ride away. Antibiotics now used on fruits trees can encourage the growth of resistant bacteria that end up in the stomach. Another source of antibiotic resistance is drug overuse in livestock. Antibiotics and resistant bacteria can enter waterways in manure runoff. Fluoroquinolones, a new class of antibiotics, were approved by the Food and Drug Administration in 1995 for use in poultry drinking water. Now, turkeys and chickens are turning up in U.S. supermarkets harboring Campylobacter, the most common cause of foodborne disease that is resistant to Fluoroquinolones. If farmers were encouraged to provide cleaner barns, better feed and more floor space per animal, the need for antibiotic use during animal production would be lessened.

Misuse of antibiotics by humans is another cause of pathogen resistance. The Center for Disease Prevention estimates that some 50 million of the 150 million outpatient prescriptions for antibiotics every year are unnecessary (www.cdc.gov/ncidod/ar; www.healthsci.tufts.edu/apua).

Take action to retard the growth of antibiotic-resistant pathogens and encourage clients to:

- Avoid asking for antibiotics for nonspecific and viral illness.
- Wash all raw fruits and vegetables thoroughly, and wash hands before and after preparing food.
- Choose meat that's labeled "no antibiotics used," such as 100% certified organic.
- Eat less or no meat, poultry and animal products.
- Avoid the use of antibacterial soaps and other products containing triclosan (Microban) unless treating a serious illness.
- Write the Federal Drug Administration to stop sub-therapeutic use of antibiotics in livestock (Commissioner, U.S. Food & Drug Administration, 5600 Fishers Lane, Room 1471, Rockville, MD 20857).

Genetically-Engineered Foods are another threat to the food supply and infectious disease survival. Long-term studies on the safety of genetically-engineered (GE) foods have not been conducted. GE foods could create superweeds, increase pesticide resistance and harm nontarget species that help maintain global balance. The Monarch butterflies are already suffering. There is no law that forces food producers to provide information about which foods have been genetically-engineered, but they are already on the shelves, in powdered milk, some cookies and candy bars, and soybean products (Ikramuddin, 1999). Make your opinions about this procedure known. For a sample letter, see www.mothers.org.

Global climate change due to greenhouse effect is hypothesized to change the prevalence and spread of infectious disease, also (Chan et al., 1999). Emissions from automobiles are believed to be the single greatest contributor to the greenhouse effect and global warming. As wellness role model, you can do your part to lower car emissions by carpooling, make your next car an electric model and walking or bicycling to your destination whenever possible and encouraging clients to follow your example. Up to 90 percent of the energy used in washing clothes goes to heating the water; do your wash in cold water since it doesn't affect cleaning.

Radiation and Electromagnetic Fields

Cell phones and other wireless devices and motorized items produce radiation and electromagnetic hazards. One study (Li et al., 1999) concluded that certain intensities of 50 Hz magnetic fields can act as cancer promoters, be additive with other promoters in cancer promotion, or both.

Cellular phones emit about 800–900 mHz of microwave radiation. Newer personal communication systems, which give off 1,800 to 2,000 mHz of radiation will soon be replacing cellular phones ("Cell phone risks still undetermined," 1997). Besides being potentially linked with cancer, cell phones create a ninefold increase in fatal collisions (see Accidents section of the chapter) and interfere with external pacemakers (Trigano, Azoulay, Rochdi, & Campillo, 1999).

Radon is an odorless, colorless gas produced by the breakdown of uranium in soil, rock, and water. Because radon is a gas, it can enter buildings through openings or cracks in the foundation. The gas deteriorates into radioactive solids that attach to dust particles in the air. Once inhaled, these solids have been linked with lung cancer. Contact the EPA's National Radon Hotline (1-800-SOS-RADON) for information.

In June 1999, the U.S. National Institute of Environmental Health Sciences (NIEHS) decided there was sufficient evidence to consider the invisible electromagnetic fields created by power lines and electric appliances as possible human carcinogens. With no federal funds on the horizon, NIEHS will do no further research (Olden, 1999). Action from environmentally minded individuals is needed to continue research funding.

Studies have linked childhood leukemia to electric and magnetic fields in the house but not to power lines (Green et al., 1999). A Norwegian study linked magnetic fields to breast cancer (Kliukiene et al., 1999), and electric utility workers are also at risk (Kheifets et al., 1999).

Because many household object emit far stronger fields than the 2 mG designation linked with higher cancer risk, it may be wise to call your power company to have your house measured. Their representative will recommend ways to reduce EMF emissions if necessary.

Toxic Chemical Exposure

Toxic chemical exposures occur in buildings that don't have adequate ventilation and occur as "off-gassing," or evaporation, from PVC vinyl (plastics) and paints. Pesticides are another ubiquitous source of toxic chemicals.

Sick Building Syndrome

Sick building syndrome occurs when there are too many environmental toxins and insufficient ventilation. One method of reducing the symptoms from sick building syndrome is to place plants in strategic places. Keeping a window open in the bedroom or office can also help, and certain plants can reduce toxic emissions: Boston fern, chrysanthemum, ficus, Peace lily, corn plant, dwarf date palm, dracaena marginata, English ivy, warneckei, and Gerber daisy (Sick Building Syndrome, 1994; "Plants as purifiers," 1994). Box 16.1 provides a list of nontoxic household cleaners.

PVC Plastics

Polyvinyl chloride (PVC) is a toxic substance and is widely used in flooring, wallcoverings, countertops, miniblinds, water pipes and windowframes. The manufacture and incineration of PVC create dioxins, which are known human carcinogens and are also linked to reproductive and immune disorders and respiratory disease (Huang et al., 1997; Rhomberg, 1998; Du & Wang, 1998; Beach et al., 1997). PVC off gasses phthalate plasticizers into the air. One class, DEHP, has been classified by the EPA as a probable human carcinogen and has produced damage to the heart, liver, kidneys, and reproductive systems in animal tests.

Choose natural linoleum (made with wood resin), cork flooring, or ceramic tiles as alternatives to vinyl flooring, and use cotton drapes or other natural-fiber materials at windows. Avoid wallpapers that contain plastics.

Box 16.1   Nontoxic Household Cleaners*

To clean drains: Pour 1 cup of washing soda or 1 cup of baking soda down drain; for maintenance, do weekly. (Commercial brands have toxic gases and caustic ingredients, including lye that can burn eyes and skin.)

To clean clogged drains: Mix vinegar, salt and baking soda, and pour down drain.

To clean wood furniture: Mix 1/4 cup vinegar (indefinite shelf life; odor dissipates in 1 hour) or lemon juice and a few drops of olive oil; use with a wool cloth that has static electricity to attract dust. (Commercial wood cleaners contain volatile organic compounds such as formaldehyde and petroleum distillates.)

To polish wood furniture: Rub a small chunk of beeswax into the wood then buff with soft cotton cloth; use hair dryer on low to soften hard beeswax. (Wood sealants have volatile organic compounds, including formaldehyde and solve-based products.)

To clean clothes instead of dry cleaning: Wash in cold water by hand; the agitator in washing machines causes fabric to shrink. (The perchlorehylene used in dry cleaning is a neurotoxin.)

Air freshener: Dissolve 2 tablespoons of baking soda in 2 cups of hot water and spray. This has an indefinite shelf life. (Many commercial air fresheners contain dichlorobenzene, a chemical that concentrates in body fat and is toxic to the central nervous system, kidneys, and liver.)

Mold-killing spray: Pour 2 teaspoons of tea tree oil (an essential oil available in health food stores) in 2 cups of water, shake vigorously and spray. (The commercial brands can be ripe with toxic gasses while tea tree oil is a powerful antifungal essential oil.)

Antiseptic spray: 1 teaspoon essential oil of lavender in 2 cups of water. (Essential oil don't promote the growth of drug-resistant bacteria like triclosan-based disinfectant and antibacterial soaps do.)

Oven cleaner: Sprinkle one box of baking soda on the bottom of the oven and spray with water until very damp. Spray every few hours and let sit overnight. In the morning, scoop out the baking soda and rinse the oven well. (Commercial oven cleaners have toxic fumes.)

Sink, tub, shower, counter-top cleaner: Place 1/2 cup of baking soda in a bowl and slowly pour in enough liquid soap to make a frosting-like consistency. Add 5 to 10 drops of rose or lavender essential oil if desired. Scoop the creamy mixture onto a sponge, wash the surface, and rinse. (Will dry out so only make as much as needed at the time.) As an alternative, use 1/2 cup of borax in a gallon of warm water.

Box 16.1 *(continued)*

Head lice: Lather hair with coconut-oil castile soap and work in a few drops of tea tree oil and neem oil. Rinse and rewash with the same ingredients. Do not rinse the second time. Instead, wrap a towel around the head for half an hour. Comb with a nit-removing comb, strand by strand. Dampen hair as needed. Wash and rinse the hair. Once dry, check thoroughly for any missed nits. Clean the comb, hands, bedding, and clothing. Put pillows in the freezer overnight to kill nits. (Commercial brands use pesticides, including lindane.)

*Adapted from Annie Berthold-Bond's Web site: *www.betterbasics.com*.

Paints

The smell of fresh paint comes from the evaporation, or off-gassing, of toxic petro-chemical solvents known as volatile organic compounds (VOCs). These include xylene, formaldehyde, toluene, and benzene, which are known carcinogens or neuro-toxins.

Look for paints labeled low-biocide or VOC-free. For the most chemically sensitive individuals, use milk paints and white-washes. Avoid using them in areas exposed to damp, or add vinegar to retard mold and mildew. When painting, keep windows open. Most paints take 6 weeks to fully dry and off-gas. Pregnant women and individuals with asthma or allergies should stay out of the painted areas for 6 weeks.

Houses built before 1978 (about 60 million in the U.S.) probably contain leaded paint. The National Lead Information Center and Clearinghouse (800-LEAD-FYI) lists EPA-certified Labs and licensed removal specialists where paint chips can be sent for testing. If lead is detected, seal the room off from the rest of the house during removal and wet-mop all dust with trisodium phosphate. Only High Energy Particulate filters can be used and children's toys must be washed with detergent and rinsed well (Pennybacker, 1999).

Formaldehyde

Formaldehyde is an eye, nose, and throat irritant found in many common home products. Particleboard, plywood and other pressed woods, paints, wallpapers, nail polish and permanent-press draperies contain formaldehyde. When these products are wet they give off a surge of formaldehyde 100 to 1,000 times higher than when dry. But acid-cured floor finishes and fingernail hardeners continue to emit substantial amounts of the gas after a 20-hour drying period. Dry products, including unwashed permanent-press shirts and fiberglass insulation, continue to release formaldehyde steadily over time.

What can you do to reduce formaldehyde effects for you and clients?

- Use low- or VOC-free paints and finishes, make sure there is plenty of ventilation (open windows), and leave the house for several days to allow them to off-gas.
- Wash new clothing, bedding, and draperies twice before using and avoid permanent-press fabrics.
- Request a material-safety data sheet from contractors before they apply floor finish, and avoid those with high formaldehyde levels.

- Keep new and recently remodeled homes cool, dry, and well-ventilated.
- Use solid wood or pressed wood products bonded with pheno-formaldehyde (PF), which has lower emissions.
- Avoid subfloors, cabinets, shelves, paneling, laminated flooring, wood-veneer furniture, and doors made of urea-formaldehyde (UF) pressed woods.
- Cover bare pressed woods in the home with low-VOC sealants such as Livos (508-477-7955) or AFM (619-239-0321).

Pesticides

Pesticide exposure begins early. Contaminants from pesticides and industrial chemicals are present in the amniotic fluid surrounding fetuses (Foster, 1999).

Exposure to pesticides remains a major environmental health problem. Farmers have consistently higher chromosome aberrations and significantly abnormal DNA-repair responses as determined by challenge/assay method (Sierra-Torres, Cajas-Salazar, Shipp, & Legator, 1999).

There is now unequivocal evidence that a wide variety of chemicals capable of disrupting the endocrine system are present in our waters. These range from natural and synthetic estrogens to industrial chemicals such as pesticides and dishwashing detergents and contraceptives that can mimic endogenous hormones. There are enough examples of the masculinization of female mollusks exposed to the anti-fouling agent TBT (tributyltin), and the feminization of male fish exposed to estrogenic chemicals in effluent from sewage-treatment works to demonstrate that adverse effects are occurring (Sumpter, 1998).

Endosulfan, dieldrin, toxaphene, and chlordane, are all pesticide chemicals known to activate agene that makes estrogen in humans. When tested individually, their estrogenic effect is almost inconsequential, but when mixed, their potency jumps 500–1,000 times and their effects are additive (Arnold et al., 1996).

The number of substances that mimic the action of endogenous estrogens is increasing rapidly. These endocrine-disrupting chemicals are not restricted to pesticides. Several different compounds used in the food industry, in plasticizers, and in dental restorations are also estrogenic (Oles et al., 1999).

Investigation of chemical exposure as a possible etiologic factor for breast cancer has not been a research priority in the United States. This is disturbing given the evidence from animal studies showing that environmental chemicals cause cancer and reproductive dysfunction (Wolff, 1995). This may not be so surprising because many of the companies who make the chemicals also run the treatment centers. For example, the primary sponsor of Breast Cancer Awareness Month, AstraZeneca, is a British-based multinational giant that manufactures the cancer drug tamoxifen as well as fungicides and herbicides, including the carcinogen acetochlor. Astra-Zereca also operates the Salick cancer-care centers (Batt & Gross, 1999; Sloan, 1999).

The fact that breast cancer risk is strongly associated with reproductive hormones is a further clue that environmental chemicals should be investigated. Besides cancer, specific outcomes that need to be explored are reproductive dysfunction, immunotoxicity, and neurotoxicity (Wolff, 1995). Try some of the measures in Table 16.1 as alternatives to toxic pesticides.

TABLE 16.1   Alternatives to Toxic Pesticides

Alternative	Examples
Natural repellents	Hang a bouquet of dried tomato leaves to repel mosquitos, flies, and spiders. Place dried lavender, cedar chips, or rosemary in bags to deter moths. Sprinkle crushed catnip on ant trails and fill cracks with white glue. Vinegar, cayenne pepper, citric extracts, cinnamon, cream of tartar, and salt may also work. Use citronella and lavender oil to repel biting insects. Plant marigolds, nasturtiums, and cloves of garlic in gardens and near doorways to repel insects. Use boric acid to control ants and cockroaches; spread under refrigerator and stove and around ductwork, allowing 2 weeks for it to work. Leave spiders alone because they eat other insects; or trap them in an inverted jar and throw outside. Use a mousetrap or a cat to catch mice. Wipe surfaces where you see ants with vinegar and sprinkle the entry points with paprika or chili powder. Protect from tick bites by adding 2 teaspoons of rose geranium or palmerosa essential oil in 2 cups of water; spray, using precautions to protect the eyes. Keep fleas away from pets: try a flea collar made with the herb pennyroyal; wash pet bedding and vacuum frequently; bathe pet often; dump captured fleas in soapy water; at night set a gooseneck lamp on the floor above a bowl of soapy water to attract fleas who will drown. To keep flies and mosquitoes away, repair screens, eliminate standing water, seal garbage containers, cover and seal foods, hang fly-paper. Mix 4 parts eucalyptus oil with liquid laundry detergent to kill mites in bedding and clothing.
Choose plants over grass	Xeriscape™ by planting native trees, vines, hedges and flowers instead of grass to deter insects and to conserve water and energy, which keeps the house cool in summer and warm in winter.
Protect plants	Spray trees and plants with liquid soap, garlic, and/or cooking oil (1 tablespoon/pint of water). To conserve moisture and regulate soil temperature: mulch with hay or straw, grass clippings (instead of putting them in your garbage), cocoa bean hulls, leaves, pine needles, sawdust, newspaper, old carpets, black plastic, stones (earthworms will rub against them and add minerals to your soil).

(continued)

TABLE 16.1 *(continued)*	
	Plant the following to outwit insects: marigold, calendula, nasturtium, geranium, chrysanthemum, chives, onions, garlic, sage, savory, coriander.
	Handpick and remove first-generation insects in the early morning when they're slow and not alert; wipe eggs off leaves with a wet tissue and cover with flour or a fine dust of ashes.
	Feed and encourage wasps, birds, toads, and salamanders—they eat other many insects.
Buy and grow organic foods	Buy more organically grown (no pesticides used) fruits and vegetables and encourage your store manager to carry them.
	Grow at least a small portion of your salad greens and herbs in small pots indoors, in flower boxes, or on your deck, including cherry tomatoes, parsley, and arrugala and other hearty greens.

The foregoing information was adapted from Annie Berthold-Bond. (1999). "Better Basics for the Home: Recipes for greener living." *News on Earth, 2*(8), 1–4. Jeanie Darlington. (1970). *Grow Your Own*. Berkeley, CA: Bookworks. Michael Castleman. (1997). "Killer Bug Killers." *Mother Jones*. (September/October), 25–26.

Accidents

Accidents are a leading cause of death for those between 1 and 37 years of age (National Safety Council, 1998). Motor vehicles are the major cause of death, many of which would not occur if seat belts were worn by passengers and helmets by motorcyclists, if the speed limit was observed, and if drinking and driving were avoided. Falls, drownings, and burns are the major causes of other preventable accidents. Workers who report occupational hazard exposures are at greater risk for both binge drinking and drinking and driving (Conrad, Furner, & Qian, 1999). Statistically adjusting for other collision variables, cell phones are associated with a ninefold increased risk for a fatal traffic collision (Violanti, 1998).

Two actions you can take to reduce accidents are (a) to serve as a wellness role model and practice safe behaviors and (b) to participate in school, worksite, and community education campaigns to reduce accidental injury and death and curb risk drinking among workers.

Noise

Noise is a major problem in many settings. Some of the most problematic sites for noise are the home (airplane, automobile, equipment noise), nursing homes, medical centers, and the worksite. Policies protecting against environmental noise need to be informed by scientific understanding and psychological and social factors, not just mathematical models (Staples, 1997).

Over 30 million workers are exposed to hazardous noise at the worksite. Continual exposure to high noise levels damages and destroys hearing cells within the ear, making noise-induced hearing loss an irreversible impairment. The law requires hearing-conservation programs for workers in industrial settings in which noise exposures equal or exceed 85 dB. Workers in construction and agriculture may not be covered by these programs. Engineering or administration controls are the first line of defense. When these fail, passive hearing protection devices must be used, including earmuffs, canal caps, and ear plugs (Lusk, 1997). As a wellness role model, you can have a major effect by promoting increased use of hearing protection devices.

Environmental Health Assessments

Environmental health assessments will help you and clients identify environmental exposures.

Client Exposure History

A client exposure history can provide useful information for you and for the client. Some questions to ask to help identify environmental exposures include the following:

1. What are your current, past, and longest held jobs?
2. Have you ever been exposed to any radiation, chemical liquids, dusts, mist, or fumes?
3. Do you see any connection between your current symptoms and your home or work activities?
4. Has anyone else in your home or work environment complained of the same problem?
5. When you use chemicals at home or work, what kind of ventilation is there?
6. What precautions do you take when handling chemicals at home or work?
7. What hobbies do you and your family members have?
8. Where do you live and work?
9. What type of home insulation, heating and cooling systems do you have?
10. What home cleaning agents do you use?
11. What pesticide exposure have you had?
12. Where do you get your drinking water?
13. What foods do you eat?
14. Has there been any renovation or remodeling at work and home?
15. Have you been near any hazardous waste or spill?
16. What jobs do the other members of your family have? (Agency for Toxic Substances, 1992)

Environmental Impact Assessment

Environmental impact assessment denotes the attempt to predict and assess the impact of development projects on the environment. Key elements of an integrated environmental health impact assessment model include:

- project analysis
- analysis of the status quo (regional analysis, population analysis, and background situation)
- prediction of impact (prognosis of future pollution and prognosis of health impact)
- assessment of impact
- recommendations
- communication of results
- evaluation of the overall procedure

You may not be involved in health impact assessments, but you need to begin to find ways to be part of this kind of action. It may be too late to work preventively once environmentally unsound projects have been implemented. The building of medical centers, community clinics, and hospitals are examples of projects that need nurses' input, but so are high-rise apart-

ments and other buildings that impact water, soil, and air quality

POLITICAL AND LEGAL ACTIONS

As a wellness role model, it is important to
think about and plan action to help reduce
the driving economic and social forces that
generate environmental health threats
(Corvalan, Kjellstrom, & Smith, 1999).
Speaking up about an environmental
health issue may be your entrée into the
world of politics and influence. Wield your
power by voting and by letting your representatives know where you stand on important health care issues such as
environmental wellness.

Call or write your legislators. A handwrit-
ten letter is often better received than E-
mail or a signed form letter. Describe the
issue, any bills currently being debated, and
their effect on you and clients. Call your
state professional association or search the
Internet for the bill's reference number.
Let representatives know that you live in
their district and they will be especially at-
tentive to what you have to say; they know
that each letter or phone call may represent
many potential votes. Look in your local
phone book for the local phone number
of your representatives or search on-line
for state or federal e-mail addresses. Find
out where your legislators have their local
offices and visit them there (Miller, 1999).

Becoming an informed advocate is not
easy. Campaigns or research that appear to
be health-promoting may be sponsored by
companies who are major polluters (Batt &
Gross, 1999), and serving as a wellness role
model may require a change of lifestyle.

Right-to-health laws are another area in
which to take reasoned action. Clients must
be informed about how their environment
affects their level of health and wellness.

Public Interest Research Groups (PIRG)
have launched a "Toxics Right-to-Know
Campaign" that seeks to require:

- Full disclosure by all polluting industries like oil, gas, sewage treatment,
  mining, incinerators, and utilities
- Public reports on small toxic releases
  that carry large health risks (dioxins,
  mercury, and other heavy metals that
  are known or suspected to cause cancer, neurological damage, and birth
  defects)
- Reporting by industries of all toxics
  they use and any possible exposure to
  toxic chemicals in the workplace, including transportation of chemicals
  through communities and placement
  of chemicals in consumer products
- Disclosures by the manufacturers of
  children's products of the presence of
  substances that cause cancer, reproductive damage, and neurological
  harm (PIRG, 1997).

Think about how right-to-know issues
can be brought home to decision makers
and social institutions so they will begin to
consider the environmental effect on
health and wellness. Also, find a way to collaborate with human rights and environmental movement representatives to work
together more effectively to enhance wellness (Iles, 1997).

If the federal government is to successfully protect the public from the adverse
effects of the environment, its policies will
need to be informed by scientific understanding, not by an overreliance on mathematical modeling of average group
responses (Staples, 1997). Humans are
unique beings who may respond quite differently to different environmental stressors, and government policies need to take
these unique responses into account. Col-

lecting environmental research findings and presenting them to appropriate governmental sources can be an effective way for you to proceed.

As a wellness advocate, it is important for you to be involved personally and professionally in political and legal actions to keep the environment safe. A good way to become more aware of toxic contaminants in water, land, and air is to contact your state's Public Interest Research Group (PIRG). Connect on-line to *http:www.pirg. org* and find out what activities, information, and needs are available in your state.

EVALUATING ENVIRONMENTAL ACTIONS

Use the following questions to help yourself or others evaluate environmental actions:

1. What sense of connection do you feel between yourself and the environment?
2. What resources do you need to seek out to help you make environmentally sound decisions?
3. What benefits have you received from the environment?
4. In what ways are you one with the environment?
5. If you listen closely, what is the environment telling you about its needs?
6. In what ways is your environment threatened?
7. How can you partner with your environment to achieve balance?
8. What ways do you need to change your life to create a path of simplicity and environmental quality?
9. How do you feel about the environmental path of action you have decided to take?
10. What other assistance do you need to attain your preferred path of environmental action?

WEBSITES

American Association of Occupational Health Nurses: *www.aaohn.org*

American Council for an Energy-Efficient Economy: *www.aceee.org/greenercars/index.htm*

Association of Occupational and Environmental Clinics: *http:// occ-env-med.mc.duke.edu/oem*

Department of Energy, Office of Energy Efficiency: *www.eren.doe.gov/ee.html*

Environmental Protection Agency: *www.epa.gov*

Environmental Defense Fund: *www.edf.org*

www.scorecard.org will tell if you live near polluting facilities, what chemicals those facilities are releasing into your community and whether or not those chemicals may cause a particular health problem; can send prepared E-mails to decision makers in your state and to the Environmental Protection Agency; provides resources for networking with environmental groups and virtual volunteering opportunities

Friends of the Earth: *www.foe.org*

Habitat for Humanity International: *http://www.habitat.org*

Legislative Advocacy and Elder Issues: *www.aarp.org*

Mothers and Others for a Livable Planet: *www.mothers.org*

Natural Resource Development Corporation: *www.nrdc.org* (check Legislative Watch for information on pending riders and how to contact your representatives and the White House)

Occupational Safety and Health Administration: *www.osha.gov*

Physicians for Social Responsibility: *http://www.psr.org*

Public Interest Research Group: *www.pirg.org*

Rocky Mountain Institute: *www.rmi.org*

Sierra Club: *www.sierraclub.org*

Union of Concerned Scientists: *www.ucsusa.org*

REFERENCES

Agency for Toxic Substances. (1992). *Taking an exposure history*. Atlanta, GA: U.S. Department of Health and Human Services, Public Health Service.

Arnold, S. F., Klotz, D. M., Collins, B. M., Vonier, P. M., Guillette, Jr., L. J., & McLachlan, J. A. (1996). Synergistic activation of estrogen receptor with combinations of environmental chemicals. *Science, 272*(5267), 1489–1492.

Ballester, D. F., Tenias, J. M., & Perez-Hoyos, S. (1999). The effects of air pollution on health: An introduction. *Rev. Esp. Salud Publica, 73*(2), 109–121.

Basen-Enquist, K., Hudmon, K. S., Tripp, M., & Chamberlain, R. (1998). Worksite health and safety climate: Scale development and effects of a health promotion intervention. *Preventive Medicine, 27*(1), 111–119.

Batt, S., & Gross, L. (1999, September/October). Cancer, Inc. *Sierra, 36,* 38–41, 63.

Beach, J. R., Raven, J., Ingram, C., Bailey, M., Johson, D., Walters, E. H., & Abramson, M. (1997). The effects on asthmatics of exposure to a conventional water-based and a volatile organic compound-free paint. *European Respiratory Journal, 10*(3), 563–566.

Binder, S., Levitt, A. M., Sacks, J. J., & Hughes, J. M. (1999). Emerging infectious diseases: Public health issues for the 21st century. *Science, 284*(5418), 1311–1313.

Bullinger, M., Hygge, S., Evans, G. W., Meis, M., & Mackensen, S. (1999). The psychological cost of aircraft noise for children. *Zentralbl Hyg Unweltmed, 202*(2–4), 127–138.

Cell phone risks still undetermined. (1997, September). *Advance for Nurse Practitioner,* 20A.

Centers for Disease Control and Prevention. (1993). It's time to stop being a passive victim. Atlanta, GA: Government Printing Office.

Chan, N. Y., Ebi, K. L., Smith, F., Wilson, T. F., & Smith, A. E. (1999). An integrated assessment framework for climate change and infectious diseases. *Environmental Health Perspectives, 107*(5), 329–337.

Cole, D. J., Hill, V. R., Humenik, F. J., & Sobsey, M. D. (1999). Health, safety and environmental concerns of farm animal waste. *Occupational Medicine, 14*(2), 423–428.

Conrad, K. M., Furner, S. E., & Qian, Y. (1999). Occupational hazard exposure and at risk drinking. *American Association of Occupational Health Nurses Journal, 47*(1), 9–16.

Corvalan, C. F., Kjellstrom, T., & Smith, K. R. (1999). Health, environment and sustainable development: Identifying links and indicators to promote action. *Epidemiology, 10*(5), 656–660.

Du, C. L., & Wang, J. D. (1998). Increased morbidity odds ratio of primary liver cancer and cirrhosis of the liver among vinyl chloride monomer workers. *Occupational Environmental Medicine, 55*(8), 528–532.

Eife, R., Weiss, M., Barros, V., Sigmund, B., Goriup, U., Komb, D., Wolf, W., Kittel, J., Schramel, P., & Reiter, K. (1999). Chronic poisoning by copper in tape water: I. Copper intoxications with predominately gastrointestinal symptoms. *Europe Journal of Medical Research, 4*(6), 219–223.

Environmental Protection Fact Sheet. (1999). No author. Methyl parathion restricted. Washington, DC: Environmental Protection Agency.

Fackelmann, K. A. (1992). Chlorin-cancer connection. *Science New,* (July 11), 23.

Fit to drink. (1999). No author. *Consumer Reports* (October), 52–55.

Foster, W. G. (1999, June). Pesticide contaminants in amniotic fluid. Research results presented to the Annual Meeting of the Endocrine Society, San Diego, CA.

Fox, N. (1999). Who's to blame when antibiotics don't work. *The Green Guide* (September), 1–3.

Frazer P. (1999). Fluoridation increases lead absorption in the blood. *News on Earth,* *1*(11), 1.

Free, K. (1999). The poor children of a wealthy nation. *Habitat World* (October/November), 2–3.

Fried, P. A., Watkinson, B., & Gray, R. (1998). Differential effects of cognitive functioning in 9- to 12-year olds prenatally exposed to cigarettes and marihuana. *Neurotoxicology Teratology, 20*(3), 293–306.

Friedmann, H. (1999). Limits and uncertainties—with special regard to radon measurements. *Health Physics, 77*(3), 309–312.

Glueck, C. J., Freiberg, R. A., Crawford, A., Gruppo, R., Roy, D., Tracy, T., Sieve-Smith, L., & Wang, P. (1998). Secondhand smoke, hypofibrinolysis, and Legg-Perthes disease. *Clinical Orthop, 352*(July), 159–167.

Gomez-Jacinto, L., & Moral-Toranzo, F. (1999). Urban traffic noise and self-reported health. *Psychological Reports, 84*(3 Pt 2), 1105–1108.

Green, L. M., Miller, A. B., Villeneuve, P. J., Agnew, D. A., Greenberg, M. L., Li, J., & Donnelly, K. E. (1999). A case-control study of childhood leukemia in southern Ontario, Canada, and exposure to magnetic fields in residencies. *International Journal of Cancer, 82*(2), 161–170.

Huang, C. Y., Huang, K. L., Cheng, T. J., Wang, J. D., Hsieth, L. L. (1997). The GST T1 and CYP2E1 genotypes are possible factors causing vinyl chloride induced abnormal liver function. *Archives of Toxicology, 71*(8), 482–488.

Ikramuddin, A. (1999a). Nestle's genetically engineered food ingredients. *The Green Guide, 71,* 5.

Ikramuddinm A. (1999b). Indoor air alert. *The Green Guide, 72,* 6.

Iles, A. T. (1997). Health and the environment: A human rights agenda for the future. *Health and Human Rights, 2*(2), 46–61.

Institute of Medicine. (1995). *Nursing, health & the environment.* Washington, DC: National Academy Press.

Kaferstein, F., & Abdussalam, M. (1999). Food safety in the 21st century. *Bulletin of the World Health Organization, 77*(4), 347–351.

Kheifets, L. I., Gilbert, E. S., Sussman, S. S., Guenel, P., Sahl, J. D., Savitz, D. A., & Theriault, G. (1999). Comparative analyses of the studies of magnetic fields and cancer in electric utility workers: Studies from France, Canada, and the United States. *Occupational Environmental Medicine, 56*(8), 567–574.

Kliukiene, J., Tynes, T., Martinsen, J. I., Blassaas, K. G., & Andersen, A. (1999). Incidence of breast cancer in a Norwegian cohort of women with potential workplace exposure to 50 Hz magnetic fields. *American Journal of Indian Medicine, 36*(1), 147–154.

Li, C. M., Chiang, H., Fu, Y. D., Shao, B. J., Shi, J. R., & Yao, G. D. (1999). Effects of 50 Hz magnetic fields on gap junctional intercellular communication. *Bioelectromagnetics, 20*(5), 290–294.

Lukes, E., & Johsnon, M. (1999). Hearing conservation: An industry-school partnership. *Journal of School Nursing, 15*(2), 22–25.

Lusk, S. L. (1997). Noise exposures. Effects on hearing and prevention of noise induced hearing loss. *American Association of Occupational Nurses Journal, 45*(8), 397–410.

Masters, R. D. (1999). Fluoridation increase lead absorption in the blood. *International Journal of Environmental Studies,* (September), 62–64.

Mobile-home bills need more teeth. No author. (1999). *NRTA Bulletin* (September), 28.

Miller, K. M. (1999). Making a legislative impact. *American Journal of Nursing, 99*(3), 54.

Newmann, T., & Ruga, W. (1995). How to improve your unit's environment. *American Journal of Nursing, 95*(April), 63–65.

Olden, K. (1999). EMF Research and Public Information Dissemination (RAPID) Program. Washington, DC: The National Institute of Environmental Health Sciences. A report to Congress, June.

Parat, S., Perdrix, A., & Baconnier, P. (1999). Relationships between air conditioning, airborne microorganisms and health. *Bulletin of the Academy of National Medicine, 183*(2), 327–342.

Pennybacker, M. (1999). Old home renovation. *The Green Guide, 69,* 1–3.

PIRG. (1997). [On-line]. Available at http://www.pirg.org/enviro/toxics/rtk/index.htm#solution.

Plants as purifiers. (1994). *Aesculapius, 3*(2), 6.

Rhomberg, W. (1998). Exposure to polymeric materials in vascular soft-tissue sarcomas. *International Archives of Occupational Environmental Health, 71*(5), 343–347.

Schnelle, J. F., Alessi, C. A., Al-Samarrai, N. R., Fricker, R. D., Jr, & Ouslander, J. G. (1999). The nursing home at night: Effects of an intervention on noise, light and sleep.

Schuster, E. (1997). Environment. In B. M. Dossey (Ed.), *American holistic nurses' core curriculum* (pp. 164–169). Gaithersburg, MD: Aspen Publishers.

Sick Building Syndrome. (1994, April). *Waterloo Gardens,* 17.

Sierra-Tores, W. W., Cajas-Salazar, N., Shipp, B. K., & Legator, M. S. (1999). Cytogenetic effects from exposure to mixed pesticides and the influence from genetic susceptibility. *Environmental Health Perspectives, 107*(6), 501–505.

Sloan, A. (1999). Breast cancer update. *The Green Guide, 71,* 6.

Smith, K. R., Corvalan, C. F., & Kjellstrom, T. (1999). How much global ill health is attributable to environmental factors? *Epidemiology, 19*(5), 573–584.

Staples, S. L. (1997). Public policy and environmental noise: Modeling exposure or understanding effects. *American Journal of Public Health, 87*(12), 2062–2067.

Stenhammar, L. (1999). Diarrhea following contamination of drinking water with copper. *European Journal of Medical Research, 4*(6), 217–218.

Sumpter, J. P. (1998). Xenoendocrine disrupters—environmental impacts. *Toxicology Letters, 28*(102–103), 337–342.

Tapia Granados, J. A. (1998). Reducing automobile traffic: An urgent policy for health promotion. *Review Panama Salud Publications, 3*(4), 227–241.

Trigano, A. J., Azoulay, A., Rochdi, M., & Campillo, A. (1999). Electromagnetic interference of external pacemakers by walkie-talkies and digital cellular phones: Experimental study. *Pacing Clinical Electrophysiology, 22*(4Pt1), 588–593.

Violanti, J. M. (1998). Cellular phone and fatal traffic collisions. *Accident Analysis Prevention, 30*(4), 519–524.

Wells, M., Stokols, D., McMahan, S., & Clitheroe, C. (1997). Evaluation of a worksite injury and illness prevention program: Do the effects of a reach out training program reach employees? *Journal of Occupational Psychology, 2*(1), 25–34.

Zahm, S. H., Ward, M. H., & Blair, A. (1997). Pesticides and cancer. *Occupational Medicine, 12*(2), 269–289.

CHAPTER 17

Complementary Health Care Practices

Nancy Oliver

YOUR ROLE IN RELATIONSHIP TO COMPLEMENTARY THERAPIES

Today you feel more confident! Community knowledge is making sense. You are learning many new things and you are excited and motivated to learn more. Community members contact you for information about complementary and holistic practices.

"Does acupuncture really work? Will it get rid of the pain in my knee?" asks a 71-year-old grandmother.

An older man who recently had a blood clot seeks your advice: "I read about problems with mixing herbal remedies and medicines in the paper today. Is it safe to take gingko biloba when I am still taking this Coumadin?"

You hear the children crying in the background on the phone before you hear: "These three kids are forever fighting. I am really stressing. What can I do to help them . . . and me?"

The last message is from a colleague being treated for cancer. "Hey, thanks for recommending that guided imagery tape for my chemotherapy treatment. I didn't have nearly as much nausea this time."

As a community practitioner you may be expected to respond as a knowledgeable resource as more and more people use complementary therapies. Many individuals are adding complementary methods to their medical regimens without notifying their primary health care provider. Working in the community, you have the perfect opportunity to access information about community health practices, to enter into partnerships and develop collaborative and meaningful health and wellness programs. This new role is in direct response to the call for communities to take responsibility for their health, one of the goals of *Healthy People 2010* (U.S. Department of Health and Human Services [DHHS], 1998).

Defining Complementary Therapies

Complementary therapies refer to any practices and interventions that are used to enhance physical, emotional, social, and spiritual health. The variety of practices is broad and ranges from drugs and diets to food supplements, mental exercises, hands-on techniques, and lifestyle regimens. Complementary health practitioners come from many disciplines and traditions—acupuncture, guided imagery, chiropractic, yoga, hypnosis, biofeedback, aromatherapy, homeopathy, relaxation techniques, reflexology, traditional Chinese medicine, macrobiotics, hypnotherapy, herbal medicine, naturopathy, iridology, Ayurvedic medicine, and various schools of massage, among others.

Helvie's Energy Theory provides a framework for understanding the concept of energy that is common to all of these practices (Helvie, 1999). Complementary health practitioners work with the body's energy to improve the flow and maintain or restore balance by using the techniques and science of the particular discipline. Helvie uses systems theory to explain the importance of internal and external environment on the individual who is considered an open system. The external environment includes all energy sources outside the individual, which he subdivides into chemical, physical, biological, or psychosocial. By using this framework, community practitioners can identify complementary services and resources as environmental energies and assess the community balance from an energy perspective.

Complementary Practices: Advocate, Skeptic, or Foe?

Community practitioners are expected to be responsible resources for complementary health practices and your attitude and beliefs about complementary health practices must be considered. Do complementary practices fit into your belief system? What do you think about the relationship between physical, emotional, social, and spiritual health? Would you go to a complementary health practitioner such as an chiropractor or doctor of Oriental medicine? It will be important to examine your position on these issues in order to best support your clients and meet the needs of the community. The questions listed in Box 17.1 provide an opportunity for self-reflection. Your responses will stimulate you to explore certain areas in more detail. Sharing your responses with colleagues will help you to develop increased awareness about areas in which you may be skeptical.

Recognizing Scientific Challenges

Defining and classifying complementary practices is a challenge for consumers, researchers, insurance providers, and health professionals. Establishing the usefulness of the therapies is equally challenging, and there is an increase in research efforts to determine which approaches have value, which are useless, and which may be dangerous (Eskinazi & Muehsam, 2000). To provide the best information about complementary practices, the community practitioners must be aware of the related research and scientific foundation for the practices.

The National Center for Complementary and Alternative Medicine

In 1992 the Office of Alternative Medicine, now known as the National Center for Complementary and Alternative Medicine (NCCAM), at the National Institutes of Health (NIH) was developed for the explicit purpose of facilitating the study of complementary treatment modalities and to disseminate information about them to both practitioners and the public. Information about NCCAM resources can be found in Box 17.2.

Box 17.1   Complementary Health Care Practices: Self-assessment

Directions: On a separate piece of paper write down your response to each question. Provide as much detail as possible.

1.   Are you currently using any complementary practices? If yes, describe the practices and reasons for them in detail.
2.   Have you ever used complementary practices? Include all practices, reasons for using them, and results. Why did you stop using them?
3.   Have you ever visited a complementary health care practitioner (chiropractor, massage therapist)? Include all details, number of times, reason, results, and why you stopped.
4.   If you have never gone to a complementary health care practitioner, why not?
5.   Before going to a complementary health care practitioner, what things would you want to know?
6.   Are you skeptical about using complementary practices? If yes, list your concerns.
7.   Do you think there is sufficient evidence to support the use of complementary therapies? How will this response influence your use of complementary practices? How will this response influence your dialogue with clients about complementary therapies? What are the main issues to consider and why?
8.   How important is it that you share your pattern of complementary health practices with your physician or primary health care provider? Why?
9.   How important is it that your clients share their patterns of complementary health practices with their physicians or primary health care providers? Why?

Box 17.2   NCCAM's Resources

NCCAM's Clearinghouse:

Contact for information regarding NCCAM or any aspect of CAM.
Toll-free number: 1-888-644-6226 between 8:30 a.m. and 5:00 p.m., EST, Monday through Friday.
E-mail: Nccam@altmedinfo.org
NCCAM's Web site is *http://nccam.nih.gov.*

Publications:

Complementary and Alternative Medicine at the NIH.
Acupuncture Information and Resources Package (Z-01) describes clinical trials and lists references and publications.St. John's Wort (Z-02) describes uses and actions, sources and references.

For free copies, call the NCCAM Clearinghouse's toll-free number: 1-888-644-6226.

To assist in the study of complementary and alternative medicine (CAM), the NCCAM developed a classification system of seven major categories:

- Mind-body medicine
- Alternative medical systems
- Lifestyle and disease prevention
- Biologically-based therapies
- Manipulative and body-based systems
- Biofield
- Bioelectromagnetics

These may be useful in categorizing resources from the community-based assessment data or in designing research studies or community educational programs, but it is the first category, mind-body medicine, that has direct implications for holistic health and wellness. There are three subcategories: mind-body systems, religion and spirituality, and social and contextual areas. Some of the therapies are identified as CAM, others as behavioral medicine, and there is an "overlapping" designation for another group (see Box 17.3). This classification system will continue to change as advances in research and science continue.

The practices listed as CAM modalities in the category of mind-body medicine in Box 17.3 are difficult to study using a causal model and traditional methods of scientific inquiry. For example, yoga and Alcoholics Anonymous usually involve groups of people sharing common experiences. Here is an opportunity for community practitioners to expand their researcher roles and creatively study individual, group, and community patterns and responses related to preserving health and wellness.

There is an increase in research data supporting the effectiveness of many CAM modalities, which focus mainly on determining the effectiveness of a particular therapy in the treatment of symptoms or chronic con-

ditions. Community practitioners must be aware of the most recent research endeavors in order to share the information with clients. To illustrate the scope of research in these areas, a summary of funded studies by NCCAM is presented in Box 17.4. These studies may also stimulate your creative research juices.

Studies of health patterns related to the category of alternative medical systems—which includes medical systems developed outside of the United States or indigenous systems such Native American medicine and Curanderismo—are limited. Belief that the use of complementary therapies is "widespread in this country and particularly common among minority groups" as cited in *Healthy People 2010* (DHHS, 1998, pp. 13–19) supports the need for community-based studies of complementary practices.

COMPLEMENTARY THERAPIES IN THE COMMUNITY

To further illustrate the increased interest in complementary therapies by the general public, health care practitioners, the government, insurers, and academia:

- One third to one half of the American people use at least one complementary therapy in addition to their regular medical care (Eisenberg et al., 1993; Elder, Gillcrist, & Minz, 1997).
- The budget of the NCCAM increased from $7.4 million in fiscal year 1996 to $50 million for 1999, and a 37% increase to $68.7 million has been appropriated for fiscal year 2000 (National Center for Complementary and Alternative Medicine Clearinghouse, 1999). Some states like Washington State are requiring all health insurers to add coverage of CAM treatments

---

Box 17.3   NCCAM's Classification of Alternative Medicine Practices for Mind-Body Medicine

Subcategory: Mind-Body Systems

CAM	Behavioral Medicine	Overlapping
Yoga	Psychotherapy	Art therapy
Internal qi gong	Meditation	Music therapy
Tai chi	Imagery	Dance therapy
	Hypnosis	Journaling
	Biofeedback	Humor
	Support groups	Body psychotherapy

Subcategory: Religion and Spirituality
Practices in this subcategory includes nonbehavioral aspects of spirituality and religion and includes only CAM modalities:

CAM

Confession
Nonlocality
Nontemporality
Soul retrieval
Spiritual healing
"Special" healers

Subcategory: Social and Contextual Areas
Included in this subcategory are social, cultural, symbolic and contextual practices that are either designated as CAM or Overlapping:

CAM	Overlapping
Caring-based approaches (for example, holistic nursing, pastoral care)	Placebo
Intuitive diagnosis	Explanatory models
	Community-based approaches (for example, Alcoholics Anonymous, Native American "sweat" rituals)

---

to their coverage of standard medical care (Millbank Memorial Fund, 1998).

- Blue Shield of California and other insurers are offering alternative services discount programs and most of the largest health maintenance organizations (HMOs) in California offer optional acupuncture and chiropractic care (Millbank Memorial Fund, 1998).
- There is an increase in best-selling books and Web sites about complementary therapies for both the general

---

Box 17.4   NCCAM Research Awards for Fiscal Year 1999 (Awarded jointly with other NIH Institutes and Centers)

Biomechanics:
  Biomechanical effect of acupuncture needling
Cancer:
  Self-transcendence in breast-cancer support groups
Cardiovascular diseases:
  Acupuncture and hypertension: efficacy and mechanisms
  Effect of high-dose Vitamin E on carotid atherosclerosis
  Effects of meditation on mechanisms of CHD
General medicine:
  Melatonin and cerebral blood flow autoregulation
Mental health:
  A placebo-controlled clinical trial of a standardized extract *Hypericum perforatum* in
    major depressive disorder
  Acupuncture in the treatment of depression
  Acupuncture treatment of depression during pregnancy
  Ginkgo biloba prevention trial in older individuals
  Omega-3 fatty acids in bipolar disorder prophylaxis
  Oxidative cell injury in first episode psychotic patients
Neurology:
  Melatonin for sleep disorders in Parkinson's disease
  Neuroprotective agents from Oriental medicines
Pain:
  Acupuncture for dental pain: Testing a model
  Efficacy of acupuncture in the treatment of fibromyalgia
  Evaluating the efficacy of acupuncture for back pain
  Nonpharmacologic analgesia for invasive procedures
  Pilot study of acupuncture in fibromyalgia
  RCT-acupuncture safety/efficacy in knee osteoarthritis
  Study of the efficacy of glucosamine and glucosamine-chondriotin sulfate in
    knee osteoarthritis
  Usual care versus choice of alternative Rx for low back pain
Urology:
  Saw palmetto extract in benign prostatic hyperplasia

---

public and the professional community.

- More than 34 of the nation's 125 plus medical schools have added complementary therapy elective courses to their curricula.

What kinds of evidence of increased interest in complementary therapies can you identify in your community? Do your colleagues, neighbors, friends, or relatives discuss complementary therapies? What do they say?

Patterns of Use

People are becoming more expert and independent at caring for themselves. They are designing creative health and wellness plans that include complementary practices, usually without consultation with health care professionals. To aid in the treatment of chronic conditions, Eisenberg and others (1993) found that individuals used complementary therapies for the following conditions:

Allergies	Digestive problems
Anxiety	Headache
Arthritis	High blood pressure
Back problems	Insomnia
Depression	Sprains or strains

The complementary therapies identified by participants in the Eisenberg study included imagery, spiritual healing, commercial weight-loss programs, lifestyle diets (e.g., macrobiotics) and those listed in Box 17.5.

Eisenberg et al. (1993) was a landmark study that provided the basis for the continued interest in complementary therapies from a medical perspective. Disease prevention and healthy lifestyles are major components of complementary therapies; however, healthy behaviors are rarely studied, which is another research challenge for community practitioners.

Accountability

Protecting consumers from being harmed by complementary treatments must be a high priority for community practitioners as well as for health plans, other health care professionals, and the general public (Millbank Memorial Fund, 1998). Regulations for professions and occupations vary from state to state. As a responsible community practitioner, you will be required to examine your state's licensing, certification, and registration practices related to complementary therapists such as acupuncturists, massage therapists, and homeopaths. Changes are occurring to meet the public demands for complementary services and state boards will need input from knowledgeable consumer advocates such as community practitioners.

The 13th goal of *Healthy People 2010* is directed at ensuring the safest and most effective possible use of medical products (DHHS, 1998). Objective 13-7 is directly related to complementary therapies and calls for primary care providers to question clients about the use of complementary health care practices and to enter the information into the patient's permanent record. Responsibility for accessing and documenting information about complementary practices is given to the primary care providers.

Consumer Characteristics

Who uses complementary modalities? If we ask ourselves this question, one response might be "people from specific ethnic and cultural groups." The importance of recognizing, understanding, and honoring traditional beliefs about health, healing, and disease is always a concern of health care providers. Asking about the use of cultural health practices is not always included in health care assessments. Recognizing the relationship of acculturation to health care decisions will be helpful for community practitioners involved in culturally and ethnically diverse communities. Patcher (1994) found that cultural practices were more likely to be used by people who (a) are recent immigrants to the mainland

Box 17.5   Resources for Information About Acupuncture, Chiropractic, and Homeopathy

Acupuncture and Acupuncturists

American Academy of Medical Acupuncture
  5820 Wilshire Boulevard
  Los Angeles, CA 90036
  (213) 937-5514
  www.medicalacupuncture.org/aama.htm

American Association of Oriental Medicine
  433 Front Street
  Catasauqua, PA 18032
  (610) 266-1433
  www.aaom.org

National Commission for the Certification of Acupuncturists
  P.O. Box 97075
  Washington, DC 20090
  (202) 232-14404
  acupuncture.com/TCMSchools/NCAA.htm

Chiropractic and Chiropractors

American Chiropractic Association
  1701 Clarendon Boulevard
  Arlington, VA 22209
  (703) 2776-8800
  www.amerchiro.org

International Chiropractors Association
  1110 North Glebe Road, Ste. 1000
  Arlington, VA 22201
  (703) 528-5000
  www.chiropractic.org

World Chiropractic Alliance
  2950 North Dobson Road, Ste. 1
  Chandler, AZ 85224
  (800) 347-1011
  www.choicemall.com/worldchiropractic

Box 17.5   **(continued)**

Homeopathy and Homeopaths

International Foundation for Homeopathy
    2366 Eastlake Avenue East, Ste. 325
    Seattle, WA 98012-3366
    (206) 324-8230
    www.healthy.net/pan/pa/homeopathic/ifh/index.html

National Center for Homeopathy
    801 North Fairfax, Ste. 306
    Alexandria, VA 22314
    (703) 548-7790
    www.healthy/net/nch

United States; (b) live in ethnic enclaves; (c) prefer to speak in their native tongue; (d) were educated in their country or origin; (e) migrate back and forth to the country of origin; (f) are in constant contact with older individuals who maintain a high degree of ethnic identity.

American-born, English-speaking, middle-class people with college educations also use complementary therapies (Hufford, 1997). These characteristics are consistent with the findings from the study by Eisenberg and others (1993) in which the use of complementary therapies was significantly more common among people 25 to 49 years of age; significantly less common among Blacks than among Whites, Hispanics, and Asians; and significantly more common among persons with some college education and among people with annual incomes of about $35,000 rather than lower incomes. The following explanation by Jonas (1997) provides valuable insights into the use of complementary practices:

Individuals do not appear to seek out alternative practices because they are disillusioned with conventional medicine in general, or harbor increasing anti-science sentiments, or have a general attraction to CAM (Complementary and Alternative Medicine) philosophies and health beliefs, or represent a disproportionate number of uneducated, poor, seriously ill, or neurotic patients. Community members use alternative practices because it is part of their social network, or they are not satisfied with the process or results of their conventional care. (p. 34)

It can be concluded that many individuals use some type of complementary modality and the wise community practitioner would question all people.

Case study: Community practitioner as expert resource

Frederic Gordon is a licensed massage therapist who has volunteered at a local community senior center for the past 8 months. The older adults had been very generous in sharing their time, patience, and support with Fred and his family during what he describes as the "fall of my grandfather." Fred schedules 30-minute massages between 1:00 and 5:00 p.m. on Tuesday afternoons and has "four regular customers and a variety of others." An increas-

ing number of older adults are scheduling appointments for individual sessions at the clinic where Fred practices.

Fred calls you to discuss his concern about a pattern that is developing. He relates that about a dozen of the seniors whom he sees weekly or biweekly have shared with him their decrease in stress and muscle tension and how they feel so much better. This validates his effectiveness and he is pleased. However, the group members talk among themselves and have also shared their experiences. One 72-year-old woman announced that she had discontinued taking her "water pill for high blood pressure." Based on this behavior two women and four men decided to reduce or eliminate taking their "blood pressure pills." Individual reports confirmed this behavior. Fred urged the individuals to immediately share the changes with their primary health care provider. Upon follow-up he discovered that only three had attempted to share the benefits of the massage and the change in medication schedule with their provider. Of the three, only one was supported by the primary health provider, who agreed to develop a plan to incorporate massage into the management of the client's blood pressure.

The following questions will direct you in considering different issues in this scenario:

- Do people have the right to change their medication-taking behavior?
- What is the primary care provider's responsibility related to patients' integrating massage therapy into their health care practices?
- How can you help the massage therapist identify his role and responsibility?
- What can community practitioners do to educate older adults, primary care providers, massage therapists, and community about complementary practices health care practices?

Common Complementary Practices

Community practitioners will be required to have a general understanding of complementary therapies. Your expertise will develop based on your self-assessment, individual interests, experiences, and the availability of resources. Brief descriptions of three frequently used complementary practices that require complementary practitioners in addition to imagery and relaxation are included in the following section. A valuable resource is the *Encyclopedia of Complementary Health Practices* (Clark, 1999). This is a comprehensive resource for contemporary, economic, educational, legal, legislative, and health policy issues related to complementary therapies in addition to providing an introduction to an extensive number of practices and treatments.

Acupuncture

Acupuncture is a branch of traditional Chinese medicine in which health is considered a state of harmony or balance. In this system the imbalance is reflected in either excesses or deficiencies of vital life energy referred to as *qi* (pronounced and sometimes spelled *chi*). Meridians are the intricate pathways that carry *qi* throughout the body and are the focal points for insertion of the thin needles used to balance and redirect the energy flow.

Licensure of acupuncturists is regulated by the individual states and information can be accessed from your state board of examiners (Leake & Broderick, 1999). It is important to recognize that many physicians are integrating specific complementary modalities like acupuncture into their practices. They are completing extensive acupuncture training courses, for example, in order to offer more options for pain management to their clients. Other issues to consider such as those related to efficacy, biological effects, and integration of acupuncture into the health care system are included in the NIH Consensus statement on acupuncture (NIH, 1997). For additional resources see Box 17.5.

Chiropractic

Chiropractic practitioners consider health to be a state of balance, especially of the nervous and musculoskeletal systems. Disease is thought to be caused by misalignment of the spinal vertebrae, which leads to dysfunction of nerves, blood vessels, and organs. Chiropractic diagnosis and treatment are focused on reducing pain and improving function of the neuromusculoskeletal system of the body.

Chiropractic therapy should be obtained from health care professionals who have graduated from one of the American chiropractic colleges. Resources for information about chiropractic therapy and chiropractors is located in Box 17.5.

Homeopathy

There are two basic concepts that provide the foundation for homeopathy. The first is the law of similars, which means that "like cures like." In other words, a natural substance that produces a given symptom in a healthy person would cure it in a sick person. The second concept is that less is more, or the law of infinitesimals. The natural substance that caused the symptoms is diluted many times over with the intended result being the more dilute the solution, the more effective the remedy. Homeopaths treat both acute and chronic health problems and use the remedies to prevent disease and promote health in people who are not sick. Remedies are prescribed after an extensive assessment of physical, emo-

tional, and mental symptoms. Homeopathic remedies are also available in neighborhood pharmacies and from mail-order companies without consultation with a homeopathic practitioner. Homeopaths are trained through different educational programs, and information can be obtained from the resources in Box 17.5.

Complementary practices do not always require visits to practitioners. Practices such as imagery and relaxation techniques can be learned and practiced independently, depending upon the purpose and goal of the therapy.

Imagery

Imagery refers to our ability to develop an image, picture, or other sensory experience (taste, feeling, sound) either spontaneously or in response to a suggestion. The images may be seen in "the mind's eye" in response to, for example, the reported traffic jam you hear on your radio as you are turning onto the freeway ramp. You may clearly "see" the rows of stationary cars before you actually join them. The ability to use our inner resources to develop imagery for health and healing can be achieved through guidance and practice. Achterberg, Dossey, and Kolkmeier (1994) provide detailed descriptions for teaching clients to develop their own healing rituals through the use of imagery.

Different types of imagery require different levels of practitioner involvement. For example, the technique of interactive guided imagery (IGI) developed by Martin L. Grossman, M.D., and David E. Bresler, Ph.D., is a highly specialized approach to healing in which a trained therapist (guide) assists the client to a relaxed state and then engages in an active dialogue to arrive at a mutually established goal, for example a decrease in anxiety level before stressful events (Grossman & Bresler, 1998).

Through training and experience imagery can become a valuable tool for health and wellness. There are audiotapes and programs available to assist in developing the skills for using imagery in our own personal life. The exercise in Box 17.6 will give you an idea of how imagery can be helpful to change experiences related to the familiar drama of "Not having enough time." Frequent use of the technique will also result in the image occurring spontaneously when you say the words "I have all of the time that I need."

Relaxation Techniques

Relaxation is directly related to stress. Achieving a state of physical and mental quietness is the goal of relaxation. Providing opportunities for our bodies and minds to be in a tension-free state has many benefits including increased energy, creativity, and balance; decreased pain and anxiety; improved immune system function; facilitated sleep and rest; improved sense of well-being (Anselmo & Kolkmeier, 2000). There are many pioneers in the field of relaxation like Herbert Benson (1984) and J. Kabat-Zinn (1990) whose works provide rich resources for study and practice. Please refer to Box 17.7 for additional resources.

There are many different types of relaxation exercises including autogenic training, biofeedback, hypnosis, meditation, and progressive muscle relaxation. It has been suggested that the best way to learn about relaxation is through direct experience (Anselmo & Kolkmeier, 2000). Com-

---

Box 17.6   Imagery Exercise: "I Have All the Time I Need"

Directions: Accessing our imaginations requires a quiet environment and a quiet body and mind. You will be expected to move into a relaxed state, so practicing relaxation is essential. Once you have achieved a state of relaxation, begin to:

1.   Think about a specific activity or event that is causing you to feel that you will not have enough time to complete it.
2.   Add as many details to the event as possible, paying attention to the physical and emotional sensations that you may be feeling.
3.   Focus on your hands. Are they shut tight or wide open?
4.   Open your hands wide and let yourself image what time would be like if you were holding it in your hands. Feel the weight of time—take in as much time as you need. Balance the time in both your left and right hands. See and feel this valuable gift of time—enjoy the experience—of holding time in your hands.
5.   Now bring the image of the event that needs this time into your focus. Use your hands to move the time around the image. See the changes in yourself as you move time in—what does your body feel like now? Put as much time into the picture as you need. You have all the time that you need.
6.   When you are ready, open your eyes and remember the feeling. Be mindful of the event and the time required and see how it goes.

Practice with this time exercise will result in more time on your hands!

Box 17.7   Relaxation Resources

The Relaxation Response
> The Mind Body Medicine Institute
> Division of Behavioral Medicine
> New England Deaconess Hospital
> 185 Pilgrim Road
> Boston, MA 02215
> (617) 732-9530

Biofeedback Workshops
> Association for Applied Psychophysiology and Biofeedback
> 10200 West 44th Avenue #310
> Wheat Ridge, CO 80033
> (303) 422-8436

Mindfulness Meditation
> Stress Reduction Clinic
> University of Massachusetts Medical Center
> Worcester, MA 01655
> (508) 856-1616

Yoga, Relaxation, Qi Gong
> Check local holistic education institutes, universities, continuing education programs, Chinese energy medicine centers, yoga ashrams, and health food stores for resources in your area.

---

munity practitioners are role models for health and wellness in the community. You are encouraged to develop your own relaxation program by identifying the relaxation resources in your community and using these to develop and maintain your self-care relaxation skills.

The telephone meditation in Box 17.8 is adapted from the work of Tich Nhat Hanh (1991). This technique is useful because it is attached to a familiar sound the occurs during the day—the telephone ringing. By following the steps in the exercise you will be entering a mindful, relaxed state for a few minutes each time you respond to the call of the telephone. You will become consciously aware of your ability to move easily into a quiet, happy state. The breathing technique uses the in-and-out exercise in which these four lines are repeated as we breathe in and out:

> Breathing in, I calm my body.
> Breathing out, I smile.
> Dwelling in the present moment,
> I know this is a wonderful moment!

Tich Nhat Hahn suggests that your breath is used to calm your body and encourages us to practice feeling the calmness in our bodies when we breath in. When you breathe out and smile, all the muscles in your face are used and it becomes easier to smile frequently. Being in the present

---

Box 17.8   Telephone Meditation

Directions: Practice the in-and-out breathing technique using calm and a smile when breathing so it is natural and you enjoy it. Now, when the phone rings follow these steps.

1.   The first ring reminds you to breathe in and feel calm. Breath out and smile.
2.   Repeat this breathing pattern with the second and third rings.
3.   When you pick up the receiver be sure that you continue to feel calm and that your smile is present. Notice how your voice sounds when you are smiling.
4.   Share the practice with others.
5.   Congratulate yourself for developing this practice of mindful meditation and enjoy the decrease in stress that you will experience.

---

moment helps us to focus our attention to the present, and the last phrase allows us to recognize the wonder of the moment. With practice, the words *calming, smiling, present moment,* and *wonderful moment* can be used to evoke the same calming and grounding response. Practice with this technique will help the telephone meditation become a natural part of your daily self-care activities.

COMMUNITY RESOURCE ASSESSMENT

It is important to remember that many complementary practices are aimed at preventing illness rather than treating it, and complementary practitioners such as acupuncturists or chiropractors may be located in health centers rather than medical clinics. On the other hand, vitamins and herbal therapies are available for purchase from a variety of sources including local grocery stores. Indigenous healers such as shamans and currandaros may be more difficult to locate. Learning about your community's complementary health resources will require a creative combination of the basic community assessment skills of observation

and interview. Equally challenging will be the identification of patterns of complementary practices in the community.

Community Characteristics

Before beginning any community assessment we must have some descriptive data about the community. You will be expected to review measurement data, which refers to community assessment information such as population statistics, population indices, morbidity and mortality rates, census statistics, and epidemiological data that has been collected and quantified (McCarthy & Mandle, 1998). Sources of health information data may be available from community libraries; town, city or state public health departments; environmental protection agencies; and community health-related organizations.

The census report data will provide information about the community's ethnic and cultural diversity. Census tract data can be obtained from local governmental agencies such as city hall or the planning office and may be useful in identifying target areas to be visited.

Complementary Resources in the Community

The following steps will be useful to you as you begin to explore your local complementary resources:

1. Learn about the laws and regulations for complementary therapies in your state: (a) Consult with your state health commissioner and learn about complementary policy mandates and legislation, and (b) Identify centers or schools in your community that offer credentialing courses in complementary practices; visit agencies and assess the variety of offerings and practices.

2. Assess community activity with regard to complementary practices: Find out if there are freestanding complementary centers in your community, including ethnic and cultural health centers. How do they operate? Who are their practitioners and clients? Interviews with key people will be important.

3. Identify level of interest in the community: Are there community education conferences or seminars related to complementary practices? What are they and who offers them? Community health agencies, neighborhood newspapers, and local parks and recreation departments may be valuable resources to explore as well as health-food stores and pharmacies.

Patterns will develop as you compile your community resource information. The more information you can collect, the more complete the picture will be of your community's involvement in complementary health care. Patterns of practices will emerge as you develop relationships with complementary health care providers. You will learn about the conditions and uses of the different therapies by interviewing and observing both practitioners and clients. Your role as a community practitioner will be enhanced through these relationships, and these valuable connections will be important for your community education programs.

Educational Program

You will be expected to develop an educational program about complementary therapies that will be meaningful to your community. The information collected in your community resource assessment will provide a background about available resources and patterns of complementary practices. Based on this information an educational program could be designed to bring together a group of complementary practitioners to discuss their therapies with the goal to increase community members involvement in their own health care.

Imagine that the resources in your community included a yoga instructor at the community YMCA, a Doctor of Oriental Medicine at the health-food store, and two chiropractors in private practice in a clinic with one full-time massage therapist. What kind of program would you develop to help the community members increase their knowledge about these practices? What would the important issues be? What would the benefits be of the program? It is important to remember that introducing complementary practices may require a series of interrelated programs that would take planning and cooperation from all those involved. The role of the community practitioner would also include being a facilitator and evaluator.

As you continue to monitor the patterns of complementary practice use in your community, you will develop long-range program goals. Consider that the 40-something users of complementary practices will be 60- and 70-something in 20 and 30 years. What will their needs be, based on their current practices? There are many opportunities for community involvement in complementary practices that will enhance the health and wellness of the individuals and the community. The creative community practitioner will be a visionary in recognizing the potential and influencing the community's health with a plan for a preferable future where access to complementary practices is available to all.

REFERENCES

Anselmo, J., & Kolkmeier, L. G. (2000). Relaxation: The first step to restore, renew, and self-heal. In B. M. Dossey, L. Keegan, & C. E. Guzzetta (Eds.), *Holistic nursing: A handbook for practice* (pp. 497–535). Gaithersburg, MD: Aspen.

Achterberg, J., Dossey, B., & Kolkmeier, L. (1994). *Rituals of healing: Using imagery for health and wellness.* New York: Bantam.

Benson, H. (1984). *Beyond the relaxation response.* New York: Times Books.

Clark, C. C. (Ed.). (1999). *Encyclopedia of complementary health practices.* New York: Springer.

Eisenberg, D. M., Kessler, R. C., Foster, C., Norlock, F. E., Calkins, D. R., & Delbanco, T. L. (1993). Unconventional medicine in the United States: Prevalence, costs, and patterns of use. *The New England Journal of Medicine, 328,* 246–252.

Elder, N. C., Gillcrist, A., & Minz, R. (1997). Use of alternative health care by family practice patients. *Archives of Family Medicine, 5,* 181–184.

Eskinazi, D., & Muehsam, D. (2000). Factors that shape alternative medicine: The role of the alternative medicine research community. *Alternative Therapies, 6,* 49–53.

Grossman, M. L., & Bresler, D. E. (1998). *Interactive guided imagery: Clinical techniques for brief therapy and mind/body medicine* (7th ed.).

Mill Valley, CA: Academy for Guided Imagery.

Hahn, Tich Nhat. (1991). *Peace is every step: The path of mindfulness in everyday life.* New York: Bantam Books.

Helvie, C. O. (1999). A theory for complementary health practitioners. In C. C. Clark (Ed.), *Encyclopedia of complementary health practices* (pp. 5–12). New York: Springer.

Hufford, D. J. (1997). Cultural diversity, folk medicine, and alternative medicine. *Alternative Therapies, 3*(4), 78.

Kabat-Zinn, J. (1990). *Full catastrophe living: Using the wisdom of your body and mind to face stress, pain, and illness.* New York: Bantam-DoubledayDell.

Jonas, W. B. (1997). Alternative medicine. *Journal of Family Practice, 45*(1), 34–37.

Leake, R., & Broderick, J. E. (1999). Current licensure for acupuncture in the United States. *Alternative Therapies in Health and Medicine, 5*(4), 94–96.

McCarthy, N. C., & Mandle, C. L. (1998). Health promotion and the community. In C. L Edelman & C. L. Mandle (Eds.), *Health promotion throughout the lifespan* (pp. 171–191). St. Louis, MO: Mosby.

Millbank Memorial Fund. (1998). *Enhancing the accountability of alternative medicine.* New York: Author.

National Center for Complementary and Alternative Medicine Clearinghouse. (1999). Congress provides the NCCAM with FY 2000 budget increase. *Complementary and Alternative Medicine at the NIH, VI*(1), 4.

National Institutes for Health. (1997). Acupuncture. *NIH consensus statement, 15*(5). Washington, DC: Author.

Patcher, L. M. (1994). Culture and clinical care. *Journal of the American Medical Association, 271*(9), 127.

U.S. Department of Health and Human Services. (1998). *Health people 2010 objectives: Draft for public comment.* Washington, DC: U.S. Government Printing Office.

PART **IV**

Interaction Skills

CHAPTER 18

Advanced Communication Skills With Individuals and Groups

Carolyn Chambers Clark

SELF-AWARENESS

Facilitating wellness in others demands that you be a skilled communicator who listens and observes, then feeds back important information and assists in problem-solving and support. The only way you can do all these things is if you have a high level of self-awareness, so that when you interact with clients you are not operating out of negative patterning from previous relationships. Facilitating wellness involves exhibiting specific communication characteristics (Hover-Kramer, 1997):

- self-esteem
- confidence
- sense of self-worth
- positive outlook
- flexibility, but not overcompliance
- sense of purpose
- goal orientation
- directness
- ability to find a common ground
- caring without being too eager to please

- honesty
- respectful of self and others

Centering to Enhance Communication

One way to ensure better communication with clients is to learn and regularly practice centering yourself in the present moment. See Box 18.1 for directions for centering. When you are centered and relaxed, your voice can carry the message that you care, that you have time for clients and that they are safe with you (Quinn, 1997).

Examining Your Part in Blocking Effective Communication

Centering will allow you to sidestep many of the common blocks to listening that appear in Table 18.1. Use this information to enhance your self-awareness by studying what you say to see which of these blocks may be reducing your communication effectiveness.

Box 18.1   Directions for Centering

- Quietly become aware of your breathing.
- Without effort, let your breathing move gently to your abdominal area.
- Be aware of an enveloping stillness
- Let personal insights emerge as you tune in to the client's communication and energy.

Based on p. 19, *Accepting your power to heal—The personal practice of therapeutic touch* by Dolores Kreiger. Santa Fe, NM: Bear & Company.

TABLE 18.1   Blocks to Listening

Block	Definition
Comparing	Only partially listening to clients because of trying to assess who is smarter, more competent, more emotionally healthy, or suffering more
Mind-reading	Trying to figure out what clients really mean rather than just listening to what is being said
Rehearsing	Going over in your mind what you plan to say next rather than listening to what clients are saying
Filtering	Listening to only the part of clients' messages that you are comfortable hearing
Judging	Mentally or verbally labeling client statements as irrational, stupid, manipulative, etc.
Dreaming	Losing focus because something client says triggers a chain of private associations
Identifying	Focusing on your own pain, anxiety, anger, or whatever emotion or sensation clients bring up
Advising	Suggesting what should be done rather than asking clients for their ideas
Sparring	Looking for ways to disagree, discount, or put down what the client says
Being right	Unable to listen to criticism because mistakes cannot be acknowledged
Derailing	Changing the subject when bored or uncomfortable, joking or quipping
Placating	Agreeing with everything to be pleasant and nice

Abstracted from McKay, Davis, & Fanning, Messages, *The Communication Book*, 1995, Oakland: New Harbinger.

Examine Your Assumptions

It is difficult, if not impossible, not to make generalizations. Making assumptions about what clients may mean can close your mind to the real significance of what is being said. To reduce the misunderstanding that assumptions can cause, start to study the conclusions you draw about clients (Avery, Auvine, Streibel, & Weiss, 1981). Be aware that assumptions are speculation that need to be checked out with clients. For example, you might say, "As I understand it, you don't want to discuss your anger at this time, is that accurate?" By checking out your assumptions with clients, you offer them the opportunity to provide you with new information or explanations. At the same time, you increase their understanding of clear communication processes by role-modeling how to check out assumptions with others.

EMPATHY

Empathy is the ability to communicate at least as much feeling and meaning as the speaker has communicated. The following examples are the five levels of empathy (Carkhuff, 1969):

Level 1: You communicate no awareness of the expressed surface feelings of the client and you are not really focusing on what the client is saying.

Level 2: You communicate your own understanding of what the client is experiencing, but it is not congruent with the client.

Level 3: Your expressions are essentially interchangeable with the client's (paraphrasing what was said). You are trying to understand, but only hear or see the superficial meaning.

Level 4: Your communication adds noticeably to the expressions of the client, communicating a level deeper than the client was able to express. You think you understand what the client is saying and try to express it.

Level 5: Your communication adds significantly to the feeling and meaning of the client in such a way that you accurately express feelings that are levels below what the client is able to express. You

are tuned in to the client's wavelength totally.

Example:

Client: "I'm a little upset that this community doesn't support us when we take a stand to get a better environment. They say they will, then they stay silent. Why don't they make up their minds? Half the time they don't even listen to me when I talk about it, and half the time they don't read the information I give them or they misplace it." (Angry facial expressions and tone of voice; right hand pounding the palm of the other hand.) "I really thought they wanted a better life." (Confused look on face.)

Level 1: response: "Why don't we talk about last week's minutes?"

Level 2: response: "Maybe everyone is busy with their own problems."

Level 3: response: "You're a little upset because the community doesn't pay attention to your information on improving the environment."

Level 4: response: "Your community doesn't seem to support your exercise program and that is really upsetting for you."

Level 5: response: "You're really angry that your community isn't helping one bit with your environmental plan. The way they keep changing their reactions is confusing and you wish they'd make up their minds to support you and stick to it."

Guidelines for communicating effectively with clients include the following (Carkhuff, 1969; Scandrett-Hibdon, 1997):

1.   Concentrate totally on what clients are saying and the intensity of their verbal and nonverbal expressions.

2.   Use words that are in tune with the client's words.

3.   Respond with a feeling tone that is similar to client's.

4.   Respond frequently after you start to understand clients; the more active you are, the more likely it will be that clients will take an active role in their wellness process.

5.   Fill in what is missing from client's verbal expression, based on a clear understanding of their nonverbal expressions.

6.   Communicate in a genuine and spontaneous manner. Trust your feelings.

7.   Make communication between you and clients concrete by asking for specific details and specific instances of what is blocking movement toward health and wellness: "Give me an example of the last time your community didn't support you. What exactly was said and what did they do?"

8.   Disclose personally relevant material that provides role-modeling of how to attain wellness. "When I tried to get a community to take a stand, I felt frustrated, but I eventually was successful. I believe you can be, too, and I'm going to help you."

9.   Be genuine and share moment-to-moment experiences to help clients understand how relationships work. "We're all a little anxious because this is our first discussion with each other and that's okay. Let's talk about what could make us more comfortable" or "I want to help you, but when you brandish that chair at me, I feel afraid, and then I can't be helpful."

10.   Confront verbal and nonverbal discrepancies in client's communication: "You are smiling, but I hear you saying you're angry."

11.   Focus on what clients are really trying to tell you that they cannot tell you directly: "I hear your frustration with trying to lose weight and you're wondering if I can really help you."

12.   Show respect for clients by communicating the belief that they know what is needed, have the ability to make their own decisions, and have the resources and strengths to take action.

13.   Focus on the relationship and what is happening in the here and now: "I sense you want me to decide for you, but I can only help you take a look at possible plans."

14.   Assist with problem-solving by helping clients specify goals: "What specifically do you want to change?" and "How will you know when you've met your goal?" and "When do you plan to meet your goal?"

15.   Help clients brainstorm: "What are some ways you can meet your goal?" and "Let's think of all possible ways you could meet your goal and not limit or judge any methods for now. Let's just have fun with it."

16.   Help clients evaluate alternative ways to meet their goals: "Let's take a look at the three ways you could meet your goal and see what the gain and cost of each is" and "You've decided on a path to your goal, but keep in mind there are other alternatives for you to use later if you wish."

17.   Ask clients to plan small steps to their goal to build in success: "Let's think about some small steps you can take to your goal so you can experience success as you move along" and "Picture yourself meeting your goal and see if that's what you really want" and "How do you think you might sabotage your plan?" and "What steps can you take so you don't sabotage your plan?"

ASSERTIVENESS

Assertiveness includes being able to stand up for your rights while being respectful of others' rights. "I-messages" are used to indicate you are responsible for your statements: "I feel angry" not "You make me angry." Some "we-messages" can also be assertive if they imply collaboration: "We can talk about this and work it out."

Being assertive is a useful skill when promoting health and wellness. Acting assertively allows you to role-model healthy behaviors for clients. You will be more assertive when you refrain from blaming others, stick to the point of the discussion without changing topics, use open and direct body communication, speak firmly, make sure your gestures match your words, and make frequent and direct eye contact (unless dealing with participants from cultures who avoid direct eye contact).

Assertiveness Procedures for Dealing with Criticism

Leaders cannot avoid criticism. Some strategies for dealing with criticism include: acknowledging, clouding, agreeing in part, agreeing in probability, or agreeing in principle, and assertive probing (McKay, Davis, & Fanning, 1995).

Acknowledging

Whenever you are criticized, the assertive thing to do is to acknowledge that you've received the message: "You're right, I am late for the meeting." Or "Yes, I did forget to follow through on that. I will do so by tomorrow." There is no need to apologize at length; a simple "I'm sorry" will do if you genuinely feel it; otherwise don't apologize if you don't mean it because being assertive means you are being authentic. Likewise, excuses don't fit with an assertive presentation. They are carryovers from childhood when explanations and apologies were demanded. As an adult, you have the right to choose whether you want to give an expla-

nation or apologize. It is not often useful to give an explanation or apology because it provides more ammunition for whoever is being critical.

Clouding

Clouding works well when nonconstructive, manipulative criticism is received. It can allow you to stand your ground while continuing to communicate with others. Clouding requires careful listening to determine what you can honestly agree with in part, in probability, or in principle. The idea is to agree with the part of the person's statement that makes some sense, but not agree to change: "You're right, it does seem that way."

Assertive Probing

In assertive probing, you can remain in communication with the person criticizing you, but ask probing questions about their concerns: "What don't you like about what I said?" or "What is it that bothers you about the community?"

Additional Assertive Strategies

There are other assertive strategies you can use to stand up for your rights while continuing to communicate with others. Approaches that will be discussed include the broken record, content-to-process shift, momentary delay, time out, joining, and circling the attacker (Dobson & Miller, 1978).

The Broken Record

The broken record works well when clients don't hear or accept what you have to say. The first step in broken record is to clarify the limits of what can be expected. The second step is to avoid giving excuses or explanations, not giving any additional information that can become ammunition for future attacks. The third step is to use body language that supports the statement, including maintaining appropriate eye contact, standing or sitting erect, and keeping hands and arms quiet. The fourth step is to calmly and firmly repeat the chosen statement as many times as necessary until the other person acknowledges no negotiation is possible.

Example:

Client: "We want you to talk to the media for us."

You: "I understand your desire, but I believe it would be better if you talk to the media."

Client: "But you're so good at doing it. Won't you help us out?"

You: "I think it would be better if you talk to the media."

Client: "Okay, but I still think you should talk to the media."

Content-to-Process Shift

When the point of the conversation has drifted from its original topic, using the content-to-process shift to allows you to help clients get back on track: "We're off the point now. Let's get back to what we agreed to discuss."

Content-to-process shift is also helpful when voices are raised and there is anger: "We seem to be getting into a battle about this. Let's try to stick to collaborating on solutions."

Momentary Delay

Questions or statements often seem to imply a command to answer quickly. Rather than being swayed by the emotion of the moment, take a deep breath and wait until

you're ready to answer: "Let me think about that for a minute [hour, day, week]."

Time Out

Time out is similar to momentary delay, except in this approach both you and the client take time to think through a problem or come up with a solution: "Let's both sleep on this and come back tomorrow with a solution or two."

Joining and Circling the Attacker

In each attacking or conflict situation, there are six alternative ways to respond:

1. Do nothing. Do not dignify the attack when it is nonsensical or unfair. To be assertive, this must be a conscious choice, not silence that comes from fear.

2. Use deflection, absurdity, or humor. Any of these approaches can surprise the attacker and break a line of attack: "What a nice suit" (deflection); "I couldn't get the report done, I was attacked by Martians" (absurdity); "Have you heard the one about . . . ?" (humor).

3. Joining the attacker: "I don't blame you for being angry about what I did. I would be, too."

4. Fighting back: "I won't stand here and be insulted. I resent being blamed for someone else's error. We can continue arguing or use our energy to solve the problem by working together."

5. Parley: "Maybe we can figure out a way to solve both our problems by working together."

6. Withdrawal: May be the best choice when the other person only wants to fight unfairly.

CONFLICT RESOLUTION

Conflict is a natural and healthy part of community process. Be suspicious if there isn't any conflict in your group because participants may be holding back their real feelings. To handle conflict in a community group, use the following principles (Avery et al., 1981; Gillespie, 1996):

1. Bring hidden conflicts into the open by stating what you observe. If there is hidden conflict (disagreement), ask those involved what they are feeling.

2. Disagree with ideas, not people, and ask the group to do the same. If you have some operating rules they can be referred to when someone steps out of line. With feelings running high, outbursts can occur, so provide boundaries.

3. When defining an issue or problem, always share responsibility: "We have a problem and we need to find a solution to it."

4. Avoid compromising too soon; try to stay open to a creative solution that gives everyone what they most need.

5. Ask group members to state others' stands.

6. Get participants to agree on the underlying source of disagreement.

7. Ask each member to list what the other side should do.

8. Exchange lists and ask the group to decide on a compromise by having each side write down 10 questions for their opponents; the answers will provide insights that could lead to a compromise.

9. Remind team members that changing a position after receiving new information can be a sign of strength.

10. Avoid taking sides. Step back and see all sides of the issue.

11. If the conflict does not seem to be subsiding, try calling a break asking for a few minutes of silence, then ask that everyone count to 10 before responding to the previous speaker. If there is still a deadlock, suggest that the discussion be stopped and picked up again at another time, but be sure to set that time and follow through to ensure that the issue is discussed.

12. Consider setting up a special, structured process for dealing with conflict that is difficult to handle within the confines of a meeting: a special meeting or an all-day retreat that uses a neutral facilitator to help you through the rough spots.

MEDIATION

Mediation is used when two or more clients are having difficulty working together. Those involved must be willing to negotiate with you, but their feelings may be getting in the way. Use the following steps to complete mediation (Avery et al., 1981):

1. Agree on outcomes: "Do you really want to work this out?"; "Is this negotiable for all of you?"; "Are your goals compatible?"

2. Express feelings to clear the air: "Let's get your feelings out so we can then work on solutions"; "This is a safe place to express your hurt and angry feelings."

3. Check out assumptions: "What are your fears about this process?"; "What are your expectations about what will happen?"

4. Discuss perceptions: "Talk about what you see happening."

5. Critique the problem: "I want each of you to analyze the problem, not the other people"; "Please look at your own actions and tell me how they have contributed to the problem."

6. Investigate dreams: "I want you each to state what you want to happen between you"; "Wish for 100 percent of what you want"; "Let's explore all possible options."

7. Craft a contract: "Let's make an agreement or contract to do things differently"; "I'd like each of you to promise you will change the behaviors that contribute to the problem."

8. Share positive thoughts: "Tell each other what you appreciate about them and what you like about them both in general and during this mediation process."

MOTIVATION AND GOAL SETTING PRINCIPLES

Cairo (1992) developed an eight-step method for assisting clients in meeting their goals. The steps include: (a) examining your identity, (b) defining your values, (c) establishing goals, (d) developing an action plan, (e) examining various facets of motivation, (f) establishing discipline, (g) maintaining flexibility, (h) reaching an outcome.

Examining Identity

To help clients on their journey toward health and wellness, ask them to examine their strengths and weaknesses. Without undertaking this crucial step, the process of defining goals and working toward them will be flawed. Goals can be more easily built by using strengths rather than focusing on weaknesses.

Determining Values

Values are fundamental beliefs. Assist clients in identifying their personal values by assessing the following:

- their attitude toward and relationships with others
- moral issues of importance
- obligations felt to community, country, and family
- priorities for personal fulfillment

Establishing values allows clients to prioritize goals. Without this step, all goals appear equally enticing.

Defining Goals

Less than 5% of the population sets goals, even though without them individuals are apt to wander off course (Cairo, 1992). Below are some principles for setting health and wellness promotion goals:

1. Base goals on personal values.
2. Set specific goals, for example, to lose 20 pounds by December or to stop smoking by April.
3. Write goals down as evidence of a commitment.
4. Set a challenging but realistic goal.
5. Visualize attaining the goal.
6. Provide incentives to help overcome procrastination: dinner at a favorite restaurant, taking a vacation after losing 20 pounds, or buying a fishing rod after stopping smoking.

Developing an Action Plan

Clients may believe that setting goals and providing incentives may be sufficient to attaining health and wellness. Cairo (1992) points out that an action plan establishes what needs to be done to turn a goal into reality. Developing an action plan requires the following steps:

1. Create a Wellness and Health Promotion Goal Activity Page that includes actions needed to attain a goal. List activities in order of importance.
2. In a column to the right of each activity, identify who or what would help achieve the goal.

3. In the next column write down a target date for accomplishing each activity.
4. Develop a Wellness and Health Promotion Goal Activity Page for each goal that can be comfortably accomplished.
5. Spend a minimum of 5 minutes a day doing the priority activity for the top goal.
6. Concentrate on only the first activity to reduce fear of action.

Motivating Clients

Do you believe you can motivate clients to change their behavior and move forward on their journey to health and wellness? Cairo (1992) takes the position that motivation is not internal, but external. According to this model, motivation is rewarded by incentives and that is why behavior changes. Rewards can also be thought of as consequences. If a client wants or needs something badly enough, then motivation exists to obtain that something. If you want to help clients change their behavior, help them change the consequences. The best rewards are those that meet client basic needs and wants. General wants and needs include:

- love and acceptance
- satisfaction from work
- approval of others
- involvement with a group
- feedback

To the degree you are able to provide what clients want, or help them provide it themselves, clients will change their behavior toward wellness and health. Praise and recognition can often evoke client change.

Using Listening Skills to Motivate

Possibly the greatest motivator is respect. One of the best ways to communicate respect is by developing good listening skills. Effective listening takes practice, commitment, and energy. Principles for effective listening include:

1. Focus all your attention on the speaker, making that person feel important enough to be listened to.
2. Refuse to judge whatever the client says, valuing the message and making a genuine attempt to see the world through the client's eyes.
3. Shut out your own prejudices.
4. Realize that words can be deceptive and watch for clues in body language, tone, volume, and inflection.
5. Practice reflexive listening by repeating what you believe you heard the client say; for example, "You sound angry about what happened." This gives the client an opportunity to reaffirm or correct the message.
6. Resist giving advice unless it is asked for.
7. Look for statements to agree with, refusing to argue a point.
8. Make clients feel important by remembering names and things they tell you.
9. Realize that listening is a learned skill and requires practice.
10. Monitor your thoughts and exchange positive for negative ones.

Box 18.2 presents a case study that focuses on listening.

Using Encouragement as Motivation

Clients will be motivated if you enhance their self-worth (Cairo, 1992). You can in-

---

Box 18.2   Case Study Focused on Listening

A group of women in the community have been trying to lose weight, but when they feel stressed they binge. They're having trouble finding the self-discipline to stay on a food plan and exercise regularly. They are becoming discouraged.

You listen to their doubts and lack of confidence. You give them positive feedback, telling them, "I know it's frustrating trying to lose weight, but you're doing a good job. You've already lost some weight. I have confidence you can stick to your goals and lose the weight you want to lose." You assure the women that if they work at it, they will lose weight. The group seems inspired to work harder at their weight-loss plan because you listened to their frustration and motivated them by reinforcing their self-esteem and by recognizing that they are doing a good job.

---

spire others to take a risk, change behavior, or move toward their goals by offering encouragement. To be effective, encouragement should be specific. Instead of simply saying, "Good," try, "I'm impressed at how you followed through with your goal to stop smoking and overcame your frustration."

Use the following five principles when giving encouragement:

1. Assist clients in stating measurable, realistic, and meaningful goals.
2. Allow clients to participate by owning their goals.
3. Use learning situations to stimulate interest in change.
4. Motivate clients by using your own self-confidence to demonstrate possible healthy actions.
5. Ensure that clients have identified specific actions to meet their goals.

Motivating Through Feedback

When misused, feedback can serve as a barrier to client progress. When used effectively, feedback can motivate even the least motivated client. Behavior changes when consequences change (Cairo, 1992). Increase client rewards by giving more positive feedback. To get yourself started

thinking about how to use positive feedback more often, do the following:

- Jot down a list of current clients
- Write down at least 5 positive behaviors for each client
- Use this information in a 10:1 ratio to confrontation

Motivating Through Confrontation

Confrontation can be a useful approach when clients do not fulfill their agreements or are behaving in ways contrary to their goals. Confrontation can be a motivator if used correctly. Not knowing how to confront ineffective behavior in a helpful way can result in resentment or even bitterness in clients. Not confronting inappropriate behavior is the same as agreeing with it. Use confrontation to:

1. Solve problems. Point out the behavior that is inconsistent with client goals and suggest an alternative: "As I understand it, your goal is to learn to handle your anger. Instead of shouting, what about stating how you feel, using an 'I' message?"

2. Avoid personal attacks. Focus on behaviors, not labels. Describe in detail the behavior you have agreed on: "Your goal is

to stop eating ice cream, but you say you had some for dessert. Let's see how we can make a plan to keep you from eating ice cream."

3. Ask for agreement. Seek to come to an agreement with the client for change. Encourage a desire to move toward wellness. "I know you can do this, I've seen you do it before. Can we agree you'll make every effort to stop smoking?" (Cairo, 1992).

Some guidelines for using confrontation are:

1. Act promptly. Speak out right away and don't bring the issue up again unless it happens again. Rehashing is nonproductive.

2. Discuss any issues in private. Avoid embarrassing clients by pointing out inconsistencies in behavior and goals out of earshot of anyone else.

3. Be positive. Encourage clients by expressing your confidence they can meet their goals (Cairo, 1992).

BUILDING CONSENSUS

Consensus means that all involved think the decision is acceptable. They may not be totally satisfied with the outcome, but they are willing to agree to it. Consensus differs from other forms of decision-making because it stresses cooperation between those involved. The process of consensus is associated with the Quakers (the Religious Society of Friends) who developed and used these procedures for more than 300 years (Avery et al., 1981).

The advantages to using consensus procedures are:

- A quality decision is developed that has been fully examined.

- More imaginative and creative possibilities are discovered as the group attempts to meet everyone's needs.
- There is more commitment to the decision because there is more involvement in reaching it.
- Group process skills, valuing and respecting others' opinions and responsibility for the group are learned; these skills can be used in other settings.

The Lakota, a Native American group, make no important decisions unless women, men, children, and elders are all present. At some point, an older woman stands and reminds the decision makers to take no actions without considering the effects of their behavior on seven future generations (Avery et al., 1981).

The Process of Consensus

There is a specific process and specific tools and techniques that you can use to build a consensus, including agendas, or introducing items, promoting group discussion, testing for consensus, evaluating decisions, and deciding on what to do if the group cannot agree.

Agendas

A family or group prepares for developing consensus by coming together and setting an agenda. Participants must agree on what they will talk about and in what order. Writing the agreed-upon agenda on a blackboard or large piece of paper can remind the group what to discuss next and to stay focused.

Agenda items should include a clearly stated topic of discussion, the name of the person responsible for introducing the item, action to be taken (announcement, report, discussion, or decision), and estimated time needed to complete the action. It's common to underestimate the amount of time an item will require, so add a few more minutes than you think an item will take.

It is preferable to have a log or book available ahead of time, even between meetings, so participants can jot down items for the next session. Asking people to generate items in the meeting can eat up valuable time and important items may be forgotten or overlooked.

The agenda should be reviewed with the group early in the meeting to make sure the time limits are realistic and that the order of items is appropriate. Either start with difficult, divisive items and finish with unifying ones or vice versa, building trust first so that more difficult items can be tackled. Always consider which items can be discussed outside the group through special brown-bag lunch meetings, subgroups, delegated tasks, or written dialogue. In the latter case, use a special notebook for dialogues; one or more individuals generate a list of questions relevant to an issue and write them in the log. Other participants write their thoughts and feelings about the issue in the book. By the time of the meeting, the groundwork has been laid and some feelings and perspectives have already been shared (Avery et al., 1981).

Promoting Group Discussion

There are a number of ways of promoting group discussion toward consensus. One way it to begin with a review of why the particular issue is important. Another way it to provide and ask for personal statements of concerns, thoughts, or feelings about the item. A written proposal could also be the focus for discussion. Any discussion will be more fruitful if you encourage positive suggestions to improve the proposal, not just negative reactions showing its weaknesses.

The group will move along more effectively if you make sure the roles of timekeeper, recorder, process watcher, vibes watcher, and devil's advocate are filled. Be sure these roles rotate so everyone can learn the skills and contribute. The group will also come to consensus if everyone participates and no one dominates the discussion. Hand out a pile of matchsticks to all participants to limit each person's number of contributions.

Fill important group roles.   Make sure that important group roles are filled if you want to reach consensus. If one or more of these roles is missing, you may not be able to hold the group together or to remember or implement decisions that have been made.

Timekeeper.   Appoint a timekeeper or keep time yourself. Every 10 or 15 minutes, summarize what has been occurring: "We've been looking at alternatives to buying a new van for 10 minutes now. How much more time do we want to spend on this? Are most of our ideas on the table at this point?" By reminding participants and nudging them along while still being sensitive to feelings, everyone will feel encouraged to speak up. Equalize participation by using brain-storming, silence, round robin, or traveling chair, which are discussed later in this chapter.

Recorder.   It would be a shame to spend time and energy reaching consensus and then not remember the exact agreement. A recorder should have a number of responsibilities that can help the group achieve consensus and implement their decisions. The recorder's responsibilities are as follows:

- Summarize ideas from brainstorming and round robins.

- List issues to return to next session.
- Note content of major discussions.
- Record names of people who volunteered to take responsibility for action and when they will take the action.
- Read decisions to the group after they are made to check for accuracy and underline closure.
- Mark undecided items in the notes with a star for easy identification.
- Following the meeting, distribute copies of notes to participants.
- At the next meeting, summarize major points, decisions, deferred issues, and assignment reminders.

Other roles to fill. The process watcher observes the group process and brings problems to its attention. The vibes watcher samples the emotional climate of the meeting and reports it to the group. Conflicts and hidden agendas often surface when trying to reach consensus. If the vibes watcher can pay attention to what is happening, potential negative events can be spotted early and defused. The devil's advocate represents the unrepresented position during a consensus discussion and will give reasons why a decision is a bad one or why a solution won't work.

Brainstorming to identify solutions. Brainstorming encourages creative response and detachment from individual ideas by stressing quantity, not quality. Ask participants to come up with as many solutions to a problem that they can within, say, 10 minutes. Because participants are free to make spontaneous comments, they can feel free to take risks and step out of their usual roles. Be sure to tell the group this is a time to generate ideas, not criticize them in any way. This will provide a sense of safety and a time during which creative ideas will be heard and nurtured.

Silence. Silence includes pausing during a discussion and saying, "Let's take two minutes to think about this issue." This procedure gives everyone a chance to slow down. When you use silence, quick thinkers and talkers won't be able to dominate the discussion.

Round robin. A good follow-up procedure after a short silence is a round robin. In this approach, each person offers one idea or possible solution to a problem. Go around the group repeatedly until all ideas have been expressed and recorded. Participants can pass on one turn and still be included in the next round. Give the speaker an egg timer to encourage concise and focused statements.

Evaluating Decisions

Never end a consensus meeting without conducting an evaluation of what has happened. Help the group examine what went on, how well they achieved their goals, and how future sessions can be improved. Don't be tempted to hurry through the evaluation component of a consensus meeting; it can provide valuable insight for you.

Evaluations can provide a much-needed outlet for criticism and frustration about how the group or individual members behaved or for items that were not on the agenda. Sometimes participants use the evaluation to express praise, support, and positive thoughts about decisions. Encourage the group to think about what went right as well as what needs improvement. You can use evaluations at any time while trying to get to consensus, including right before a break and whenever frustration surfaces. Statements should stay focused on process issues, not on agenda items.

Written evaluations are also useful. Post near the exit a large piece of paper divided

---

Box 18.3   Evaluation Example

During a recent meeting to enhance safety in the community, the group seemed lethargic and drifted off on tangents. They did manage to make two decisions, but as the meeting ended and participants started to leave, the facilitator called for an evaluation. With some coaching from the facilitator, participants started to express their frustration with the meeting and its outcome. Some individuals were so dissatisfied that they said they had no intention of carrying out the decisions the rest of the group had made. They had stopped discussing safety in the community and remained silent, waiting for the meeting to end. Without this evaluation, participants would have left with invalid expectations of each other and without trying to solve group process problems.

---

into the following columns: positives, negatives, suggested changes. Written evaluations are most suited for long or complex meetings and can provide highly useful information for restructuring your meetings. See Box 18.3 for an example of how important evaluations can be.

Begin to implement advanced communication skills in your community work. It will help your work move more smoothly when you really listen and respond to client needs.

REFERENCES

Avery, M., Auvine, B., Streibel, B., & Weiss, L. (1981). *Building united judgment: A handbook for consensus decision-making.* Madison, WI: The Center for Conflict Resolution.

Cairo, J. (1992). *Motivation and goal-setting: The keys to achieving success.* Shawnee Mission, KS: Rockhurst College Continuing Education Center.

Carkhuff, R. R. (1969). *Helping and human relations.* New York: Holt, Rhinehart, and Winston.

Dobson, T., & Miller, V. (1978). *Giving in to get your way.* New York: Delacorte Press.

Gillespie, J. (1996). How to deal with conflict. *Communication Briefings, 15*(3), 1.

Hover-Kramer D. (1997). Relationships. In B. Montgomery Dossey (Ed.), *American Holistic Nursing Associations Core Curriculum for Holistic Nursing* (pp. 119–124). Gaithersburg, MD: Aspen.

Krieger, D. (1993). *Accepting your power to heal— The personal practice of therapeutic touch.* Santa Fe, NM: Bear.

McKay, M., Davis, M., & Fanning, P. (1995). *Messages: The communication book.* Oakland, CA: New Harbinger.

Quinn J. (1997). Transpersonal human caring and healing. *American Holistic Nursing Associations' Core Curriculum for Holistic Nursing* (pp. 13–16). Gaithersburg, MD: Aspen.

Scrandett-Hibdon S. (1997). Therapeutic communication: The art of helping. *American Holistic Nursing Associations Core Curriculum for Holistic Nursing* (pp. 102–107). Gaithersburg, MD: Aspen.

CHAPTER 19

Working With Groups

Cynthia G. Johnson and Beth R. Keely

G roups are important in solving problems in the community. You may be called on to provide support and leadership for community groups involved in health and wellness promotion. By serving as group leader and community collaborator, you will be able to achieve goals and objectives that would be impossible through individual efforts. An environment that fosters successful group collaboration will demand that you understand methods for working in groups.

In this chapter you will learn successful strategies for working with groups, methods for overcoming blocks to group process, and methods for reinforcing group strengths, self-care capabilities and group resilience.

DEFINING GROUPS, GROUP PROCESS, COHESIVENESS, SCAPEGOATING, TRANSFERENCE, AND COUNTERTRANSFERENCE

It is important to know and be able to recognize certain groups and processes to be an effective group leader. In this section, rele-

vant terms related to group work are defined.

Groups

Cookfair (1996) describes a group as an open system composed of three or more persons held together by a common interest or bond. Porter-O'Grady (1986) sees a group as a collection of individuals who must work interdependently in order to obtain and meet individual professional and organizational objectives. Whatever definition is used, there seems to be a growing awareness that groups, task forces, management groups, stress-reduction groups, and care-for-the-caregiver groups are some of the growing numbers of the professional-oriented groups you may be involved with in the community (Northouse & Northouse, 1998). Four main functions characterize an effective working group: Accomplishing its stated objectives, maintaining cohesiveness, developing a working structure, and modifying the structure to improve effectiveness. With the increasing use of groups within the community, it is necessary for you to understand the group processes.

Group Process

Group process (McLaughlin & Kaluzny, 1999) involves the work, activities, operations, and relationships designed to accomplish the goals set by the group. It is the way group members interact with one another and can include interruptions, silences, judgments, glares, scapegoating and many other behaviors. As a community practitioner, you may be called on to form, lead, direct, or participate as a member of a group for promoting health or solving a community problem. You must be familiar with the unique processes that are needed for group formation, development, and maintenance.

Several factors and conditions can shape the structure and function of a group positively or negatively. Lewin (1951) refers to these factors as driving and restraining forces.

For example, the physical environment, personal space, and seating arrangements; leadership styles and roles; methods of decision-making; group members' trust; cohesion and conformity; interpersonal attraction; and power and influence are all important areas to consider in the group process. When you lead a group, take each of these factors into account and strive to use each to help the group move forward in the most constructive fashion.

Cohesiveness

Cohesion refers to how well group members feel they belong, fit into the group, and are included by others (Cookfair, 1996). Group cohesiveness is the strength of the individuals desire to maintain their membership in the group. A group is cohesive when its members are attracted to it. Cohesiveness is the glue that holds the group together and allows movement towards the common goals. Without cohesiveness groups are usually unsuccessful. When members do not feel comfortable within a group they tend to lose interest, motivation, enjoyment, and drive and will eventually leave the group. High cohesiveness is frequently associated with increased participation and better interactions among members of the group (Northouse & Northouse, 1998).

You can use creative warm-up exercises and ice-breakers for introductions. One effective exercise is to ask each member to choose someone whom they don't know to introduce to the group. Each person spends 5 minutes getting acquainted and getting information. Then they introduce one another to the group. Beyond the introductory tasks, an effort should be made to describe clearly the reasons for the group's existence (Breckon, Harvey, & Lancaster, 1998). Box 19.1 lists some of the factors that may affect group cohesiveness. Box 19.2 shows some indicators you can use to evaluate group cohesiveness.

Scapegoating

A *scapegoat* is a person or thing made to bear the blame for the mistakes of others. In a group setting, one group member, including the leader, may be blamed for problems within the group. In scapegoating the leader and members may join together in a collaborative resistance effort, or group members may attempt to test the leader's style, patience, and goals.

As you become aware of scapegoating, manage it, try refraining from rescuing individuals, and assisting the group in recognizing their uncomfortable feelings,

Box 19.1   Factors Relating to Group Cohesiveness

Barriers: Many factors can deter cohesiveness

- Grouping of the membership: Sometimes members who have similar ideas tend to gravitate to each other and form a subgroup. If this group gets larger than the core group it can be a deterrence to meeting the goals.
- Unstable group members: These are members who may not be motivated and who attend the meetings infrequently. The group leader must be aware of this and attempt to motivate these members to bring them back as active participants.
- Autocratic leader who makes all the decisions and analyzes group members' behaviors. This is a major deterrent to successful group process. The leadership style should complement the group; a democratic style works best.

Techniques for Improving Cohesiveness

- Sharing ideas and beliefs by saying, "I read that a group in _____ had tremendous success with _____" or "In another group, we tried _____ and had some success with this method."
- Having a comfortable environment. The physical setting, lighting, temperature of the room, and seating arrangements enhance cohesiveness.
- Ask group members to write down their perceptions of themselves and others in the group.
- Compromising in areas where there are diverse opinions, for instance, by saying "Let's weigh some of the alternatives."

Enhancers

- Use a democratic style
- Size of the group: Depending on the task, an intermediate size of 8–12 is preferred. Consider a small task force for more specific tasks.
- Communication patterns: A lateral and bottom-up approach allows for more of a decentralized approach.
- Group goals: Everyone must know and understand the goals of the group. Provide the goals in writing.
- Interdependence: Members must feel the connectedness with one another. This is enhanced by developing trust.
- Trust: Trustworthy behaviors of the leader and members increase cohesiveness. Respect for one another enhances trust (Cookfair, 1996).

Box 19.2   Evaluative Indicators of Group Cohesiveness

- Group members are friendly to one another
- Group members enjoy each other and interact well
- Group members are sensitive to one another and readily praise for accomplishments
- Group members work collaboratively
- Group members developed trust for one another
- The group leader uses a democratic approach
- Group action is interdependent and shows collaborative efforts
- There is a high level of group communication
- The group accomplishes its goals
- Attendance at meetings is at a high level
- Group members have less anxiety and an increased level of participation

---

perhaps by saying, "I know that some of you might be feeling somewhat anxious" or "I sense some uncomfortable feelings in this room." Try to anticipate any scapegoating efforts by reducing stress and anxiety in the group. See chapter 13 for ways to help group members reduce their stress and anxiety. Members who begin to isolate themselves from the group or who have difficulty with socialization need to be watched very carefully. You may need to teach them social skills, ways to directly express their feelings in the group, talk to them one-on-one between group sessions, or refer them to assertiveness classes.

Transference and Countertransference

The transference and countertransference phenomena must also be considered in a group relationship. These are normal occurrences that may surface and may inhibit the effectiveness of the group.

Transference can occur in groups when feelings, attitudes, and wishes originally linked with early significant others are projected onto group members. For example,

a group member may shout and yell at you when you suggest the group meet weekly. When you ask him what happened, he says you look like his mother and that she was always "shooting off her mouth, too."

To reduce transference, explore the meaning of individual words, events, gestures, and situations and their meanings within the context of the group. Some questions to do this are: "What is it that Jerry is doing that's upsetting you?" or "What is it that I am doing to upset you?" If the group member's perceptions are accurate, modify your behavior. If not, point out how you are different by saying, for example, "I may look like your mother, but I'm a community practitioner and I want to help make this group work." Clarify sentences and statements. Give group members time to explain the issue and to realize that their reaction may be related to a different time, place, or person.

Teach group members to separate past relationships from the current ones by refocusing on the current goals and purpose of the group: "That may have been true then, but in this group we've agreed to . . . " Acting in a calm, goal-oriented way may or may not help the group member to calm down, but it will provide other group members with a model for handling behavior.

Countertransference refers to a response you might have to a client based on your life experiences. It is a psychoanalytical concept referring to the unconscious response of the practitioner to the client (O'Kelly, 1998). If a client shouts at you and you respond with anger, your response is an example of countertransference, possibly based on your experiences of being shouted at. If you felt comfortable with the anger you could stay calm, but realize that reacting in kind signals discomfort with the feeling. Everyone has countertransferential feelings at times. They only become a problem if you don't identify your own and take steps not to respond in negative ways to the group (see chapter 13 for stress-reducing measures). You might also want to talk out your feelings with a trusted colleague to ensure that you don't react inappropriately with the clients you are trying to help.

Specific indicators that signal countertransference as a problem include: uneasy feelings during or after the group meetings, being late for meetings, anxiety, irritability, or even hostility. As a group leader you must learn to recognize countertransference and consciously develop goal-directed responses when it occurs.

CHARACTERISTICS AND FACTORS AFFECTING GROUP WORK

In establishing a group, identify functional characteristics (purpose and types of groups), structural factors (the selection of members, the composition and size of the group), and interactional factors (psychological, social, and behavioral dimensions, norms, values, beliefs, relationships, and commitments). If you are not the group leader, help the group find a leader and assess the roles and basic needs of group members.

Purpose of Groups

Groups are sometimes defined according to their purpose. In collaboration with the group help it to identify its purpose. One purpose may be to give information about a particular subject. Another may be to seek or solicit information from community residents. A major purpose of a community group may be to brainstorm or to collect ideas without making any judgments. Another group purpose may be for decision-making and problem-solving. See the seven purposes for group meetings in Box 19.3.

Types of Groups

You maybe involved in one of many types of groups, and groups can be closed or open. In an *open group* new members may join and others may leave at any time; in a *closed group*, members begin the group at one time and no new members are accepted. Cookfair (1996) identified four types of groups: community development, support or self-help, educational, and focus. Additionally, most groups use task forces to accomplish certain tasks.

Community development groups are concerned with advocacy. These groups are designed to empower community residents for change. Involvement and the use of strength in numbers are two components for success. Examples of these are groups of individuals wanting to provide increased access to facilities or groups formed for grassroots policy development.

Self-help groups are formed by professionals or laypersons for the specific purpose of support or cohesiveness. Group members may require support for behavioral modifi-

---

Box 19.3   Seven Purposes for Group Meetings

1. Tell—To transmit information to a group
2. Sell—To persuade the group about an idea
3. Seek information—To solicit information about an issue
4. Brainstorm—To collect a wide variety of ideas from a group
5. Seek advice—To solicit opinions from a group
6. Problem solving—To discuss and debate to move towards resolution (Rowland & Rowland, 1997)
7. Decision making—To choose options directed towards the solution of a problem

---

cation, grief, weight management, or resocialization. You may be called on to be a facilitator or consultant for any one of these groups.

Educational groups provide education in preventive health. Examples are a diabetic class for a group of residents or a nutrition education class for health professionals or school children.

Focus groups are used to solicit information about feelings, ideas, and opinions about an issue or experience. Marketing research firms rely on focus groups to market their products. One advantage of the focus group is its synergy.

Task forces are subgroups that are charged with a specific task agreed upon by all members. The focus is the completion of a task in a specified amount of time. The leader of a task force, called a chairperson, establishes the exchange of information among members and directs the group toward task accomplishments. Table 19.1 compares the types of groups in relation to their goals and objectives, purpose, format and leadership style, and focus.

Structural factors such as the selection or election of members, composition, and size of groups are the second important area in establishing groups. They include membership, group composition, and group size.

Membership

In group formation, members either volunteer or are selected or elected. Because members often volunteer, it is important that a thorough assessment be done to identify members' age and developmental level, strengths and limitations. For example, the age and developmental levels are important in determining the length of life experience, health status, and, indirectly, the ability to find solutions to problems. Physical health status may also influence group members' ability to attend meetings and participate effectively. Each member has unique characteristics and brings a different perspective to the group. Through a selection or election process, the characteristics, interests, and, sometimes, personality are known before group formation. A thorough assessment via an interview or information sheet will prevent future barriers to the group process.

Differences in educational levels among group members can be a barrier to group work. Individuals may have college degrees but still lack knowledge in the proposed issues, in the group process, or in decision-making and problem-solving processes. It is the group leader's responsibility to perform a comprehensive assessment of the

TABLE 19.1   Comparison of Features of Five Types of Groups

Features	Community	Educational	Self-help	Focus	Task force
Goals & Objectives	Empowerment	Provide education	Support and cohesiveness	Solicit information	To achieve group's task
Purpose	Advocacy for change	Preventive health	Support for behavior modification, grief, or weight management	Get information about feelings, ideas, opinions	Perform a specific agreed upon task
Format of meetings	Open	Formal with agenda and outline	Specific format	Open, focus questionnaire	Specific and focused
Focus	Strength in numbers; change process	Give information	Elicit concerns about the issues	Obtain information	Completion of specific task
Leadership	Democratic; knowledge of the change process	Democratic; need skills in teaching	Democratic; providing resource; facilitating problem-solving	Democratic; controlled and focused to get information	Democratic; encourage exchange of information for task completion
Membership	Large groups; divided into small work groups	Small, intermediate or large group	Small groups for individualized attention	Small groups	Small groups
Group life	Usually long term	Short term	Long term	Short term	Short term

group's educational levels to enhance the effectiveness of the group.

Group Composition

Deciding on the composition of the group is the initial step in group process building. It is a collection of individuals working interdependently towards a common goal. To meet the needs and purpose of the group, members must work interdependently and collaboratively. Porter-O'Grady (1986)

identified four important criteria a group must meet to be effective:

- a strong reason for working together
- a strong basis for interdependence—a need for one another's experiences, ability, commitment, and expertise
- a commitment by each member that the outcome of working together will be more effective and meaningful than working independently
- accountability for functioning in the larger organization and achieving both organizational and group goals

Make every effort to ensure that the groups you lead meet these standards. As leader, ensure that each member has a purpose and specified function. Make the group work exciting and meaningful by placing the focus of the group on its members.

Group Size

The size of groups vary and is a very important consideration in group formation. Whether it will be large or small depends on the purpose, availability of the participants, and skill of the group leader. A minimum of three to five people is needed to allow the development of the complex relationships that characterize a group. Medium- or intermediate-size groups of five to seven members are best for problem-solving and conflict resolution. Generally, a large group of more than 10 members is useful for information giving and voting.

Small- and medium-size groups are effective as task forces to advance the goals and objectives and to facilitate the work of a larger group. If you have a large group and the purpose is to interact, you can ask the group to break into smaller groups and then reconvene to share their findings. In this case, you may want to develop a group agenda and written directions for interacting.

Interactional Factors

The third major area to consider in establishing a group are psychology, personal philosophies, values, norms, beliefs, social dimensions, and cultures. Psychologically, members who are insecure in their role or who prefer to work in isolation may feel uncomfortable sharing information or ideas in a group. Based on previous experience, members may lack trust and be suspicious of the leader or other members. These factors can impede group progress.

Group members' personal values, norms, beliefs, feelings may also affect group work. Knowledge and acceptance of the type, purpose, and goals of the group serve as a good baseline for encouraging members to express their values, interests, and feelings about the group. Encourage group members to express their personal beliefs, ideas, and attitudes about the problem and about working as a group. You can say, "We are here as a group for the purpose of. . . . We come from various backgrounds and have different past experiences working with groups. As we jointly develop our goals and define our purpose, let us strive to be open with each other. Feel free to ask any of us questions and clarify any misunderstandings."

Social Dimensions and Culture

The social environment—which includes economics, power, and authority, cultural differences, educational differences, and autonomy—can affect the group process. Members of lower socioeconomic status may feel less empowered and resent those of a higher status and vice versa. This can impede their ability to work together, which is why it is important to enhance group cohesiveness. See Box 19.1 for suggestions for enhancing group cohesiveness.

Culture affects individual behavior. Cultural differences can influence group leadership, the ability to work in groups, and commitment to group objectives. For example, persons from Eastern cultures may expect the leader to generate ideas and solutions and feel compelled to accept them, while individuals from Western cultures may expect the leader to listen to their ideas and use them.

Occupational culture is also important. Nurses and physicians may see things differently than accountants and lawyers. Keep in mind that all cultures bring unique aspects to the group. To make group members from different cultural and socioeconomic backgrounds feel wanted in the group, you must be sensitive to the cultural norms, language, social interaction patterns, space, time, and communication patterns and use them to benefit group process.

GROUP LEADER METHODS FOR OVERCOMING BLOCKS TO GROUP PROCESS

Roles of the Group, Members, and Leader

In planning the group process be sure not to squelch enthusiasm and participation by keeping the group task-focused. Group roles are of three types:

- *Group task roles* are focused on problem-related tasks which can be assumed by any member. A good example is asking a group member to take the role of recorder or coordinator.
- *Group-building and maintenance roles* are required of individuals concerned with role effectiveness and survival of the group. An example is a compromiser or a group-observer. Ask a group member to take one of these roles if the group is angry or needs feedback.
- *Individual roles* satisfy personal needs unrelated to group task or development. For example, a member can be an aggressor, clown, or information-giver (Dean, La Vallee, & McLaughlin, 1999).

Avoid a high level of individual-centered roles by reminding group members to return to the task if they bring up individual issues, and strive for more group-centered roles. Table 19.2 exemplifies the three types of group roles.

Communication Strategies Among Group Leader and Members

Communication is an important contributing factor in the psychological climate of a group. In a group you have the opportunity to use both verbal and nonverbal communication. Be clear in the messages you send and aware of the receivers. One way to do this is to ask the group frequently what they think or feel about what you said. You can also ask, "What's your reaction to what was said?" The six steps outlined in Box 19.4 can assist you as a group leader in communicating effectively with groups.

Nonverbal Communication

Clues about an individual's personality can be gleaned from nonverbal communication, which is about 55% of our communication. The dress, social habits, vocal cues, eye contact, posture, quality of voice, facial expressions, personality style, foods, and mannerisms all communicate. For successful group work, you must be cognizant of these types of communication. You can become more familiar about this through role-playing, role reversal, skits, and planned group experiences, which are then discussed afterwards with a more skilled group facilitator. You may set up role-playing around an anxiety-producing issue, then let members of the group guess what the actors are thinking, feeling, or trying to convey. During this exercise make observations about facial expressions, silence, trembling, or clenching of the hands. Atti-

TABLE 19.2   Three Types of Group Roles

Group Task Roles	Group Building and Maintenance	Individual Roles
Initiator/Contributor	Harmonizer	Aggressor
Information seeker	Compromiser	Blocker
Opinion seeker	Gatekeeper and expediter	Recognition-seeker
Information giver	Standard-setter	Self-confessor
Elaborator	Group observer and commentator	Player
Coordinator	Follower	Dominator
Orienter		Help-seeker
Evaluator/critic		Special-interest pleader
Procedural technician		
Recorder		

Box 19.4   Six Steps for Communicating with Groups

- Plan what should be communicated. This is more successful if it is a group effort.
- Analyze the environment and adjust accordingly. If the physical environment, lighting, and type of seats do not lend themselves to an ideal group environment, adjust accordingly.
- Deliver a clear and consistent message.
- Be aware of nonverbal communication clues (your dress, facial expression, etc.)
- Ask for feedback so you will know how your message was received. Ask: "Does anyone have any ideas about . . . ?" or "What do you think of this idea?"
- Clarify any misconceptions and misunderstanding by asking, for example, for further explanation.

---

tudes towards people and the situation will be revealed in posture and actions. Use role reversal and ask a group member to take the role of leader. Visual aids and demonstration can be used to illustrate ideas. Make observations about silences and body language.

Formal and Informal Communication

The formal process of communication includes written communication such as the agenda, minutes, and handouts. Direct in-formation is obtained through the group meetings and standing committees.

Informal communication has no agenda and can occur before or after group meetings. Members may meet informally in a restaurant to continue conversations about the group issue. It is equally important to explore these communication patterns within the group and with the leader. For example, you can ask subgroups within the groups to discuss positive ways for reaching consensus. Group members' communication patterns and behaviors change as the group evolves, matures, and becomes more cohesive. A comparison of group maturity and communication patterns appears in Table 19.3.

Establishing a Problem-Solving Process

Problem-solving is much more successful if the work is carried out collaboratively by all team members. Collect and review the facts, situation, or issue. Ask, What is the problem all about? Talk with the involved parties and ask questions related to the issue such as "How can we solve this?" Following a review of the issue, try to define the problem clearly. For example, if you think the problem is _____, say to the group: "I have an idea the problem is _____. What do the rest of you think?"

Planning is the second step in solving a problem. In this step, you and the group members decide on the method needed for a solution. This involves goal-setting, making judgment calls, and designing methods for resolving the problem. Ask the group: "What are some acceptable alternatives?" Write down, or have someone in the group write down, a list of possible solutions with alternatives as the group generates them. Ask the group members to consider the cost, reality of implementation, environment, and necessary time to complete each alternative. Using the process of elimination, erase each area that does not have a viable option. Next, present your findings to the group.

Implementation of the solution is the third step. After careful planning, and decision making, it is time to take action. Set up a timeline for implementing the solution. Collaborate to decide on the roles and responsibilities, the beginning and ending, and the process needed.

In the fourth step, evaluation of the process, the effects of group efforts are measured. Group members' responsibility in

TABLE 19.3 Group Maturity and Communication

Stages of Group Development	Level of Communication Among Members
Early stage	1. Goal-directed toward the leader of the group 2. Group norms communicated 3. Limited sharing of thoughts, ideas, and opinions 4. Energy level is high 5. Enthusiasm is high 6. Motivation is high 7. Members are willing to solve problems 8. Members exchange information
Middle stage	1. Members become comfortable 2. Members begin to communicate more openly 3. Evidence of the beginning stage of group cohesiveness 4. Group begins to reach agreement on goals and objectives
Mature stage	1. Group accepts norms 2. Members become comfortable dealing with conflicts 3. Members develop full trust in the leader and each other 4. Members share opinion, ideas, and perceptions more openly 5. Members support one another

evaluation should be negotiated in the same manner as other group roles and assigned or volunteered on the basis of competency. Be sure to set realistic evaluation timeframes. Table 19.4 lists some of the factors affecting group problem-solving (McLaughlin & Kaluzny, 1999).

Facilitate problem-solving by accurate assessment of the problem situation, requirements for acceptable alternatives, positive qualities of alternatives, and negative qualities of alternatives.

Group Norms

Groups develop *norms* (also called rules or standards) around situations important to the group. Norms establish acceptable group behavior and are a necessary consideration in group communication for setting the structure. They are the set of written or unwritten rules of conduct, acceptable standards, or value statements established by members of a group and apply to every member. Norms prevent chaotic behavior and assist members in predicting the behavior of others. They tell members what ought and ought not to be done and may vary in the degree to which they are accepted by the group. Some examples of group norms you might consider adopting to make a group more effective are as follows:

- Everyone's participation is essential and valuable.
- Everyone has a role in the group.
- No idea is too crazy.
- The group will seek win-win solutions.
- The group will be proactive.
- Decisions are made by consensus.
- The meetings will begin on time.

Consider writing these rules for group behavior on a handout or ask the group to take a few minutes to set their own rules. Time constraints may make the first method more feasible in some groups. Even if you write the group rules, it is still important to get group reactions and input to enhance cohesiveness and to teach the group problem-solving.

IDENTIFYING GROUP DYNAMICS

Consider spatial arrangements related to seating, leadership, and communication.

TABLE 19.4 Factors Affecting Group Problem Solving

Factors	Effects
Focus Effect	In a rut "Group-think" Tunnel vision
Self-weighing Effect	Group members participate only to the level of comfort and competence of other members
Judgment effect	Judgments are made but not expressed Judgments may not be in congruence with the leader or other group members
Group pressure for conformity	Loss of motivation
Influence of strong personalities on the group	Loss of members
Over-emphasis on group maintenance roles	Limited group participation
Pressure for speedy decisions	Less cohesiveness

Many adults prefer to sit side by side for group collaboration. If the seating arrangements infringe on an individual's personal space, it may evoke a feeling of discomfort and interfere with effective group work. The person who sits at the head of a table is perceived as the leader of the group; the person who sits closest to the group leader is perceived to have more power in the group. The spatial position a person occupies in a group has important significance to that person's chances of emerging as a group leader. The group should be queried about their comfort and other arrangements made if there is discomfort.

Communication flows when there are no physical barriers such as tables or chairs. Arranging the group in a circle with chairs close to each other also enhances group communication.

The physical environment, color of the room, and the noise levels are also important factors affecting group dynamics. Group members will probably be more productive in a well-lit, beautifully decorated room with windows and good ventilation and less productive in an unattractive room that is dark, too hot or cold, small, and poorly lit. Try to use a meeting room that is conducive to positive interaction.

Key Group-Building Activities

If the group is not functioning or is stagnant use group- or team-building techniques. Conditions that must be present for group building are as follows:

- There must be honesty among the members in order to build trust. This could be assessed by the level of comfort and communication within the group. Can members speak freely?
- There must be respect among the members. This can be assessed during the process of discussions and by the type of communication. Do members get time to respond? Do members build on one another's strengths?
- Members must leave their hidden or individual agendas at the door. Hidden agendas can be very disruptive to the group.
- Members must be willing to allow the personal insights, feelings, and ideas of each member to be expressed in a nonjudgemental, noncritical environment (Porter-O'Grady, 1986). Use some of the team building activities listed in Box 19.5.

Strategies to Move a Group Forward

Strategies to move a group forward include participatory leadership, a sense of direction, high standards, and being sensitive to the needs of the group for stimulation or a recess. Desired interpersonal skills that are important for a group leader in group meetings are listening, persuasion, negotiation, debate, consensus, decision-making, and conflict resolution. Box 19.6 lists the characteristics of a group leader that affect the movement of groups.

Listening

Active listening conveys to the group members that you are interested in and responsive to what they are saying. Encourage group members to listen to each other, too. Group members can assess active listening by your response, the manner in which you are paying attention, and the level of empathy you demonstrate. Comments to make to the group to elicit active listening include: "Everyone's ideas are important, so let's listen carefully and ask questions when we don't understand each other."

Box 19.5   Team-Building Activities: Take the Team-Building Test

Assessment and diagnostic meetings to determine:

- *Relationships:* Are there interpersonal or group conflicts? Is group members' expertise being utilized fully?
- *Tasks and responsibilities:* Were tasks defined and identified? How were tasks allocated? What are the various responsibilities?
- *Role identity, clarification, and negotiation:* Were roles defined, analyzed, and clarified? Did members negotiate their roles?
- *Group process:* Are there any specific environmental, economic problems? How are the communication patterns and decision-making processes?

Box 19.6.   Characteristics of Group Leaders

1. They motivate the group.
2. They demonstrate leadership skills.
3. They establish clear goals and purpose.
4. They provide direction.
5. They establish and work with timelines.
6. They provide feedback.
7. They keep the group together.
8. They move the group forward toward its goals.
9. They establish methods for evaluation.

Persuasion

Persuasion is widely defined as any effort to influence or change the belief, attitudes, or feelings of another person. The major purpose of persuasion is to influence change. You can learn to be a highly skilled persuader by getting the group's attention and earning its trust. The group will be persuaded more readily if you have personal and professional credibility. The image you convey, your interpersonal skills, and your ability to argue without abrasiveness contribute to being an effective persuader. Negotiation is the highest level of persuasion.

Negotiation

With successful negotiation, both parties are in agreement about the issue. Successful negotiation results in a win-win relationship. Here are some factors that you must take into consideration for successful negotiation:

- Timing is very important. Try to negotiate early in the day when the parties involved are not tired. Whenever possible choose the beginning of the week when ideas are fresh.
- Do your research. Be prepared with the facts of the issue. Have copies of

important materials to give to group members.

- Be confident when presenting your side of the issue. State the facts. Practice with a trusted colleague prior to the meeting or practice into a tape recorder or in front of a bathroom mirror.
- Make eye contact as often as possible as you negotiate. Be sensitive to verbal and nonverbal cues.
- Listen to both sides of the issue. Be open to others' ideas.
- Ask the group to negotiate: "There has to be some give and take to achieve our goals. What is each of you willing to give up so we can agree on a solution?"

Debate

Debating involves persuasion and argument. Controversial issues almost always involve some debating. As a leader you must be skilled and comfortable in engaging in effective dialogue. You must be able to take, defend, and support a position. Gather supporting materials and give a convincing talk about why you chose your position.

Reaching Consensus

The most effective decision-making processes involve consensus. Reaching consensus means developing an acceptable proposal that all team members can support and that none of the team members will oppose (Rowland & Rowland, 1997). To develop this proposal, ask the group to help you by searching the literature for information on the topic and giving you their views. Be sure to tell the group: "We need everyone's ideas to make this work." To reach consensus, all team members must feel that their opinions have been heard and fairly considered. Rowland and

Rowland (1997) outline four requirements for reaching consensus:

- active participation of all team members
- skills in communication: listening, conflict resolution, and discussion
- creative thinking
- open-mindedness and acceptance of differences

Making Group Decisions

There is a direct relationship between the group's decision performance and its ability to understand the problems and accurately assess the negative consequences of alternative choices (Rowland & Rowland, 1997). An effective decision-making process leads to successful group functioning. It is important that the leader be very explicit on the method of decision-making. An important question to ask is: Will the decisions be made by consensus or be based on facts or data? The major purpose of decision-making is to construct well-understood and well-received realistic actions toward the agreed objectives.

The characteristics of a successful decision-making process are listed in Box 19.7.

Resolving Conflicts

As a group leader you must be comfortable in the role and have the credibility to be able to intervene when conflicts arise. Conflict is a natural occurrence in any group that is attempting problem-solving and decision-making (McLaughlin & Kaluzny, 1999), and it can be good or destructive. Conflict may stimulate creativity and may motivate change in the group dynamics. Determine the level of conflict and attempt to minimize it as much as possible.

When people of different backgrounds, ideas, views of various issues get together,

---

Box 19.7   Characteristics of a Successful Decision-Making Process

- Group members have a chance to participate and are satisfied with the decision.
- Group members have adequate time for discussions before the final decisions.
- Experience and the expertise of group members are considered.
- Members feel committed and assist in implementing the decision.

---

there is an increased chance of conflict. Conflict may arise for one of the following reasons.

- Inaccurate facts
- Power
- Authority
- Knowledge of subject matter
- Lack of knowledge
- Variations in personal value system
- Variations in personality

Approaches to Conflict Resolution

Interpersonal conflict among members should be at a low level for effective functioning of the group. Members should be asked not to personalize the issues.

The POWER Listening Model developed by Williams (1998) makes the conflict more manageable and understandable for the group leader. This model consists of five areas (P – Positively frame; O – Organized; W – Wants; E – Emotions; R – Respect). See Box 19.8.

Developing Trust as a Group Leader

Trust develops as the leader demonstrates fairness. Your style in handling conflicts and issues provides the building blocks for the development of group trust. The level of trust between you and the rest of the group sets the pace for success or failure in group development and maintenance.

By listening and respecting group members' views on the issues, you will promote growth and encourage creativity and trust.

Methods for Reinforcing Strengths, Self-Care Capabilities, and Group Resilience

By reinforcing group strengths, independence, self-care capabilities, and resilience, you can help promote the health of the group. Take a look at some specific methods for accomplishing these tasks.

Maintaining Group Self-Care Capabilities

Group performance will diminish very quickly if the members believe that they do not have any influence. When subgroups work in isolation they may experience decreased motivation and commitment. Help the group maintain independent and self-care behaviors by calling them on the phone, E-mailing them, and sending bulletins on issues affecting the group.

Motivating the Group and Getting Group Validation

The group must be kept motivated at all times. This is a challenge for you as a group leader. Pay attention to inactive members, and get in touch with members who have missed a meeting. Send a steady stream of status reports during periods of inactivity. Another very important area is group input.

Box 19.8   The POWER Listening Model

<u>P</u>ositively framed: Put in a form that everyone can hear, understand, and act upon. For example, instead of saying "So you want to strangle your boss?" or even "You want her to leave you alone?" try "Are you frustrated because you want more uninterrupted time to work on this project?"

<u>O</u>rganized: Understand what each person really wants before deciding on an agreement. For example, when co-workers are fighting over work schedules, a fast compromise that leaves both unsatisfied may take more time and energy over the long run, than a mutually satisfying option that required a bit more listening to discover each person's underlying concerns.

<u>W</u>ants: Clarify the underlying concerns behind the demands. Use words that everyone can hear without feeling defensive. For example, instead of "you don't want to see his face ever again?" try "you want him to treat you with respect?" "Wants" here are defined as underlying "interests" rather than "positions" or demands. They make it possible for everyone to perceive a greater number of more satisfying options. Identify wants clearly.

<u>E</u>motions: State the feelings you sense so that the person really feels heard. Describe these feelings using nonjudgmental words so that no one feels put down. When we are aware of our own emotions, they become more manageable, and it becomes easier for us to listen and think. For example, instead of "Are you hurt because you feel she doesn't value you?" or "You're really furious because she treats you like a machine!" try "Are you angry because you want her to acknowledge the positive things you have done?"

<u>R</u>espect: Keep your intentions focused on listening to understand, rather than judging the other person. Most of what you tell others is through your unconscious body language. Avoid jargon. Find a way of listening that is effective <u>and</u> sounds natural. Consider what would be most respectful for that unique person or people in that particular situation. If what you hear isn't what they meant, try again, until they and their body language tell you that you understand their situation. Once they feel you have really heard them, then they will be better able to listen. If you are not able to listen, or the other person does not calm down, consider bringing in a mediator or other third party.

(Copyright Denise Williams, 1998. Used with permission.)

Members must have the opportunity to see how their influence has affected the group's process or outcomes. For example, when members brainstorm about issues and give suggestions in a group meeting and there is no feedback or evidence of change, they lose motivation. This may further lead to less group validation. To keep brainstorming members motivated, be sure to comment on every members contribution in a positive way. Box 19.9 presents some factors causing group failure and factors to keep the group motivated.

Enhancing Group Resilience

Team building is important in maintaining group resilience. Group resilience depends on the group's maturity level, which is a force that dictates group dynamics. How frequent are your meetings? Is distance a problem for some members? How well do the members work together? Some of the following principles of group dynamics (Knowles & Knowles, 1959) can help you understand group behavior:

- Group effectiveness is determined by the existence of clear, agreed-upon goals that mobilize a group's energies; agreed-upon plans to reach those goals; and organization and effective group process to reach the goals.
- A group tends to be attractive to individuals and commands their loyalty to the extent that the group satisfies their needs, helps meets their goals, and provides acceptance and security.

Box 19.9   Factors Causing Group Failure and Factors for Group Motivation

Factors Causing Group Failure

1. Lack of support from the leader and other members
2. Lack of communication
3. Unrealistic expectations for the group
4. Lack of motivation and enthusiasm
5. Lack of guidance and focus
6. Unrealistic deadlines
7. Power struggle among members and the leader

Factors for Group Motivation

1. Support group consensus.
2. Facilitate participation of group members by allowing them to express ideas, thoughts and opinions.
3. Provide a framework for decision-making based on the established norms.
4. Nurture collaborative relationships by demonstrating tolerance and a nonjudgmental attitude.
5. Offer support for the group's views and opinions.

- The level of input into the goals and decisions correlates to commitment to the group. If the level of input is high, so is the level of commitment.
- If members share and accept the perception that the change is needed and participate in planning, the group will be successful in implementing the change.
- The more the group members understand their own behaviors, values, norms, cultures, and group behavior, the more constructively they will be in participating in the group process.

You can also use the Cog's ladder (Pfeffer & Jones, 1974) to assess the group's operational stage. It consists of five stages of a group's development.

- Stage 1 is the "polite stage" where members get acquainted with one an-

other, share values, ideas, and experiences, and begin to get acquainted.
- Stage 2 is the "why are we here stage?" where members attempt to define the purpose, goals, objectives, tasks, and responsibilities.
- In stage 3, the "bid for power stage," members attempt to influence one another's values, ideas, and opinions and begin to compete for recognition, authority, and attention. It is important for someone to take the lead and move the group forward from ideas to the next stage.
- Stage 4 is the "constructive stage" where members begin to actively listen and are more open-minded. They attempt to accept one another's value systems. This is the working stage, and team building is very necessary here.
- The final stage is the "esprit de corps stage" where members are in high spir-

TABLE 19.5. Ten Major Evaluative Indicators of Group Functioning

Indicators	Functioning Groups	Nonfunctioning Groups
Environment/ seating	Relaxed; seating shows a working atmosphere; members are communicating	Tense; scattered seating; great amount of personal space
Goals/objectives	Clear goals and objectives understood by the members; goal attainment and group development and maintenance are emphasized	Unclear goals and objectives misunderstood by the members
Leadership Style	Democratic; everyone participates	Autocratic, authoritative leader who dominates the group; limited member participation
Communication	Open communication both lateral and vertical; top-down and bottom-up	Closed or difficult; one-way or top-down
Power	Power is shared among the group; the leader acknowledges the members' knowledge and experience	The power stays with the leader; the group members ideas are not acknowledged
Creativity	Encouraged; members are allowed to be creative and become self-actualized	Stifled and suppressed; members are reluctant about suggesting ideas; members are afraid of rejection
Cohesiveness	Encouraged by the leader's support, trust, and problem solving abilities	Not apparent; members may resist suggestions and ideas because of power struggle and control
Decision making	Members reach decisions by consensus	The leader makes all decisions; members have limited input
Problem solving	Emphasized; the leader and members accept constructive criticism to move towards goal achievement	Limited problem-solving ability; leader and members may engage in destructive criticism; barrier prevents goal attainment
Conflicts	There is a process for solving conflicts	No process in place for conflict resolution

its and begin to feel unity, mutual acceptance, high cohesiveness, and camaraderie. At this stage the group leader must give positive feedback and recognize the accomplishments of the members.

Moving from one stage to another varies from group to group. A group may be stagnant in one of the stages and may need assistance in moving forward. A group may reach stage 4 and still need to consider stage 2. On the other hand, a mature group may move very quickly to stage 5 and beyond, resulting in group thinking patterns. "Group-think" exists in a group when prob-

lems are solved according to the leader's view rather than by careful consideration of alternatives. Be careful not to stifle members' ideas and critical thinking ability. Encourage openness by continually asking for everyone's opinion. When groups are not highly verbal, use nonverbal, safe ways such as asking group members to write their ideas down anonymously on a slip of paper.

Evaluating Group Behavior

Ask the group to periodically critique its performance and self-evaluate its roles. Use an evaluation check list to assist you and other members in understanding group dynamics. Ask a different member at each meeting to observe and record the group's interactions and behaviors. At the end of each meeting allow 10 minutes to summarize and analyze the findings. The results can be used to identify group strengths and weakness and improve the group's effectiveness. Below are 13 questions that can be used to evaluate a group.

1. Does the seating arrangement allow for discussion?
2. Is everyone listening?
3. Is everyone participating in the discussion?
4. Does the leader facilitate group discussions?
5. Are the discussions focused on the issue?
6. Does the leader encourage participation?
7. Do the members look comfortable asking questions?
8. Does the leader clarify and offer explanation of the issues?
9. Does the leader summarize the major issues agreements and disagreements?
10. Does the group infuse new ideas and challenges?
11. Does the group maintain its creative capacity?

Several characteristics can be used to evaluate cohesiveness. Table 19.5 lists ten of the major evaluative indicators and compares a functioning group with a non-functioning group.

REFERENCES

Breckon, D. J., Harvey, J. R., & Lancaster, R. B. (1998). *Community health education.* Gaithersburg, MD: Aspen.

Cookfair, J. M. (1996). *Nursing care in the community.* St. Louis, MO: Mosby.

Dean, P. J., LaVallee, R., & McLaughlin, C. P. (1999). Teams at the core of continuous learning. In C. P. McLaughlin & A. D. Kaluzny (Eds.), *Continuous quality improvement in health care* (pp. 147–167). Gaithersberg, MD: Aspen.

Knowles, M., & Knowles, H. (1959) *Introduction to group dynamics.* New York: Association Press.

Lewin, K. (1951). *Field theory in social science.* New York: Harper & Row.

Loomis, M. E. (1979). *Group process for nurses.* St. Louis, MO: Mosby.

McLaughlin, C. P., & Kaluzny, A. D. (1999). *Continuous quality improvement in health care.* Gaithersburg, MD: Aspen.

Northouse, L. L., & Northouse, P. G. (1998). *Health communication: Strategies for health professionals.* Stamford, CT: Appleton & Lange.

O'Kelly, G. (1998). Countertransference in the nurse-patient relationship: A review of the literature. *Journal of Advanced Nursing, 28*(2), 391–397.

Pfeffer, J. W., & Jones, J. E. (Eds.). (1974). *The 1974 annual handbook for group facilitators.* La Jolla, CA: University Associates.

Porter-O'Grady, T. (1986). *Creative nursing administration: Participative management into the 21st century.* Gaithersburg, MD; Aspen.

Rowland, H. S., & Rowland, B. L. (1997). *Nursing administration handbook* (4th ed.). Gaithersburg, MD: Aspen.

Williams, D. (1998). POWER Listening Model. Unpublished paper. Contact author for further information: POB 2723, San Pedro, CA 90731.

CHAPTER 20

Working With Families

Janice Unruh Davidson

THE FAMILY AND HEALTH AND WELLNESS PROMOTION

This chapter will help you understand health promotion from the standpoint of the family. It focuses on ways to assess, plan, and intervene in establishing healthy behaviors, thereby helping families move toward health and wellness. It also provides an overview of current research regarding family health and wellness.

As a new century dawns, the family has emerged as a unit most uniquely positioned to affect health care reform by serving as the most foundational level of our society for fostering healthy behaviors. *Healthy People 2010* identifies the family as instrumental in fostering health promotion and disease prevention (see the Web site (*http://web.health.gov/healthypeople/2010/Draft/objectives*). Families can promote healthy behaviors by providing the context for practicing wellness throughout the developmental life of the family. They can contribute to promoting healthy and safe communities by establishing a healthy and safe environment within the home. Families can prevent health disorders by identi-

fying, isolating, and changing family behavior. You will want to familiarize yourself with determinants of family health and wellness, which are identified in Table 20.1.

UNDERSTANDING THE FAMILY

The first thing you need to know as a community practitioner who seeks to positively impact the health and wellness of the family is that your role is one of a partner. The family may very well be the most important client you have as a community practitioner, because a healthy family means a healthy community. For this reason, the family becomes your partner in creating a healthy community. There are a number of approaches you can take to understanding the family. *Family theory* is a body of knowledge that uniquely links the concepts of family development, family function, family health, family structure, and family systems together. The family is the basic social structure in every society. But families can be defined as anything from a simple system including one individual to a complex system of extended familial relationships. Ac-

TABLE 20.1   Determinants of Family Health and Wellness

Biological (physical)	Genetic inheritance
	Congenital malformation
	Mental retardation
Psychological-social (emotional)	Lifestyle
	Habits
	Violence Exposure
Cultural	Ethnographic variables of ethnicity and religion
	Demographic variables of age, gender, and family size
	Socioeconomic variables of income and education
	Affiliation variables of both formal and informal group memberships
	Influence of acculturation
Spiritual	Devotions and fasting
	Study of Scripture and great books
	Prayer and meditation

cording to *family systems* theory, the family functions as a system. This means that the behavior of one family member always affects all the other members because people are considered in systems theory to be part of their environment rather than separate from it. You will want to familiarize yourself with Bowen's family systems theory (1985), which included the eight key concepts summarized below:

- *Differentiation of self* refers to the degree to which family members develop and incorporate a separate identity within the context of the whole family. As a community practitioner, you can assess the extent of differentiation of members of the family by identifying the boundaries that exist within the family constellation. For example, a family that maintains the integrity of its boundaries is thought to be an open system if it interacts with its environment (outside the family) in healthy ways. Input allows the exchange of information coming from the larger environment into the family constellation, while throughput allows for processing of the information within the family system. Output allows for exchange of information going back from within the family constellation to the larger outside environment.

- A *triangle* typically refers to a dysfunctional coping pattern of the family that is used to deal with stress in unhealthy ways. The family is sometimes defined in systems theory as the interaction among subsystems, which collectively form a larger more sophisticated system. These subsystems include a dyad where two family members interact with one another; a triad involves the interaction of three family members. The community practitioner can observe for dysfunctional coping as evidenced by the routine application of triangles in relationships among family members whereby family members who have an unstable relationship attempt to draw in a third member in order to achieve stability. You will want to be cautious not to get triangulated yourself when working with such families.

- *Multigenerational transmission process* refers to the notion that health patterns and behavior can be passed from one generation to another through the family system. We now know that this process is not limited only to learned behavior within the context of the family, but extends also to the genetic pooling that plays an increasingly important role in determinants of family health. The best way you can assess the impact of this concept as a community practitioner is through the visual construction of the *genogram*. A genogram has been provided in Figure 20.1.

- *Sibling position* refers to the birth order of siblings within the constellation of the family. A variety of roles and behaviors have been found to be characteristic of the various orders of siblings within the context of the family. Roles refer to behaviors that are either assumed or assigned and provide structure to the family's organization, thus leading to the stability and function of the family. At times role strain occurs within the family as members encounter changes in the expected structure and operation of the system. If the roles are flexible, the family will move beyond the stressors encountered as sibling position changes within the context of the family. In your role as a community practitioner, you will want to document sibling position and roles within the family in an effort to understand better the organization of the family constellation and family member influence on health and wellness behaviors.

- *Emotional cutoff* refers to a dysfunctional coping pattern of the family that is used to deal with stress in unhealthy

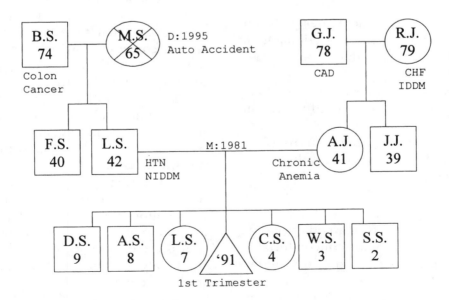

FIGURE 20.1 Family genogram.

ways. Because emotion is necessary in the family functioning as an open system, your assistance as a community practitioner is to identify patterns of dysfunction where emotion is cut off through withdrawal of affect, leading to unhealthy family behavior.

- The *nuclear family emotional system* refers to the organization of emotional system within the context of the family constellation as delimited to the nuclear family. In order to ascertain the locus of control in evaluating health and wellness behavior, you will want to assess the extent of the emotional system of the family organization to determine if it functions within the confines of the nuclear family or if it extends beyond that level to the extended family across multiple generations.

- *Family projection process* refers to a dysfunctional coping pattern of the family that is used to deal with stress in unhealthy ways through scapegoating or other unhealthy defensive alliances. As a community practitioner you will need to observe for projection among family members that leads to unhealthy family behavior.

- *Societal regression* results from dysfunction that is not averted within the context of the family and thus continues to generate the same patterns of unhealthy behaviors across multiple generations.

According to Dzurec (1995), a key indicator of *family health* is *fit*, whether positive or negative, comfortable or uncomfortable, and which is demonstrated by the family's structure, function, development, and communication patterns. You should be aware that *family structure* refers specifically to family roles and relationships, whether

nuclear, extended, or paternalistic. *Family function* can be understood as a process of continual change within the family system and between the family and the environment. According to the classic definition of family function by Smilkstein (1978), function can be viewed as a continuum from a nurturing system that is working (functional) to one that is not (dysfunctional), as family members adapt, partner (work together), grow, and demonstrate affection and resolve (or commitment) to the system. Smilkstein used these concepts to develop a tool for measuring family function, which he called APGAR. The APGAR tool as he designed it was scored according to family member responses to five questions covering these concepts with points assigned as follows: "Almost always" = 2 points; "Some of the time" = 1 point; "Hardly ever" = 0 points. Total scores were then interpreted as follows: 7–10 points = highly functional; 4–6 points = moderate dysfunction; and 0–3 points = severely dysfunctional. The tool was found to be a quick, reliable, and valid assessment of family function. As a community practitioner you may find that it is easy to identify problematic concerns or weaknesses of a family; however, it will be as important for you to also identify the strengths of a family. Similarly, you will learn in working with families that weaknesses of the family are threats to the family system just as strengths of a family serve as opportunities for healthy function.

Family structure and family function are difficult concepts to differentiate because the relationship between cause and effect are so circular. For example, family function is a consequence of family structure, but family structure exists to fulfill one or more functions of the family. You may recall that Erik Erikson (1986) in his classic work identified psychosocial tasks of individuals across the life span. With regard to the family you should be aware that Duvall and Miller (1985) applied a similar approach of psychosocial tasks to families across the life span, resulting in the family development model. As a community practitioner, you will benefit from understanding *family development* as the eight chronological stages through which the family passes, based on the age of the eldest child. The list below is a review of the stages of family development.

- Beginning family
- Childbearing family
- Family with preschool children
- Family with school-age children
- Family with teenagers
- Launching center family
- Family with middle-aged parents
- Family in old age and retirement
  Note: From Marriage and Family Development, by E. M. Duvall and B. Miller, 1985, New York: Harper & Row. Copyright 1985 by Harper & Row. Adapted by permission.

SYNTHESIZING CURRENT FAMILY THEORY RESEARCH

You will find as a community practitioner that it is helpful to keep current on the level of knowledge development with regard to family theory. The notion of family health promotion takes the concept of health promotion a step further, from the individual to the family and ultimately to the community and diverse populations. You should already be familiar with Nola Pender's Health Promotion Model (1996), which emphasizes individual health-promoting behaviors. According to Padula (1997), Pender's model made great strides in understanding health promotion, but failed to address health promotion from a family perspective. Another similar model proposed by Loveland-Cherry (1983) sought to establish links between individual health promotion and family theory, thereby addressing family health promotion. Such serve to improve systems for families' personal and public health access by facilitating understanding of health promotion from the family perspective. Understanding how such application can be made was proposed by Hartrick (1997), who observed the many evolutionary changes that have occurred over the last 15 to 20 years in health promotion and identified how family theory—which focuses on the servicing of health problems from a broader perspective than that of the individual—can enhance family capacity to promote health.

Sometimes a community practitioner will find that differentiating between family theory and family therapy is confusing. Jones and Dimond (1982) compared and contrasted family theory with family therapy in a useful review that has implications for community practice. In their comparative review, they differentiated between three basic approaches to family theory, which are (a) structural-functional, (b) interaction-based, and (c) developmental; and three basic approaches to family therapy, which are (a) structural-family, (b) interactional, and (c) multigenerational. You will notice that an important conclusion drawn by Jones and Dimond in the family wellness discussion was that family theory is health- and wellness-oriented while family therapy is illness-oriented. Our focus for this chapter is centered on family theory.

In a classic concept analysis, Weeks and O'Connor (1994) proposed a new definition of family health, focusing on connectness, energy, and hope for the future. Weeks and O'Connor (1997) went on to use this concept analysis in developing and testing a tool to assess family health, which is presented later in this chapter. But regardless of recent concept development, according to research reported by Denham (1999a), family health continues to be an ambiguous concept.

As an example, if you look at patterns of daily living from the traditional perspective, you will see emerging themes such as nutrition, exercise, sleep, work, rest, and related patterns of family life. But what about cultural differences in the definition and practice of family health? For an understanding of these cultural differences we can review Denham's research (1999a; 1999b), which evaluated family health from the perspective of cultural diversity within rural Appalachian communities. It is important to assess culture as one determinant of health because cultural definitions of health and health behavior are so variable.

Other studies have looked specifically at health and wellness from the perspective of older adults with astonishingly similar results as documented by Clark (1998) and Davidson (1988). Clark's study focused on self-care and wellness from the perspective of the individual, Davidson's on self-care and wellness from the historical perspective as evidenced across stages of family development. Both studies reveal congruence among older adults in definitions of health and healthy behavior.

As previously pointed out, it is a struggle to not look at health promoting behavior simply from the individual perspective. Toward this end, Loveland-Cherry's work (1983) examined the probability of a family's health promotion behaviors being influenced by factors relating to wellness and specific health promoting behaviors. You will want to familiarize yourself with these factors as you prepare to help families assess their health promotion needs and plan ways to meet those needs. These factors have been summarized in Table 20.2.

Health-promoting behaviors have been researched from the perspective of patterns of daily family living. For example, David-son (1989) studied health-promoting behaviors of families in a culturally diverse population. In the study population of 270 rural Mennonite families, Davidson used multiple regression analysis to examine variables that predicted health-promotion behavior. The three most predictive variables were found to be self-actualization (qualitatively validated as spirituality, including specifically "prayer, forgiveness, study of the Bible, and keeping one's eyes on the Lord"); exercise (qualitatively validated as "hard work"); and nutrition (qualitatively validated as "good food").

Other health-promoting behaviors of individuals have been proposed from the perspective of the family including family stress theory. In her classic proposal linking family theory with nurse practitioner interventions, Robinson (1997) evaluated how family stress theory impacted family health. You should be familiar with stress management, which is further explained in the following paragraph, and you will also want to understand how stress impacts health and wellness.

McCubbin and McCubbin (1993) developed a model of stress management and coping, which they identified as family resilience, which was defined as two phases: adjustment and adaptation. The adjustment phase includes interaction between the stressor and family vulnerability, topology, resistance resources, appraisal of the stressor, problem-solving strategies and coping strategies. If the family can't adjust and a crisis develops, the family moves into the adaptation phase where the family attempts to originate a new level of functioning, balance, and coherence. The extent of family resilience is thought to be the interaction that occurs between family resources, social support, and situational appraisal (past and future values, goals, priorities, and expectations). Adaptation is thought to be possible where resource and appraisal by the family

TABLE 20.2   Factors Influencing Family Health Promotion Behaviors

General Factors

- Family systems patterns
- Demographics
- Biological characteristics

Health-related factors

- Family health socialization patterns
- Family definition of health
- Perceived family health status

Behavior-specific factors

- Perceived barriers to health-promoting behaviors
- Perceived benefits to health-promoting behaviors
- Prior related behavior
- Family norms
- Intersystem support for behavior
- Situational influences
- Internal and family cues

Note: From *Family system Patterns of cohesiveness and autonomy: Relationship to family members' health behavior*, by C. J. Loveland-Cherry, 1983. Reprinted with permission.

interacts with family problem-solving and coping strategy. To learn more about positive coping strategies, Comana, Brown and Thomas (1998) reported on the effect of reminiscence therapy as a therapeutic intervention used to facilitate family coping. To use this approach, the community practitioner will function as a health partner by engaging in proactive listening and facilitating family members to identify how analogies and applications to current family problems can be drawn.

Another therapeutic strategy studied during a family crisis was that of facilitating family problem-solving. According to Cox and Davis (1999), involving the entire family in family problem-solving can serve as a positive coping strategy. Their research provides direction for community practitioners regarding potential tools available in family problem-solving assessment.

Areas of agreement and disagreement do exist in the research literature concerning family health. For example, current family research has called into question previously held assumptions that children with special needs create such extreme stressors with which families are unable to cope that the family becomes dysfunctional. According to Eddy and Walker (1999), unhappy marriages with low rewards and high costs may endure whereas families with children who have special needs may actually flourish in spite of the additional stressor found in such families. As a community practitioner working with families, you will see both extremes and have opportunities for further examination of these areas of agreement and disagreement in family theory. Other areas of agreement and disagreement coexist within the family such as is seen with different perspectives of what is important to various family members. For example, research by Olsen et al. (1999) documented that mothers tend to be more adversely impacted by negative communication dynamics while fathers tend to be more adversely impacted by income issues.

As a partner in helping families to meet their health promotion needs, you will also want to be cautious about potential adverse effects that you might have on the family. For example, Faux and Seideman (1996) documented healthcare providers who in turn demonstrated an adverse effect on the family.

Plager (1999) reported that "family legacy stories recover an understanding of family health that has become marginalized" (p. 51). Family legacy stories can be used to help families identify how health practices such as self-actualization, exercise, and nutrition have come to be, so that such behaviors can be further developed or changed. To use this approach, the community practitioner will function as a health partner by learning more about the family and each member's background to discover how their family of origin defined and practiced relevant health behaviors.

An understanding of the impact of family legacy on family health lends itself to further exploration of family rituals, as defined by Campbell (1991), which serve as usual family-interaction behaviors that help families maintain their unique identity through time despite the crises they encounter. These family routines can be identified as a mechanism for the community practitioner to use in assessing how families cope with stressors in a time of crisis. Denham (1995) researched family rituals. Her work focused attention on the needs of the entire family. Health behaviors are learned and practiced primarily in the context of the family routine. You will want to acquaint yourself with the stress-management behaviors of families and both the positive and negative aspects of coping behaviors. When the stress-management behaviors of a family do not work effectively, dysfunction of

the family as a system can occur. For example, family violence can be defined (Champion, 1998) as all forms of interpersonal violence between intimates across the life span, including verbal, emotional, physical, and sexual abuse, neglect and maltreatment. According to Champion (1998), family violence has been identified as a major public health concern facing today's society. For example, in her theoretical article she reports that a boy who grows up witnessing his father's violent behavior has a 1000% greater battering rate than those who don't witness such behavior. When working with families, you will need to find ways to assess the ability of the family to cope with stress, transition, and crisis as will be addressed in the assessment section of this chapter. You will also need to be able to plan interventions to assist families with positive coping strategies as addressed in the intervention sections of this chapter. Your efforts will be important because acute and chronic forms of family violence often lead to mental health disorders as reported by Champion (1998).

HELPING THE FAMILY ASSESS HEALTH PROMOTION NEEDS

As Hartrick, Lindsey, and Hills (1994) point out, family assessment should be comprised of four essential components including listening to the family, participatory dialogue, recognizing patterns, and envisaging action and positive change. Family assessment patterns that are specific to family wellness can follow the typology of 11 functional health patterns as defined by Gordon (1994). This provides an organized process for the identification of potential or actual family problems. The typology is as follows:

- Health perception and health management

- Nutritional–metabolic
- Elimination
- Activity and exercise
- Sleep and rest
- Cognitive–perceptual
- Self-perception and self-concept
- Roles and relationships
- Sexuality and reproduction
- Coping and stress-tolerance
- Values and beliefs
  Note: From Nursing diagnosis: Process and application, by M. Gordon, 1994. St. Louis, MO: Mosby. Copyright 1994 by Mosby. Reprinted with permission.

In a continuing education article by Hooper (1996), functional health pattern assessment is applied to families receiving home care. Although the focus of the article is illness-oriented rather than wellness-oriented, Hooper points out the benefit to the family of using family assessment to identify risk factors that are the result of family behaviors that can be self-evaluated and corrected to bring about improved health. As a community practitioner, you should be aware that specific conditions that develop at crucial times in family development will warrant more immediate family assessment. These conditions have been identified by Wright and Leahey (2000) (see Box 20.1).

There are a number of family assessment tools that can be found in the literature to assist families in assessing their health promotion needs. You will want to familiarize yourself with these various tools to determine which ones might best serve the families with whom you work. However, you will want to focus on family assessment tools that are both comprehensive but succinct because the most successful interventions are those that develop out of a family's own ability to assess itself and its health promotion needs. You will want to utilizes tools

that evaluate all determinants of health previously identified in this chapter, or combine the use of tools that measure different aspects of family health.

The FAMCHAT, a family assessment tool that measures cultural aspects of the family, was designed and tested among 131 families in 1996 by Davidson and Regier. Variables tested included ethnographic variables of ethnicity and religion; demographic variables of age, gender, and family size; socioeconomic variables of income and education, and affiliation variables of both formal and informal group memberships as well as the influence of acculturation on family cultural heritage. The Family Cultural Heritage Assessment Tool (FAMCHAT) is provided in Table 20.3 and can be used in conjunction with other family assessment tools designed to measure additional aspects of family health and wellness.

One family assessment tool that measures family health positively is the FAMTOOL, designed and tested by Weeks and O'Connor (1997). It was derived from their previously published concept analysis of family health (Weeks & O'Connor, 1994) and incorporates broadly the typology for functional assessment previously described. Content validity was established with an expert panel of judges. The FAMTOOL was tested for reliability initially with a convenience sample of 80 adults that resulted in a .90 internal consistency coefficient. Test-retest reliability was demonstrated 2 weeks later among 28 adults with a .96 stability coefficient. The tool is scored by summing response totals, ranging from 0 to 36 points, with higher points representing higher levels of family health and lower points representing lower levels of family health. The FAMTOOL is presented in Table 20.4 and can be used by the community practitioner when having the family assess their family determinants of health and wellness, in-

```
┌─────────────────────────────────────────────────────────────────────┐
```

Box 20.1   Indications for Family Assessment

— BPSS* suffering or disruption caused by a family crisis
— BPSS* suffering or disruption caused by a developmental milestone
— A family defines a problem as a family issue and there is motivation for family assessment
— A child or adolescent is identified by the family as having difficulties
— Issues that are serious enough to jeopardize family relationships
— A family member is about to be admitted to the hospital for psychiatric treatment
— A child is about to be admitted to the hospital

*BPSS = bio (physical), psychosocio (emotional) and spiritual (Wright & Leahey, 2000).

Note: From *Nurses and families: A guide to family assessment and intervention* (p. __), by L. M. Wright and M. Leahy, 2000. Philadelphia: F. A. Davis. Copyright 2000 by F. A. Davis. Reprinted with permission.

```
└─────────────────────────────────────────────────────────────────────┘
```

cluding physical, emotional, social, and spiritual measures.

FAMILY PLANNING MECHANISMS TO MEET HEALTH PROMOTION NEEDS

Although a number of approaches can be found in family literature that help families assess their health and wellness, there are few that specifically address planning mechanisms to meet health promotion needs. Planning really serves as a bridge between assessing, which many of us do, and implementing change, which fewer of us do. It takes more than just desire or follow-through. Using the change-process model originally proposed by Kurt Lewin (Matsunaga, 1975), assessing is akin to unfreezing; implementation is akin to refreezing; and planning to meet the health-promotion needs of the family seems to correlate with the moving phase of change.

Planning begins with goal-directedness. It is not enough for the family to acknowledge deficits in their health. There needs to be a desire to change, which you can foster by helping families set goals. A healthy family has the ability to acknowledge its strengths and weaknesses and is able to identify opportunities for and threats to change.

You can assist families in planning to meet their health-promotion needs by first empowering them to establish goals and then to identify mechanisms to meet those goals. Dixon (1996) describes four phases to the empowering process of families. These phases include the following:

• Professional dominated phase, which is evidenced by a high degree of trust in and dependence on the health professional
• Participatory phase, which is evidenced by increasing family member involvement and ownership of change as unfreezing begins
• Challenging phase, which is evidenced by a shift of power from the health professional to the family and moving occurs
• Collaborative phase, which is evidenced by a new family identity as refreezing begins

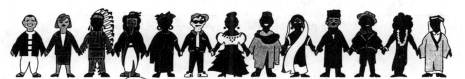

TABLE 20.3   FAMCHAT—A Family Cultural Heritage Assessment Tool

Please respond to the following questions in the space provided so that we might better serve your family:

Ethnographic variables: • Where were you born? • Are you an immigrant? • If so, how long have you lived in this country? • Have you traced your genealogy?	Ethnicity Ethnic group: Food preferences:	Religion Beliefs: Food prohibitions: Practices:	Healthcare Customs Birth: Death: Illness: Practices:
Demographic variables:	Age	Gender	Family Size
Socioeconomic variables:	Income	Education Where: Highest level:	Language Primary: —Speaking level —Reading level Secondary: —Speaking level —Reading level Other:
Affiliation variables:	Formal Group Memberships	Informal Group Memberships	
Influence of acculturation: For how many generations has your family been in this country? Do you live in an ethnic community?	Usual Verbal Communication	Usual Nonverbal Communication	

©Davidson and Regier (1996); Revised by Davidson, Regier, & Boos (2001). Reprinted with permission.

TABLE 20.4   FAMTOOL—A Family Health Assessment Tool

Please circle the number (0, 1, 2, or 3) which best describes your family:

		False	Mostly False	Mostly True	True
As a Family					
1.	We work well together	0	1	2	3
2.	We communicate effectively	0	1	2	3
3.	We share beliefs	0	1	2	3
4.	We play together	0	1	2	3
5.	We put energy into the family	0	1	2	3
6.	We value connectedness	0	1	2	3
7.	We work toward physical health	0	1	2	3
8.	We work toward emotional health	0	1	2	3
9.	We work toward social health	0	1	2	3
10.	We work toward spiritual health	0	1	2	3
11.	We value one another	0	1	2	3
12.	We have hope for the future	0	1	2	3

THANK YOU FOR COMPLETING THIS FAMILY HEALTH ANALYSIS.

Note: Published in Weeks, S. K., and O'Connor, P. C. (1997). *The FAMTOOL Family Health Assessment Tool. Rehabilitation Nursing, 22*(4), 188–191. Based on Weeks & O'Connor (1994). *Concept Analysis of Family + Health = A New Definition of Family Health. Rehabilitation Nursing, 19*(4), 207–210. Reprinted with permission.

Hulme (1999) used family empowerment as an intervention in an integrative literature review that explored its value for families of children with a chronic health condition. As a community practitioner, you will no doubt work with families who have members with chronic health conditions, but the model of empowering families can be used in meeting health-promotion needs of the family as well. You will find that a work sheet for planning is useful when empowering families to meet their health-promotion needs. The family empowerment work sheet for planning to meet health promotion needs has been developed by merging the concepts of change process and family empowerment with specific mechanisms for working with families to achieve health and wellness. It is provided in Table 20.5.

Use it in the following ways:

- Planning for family development change
- Planning for family structure change
- Planning for family function change
- Planning for family systems change
- Planning for family health behaviors change:
  - self-actualization
  - exercise
  - nutrition
  - communication

TABLE 20.5 Family Empowerment Work Sheet for Planning to Meet Health Promotion Needs

Directions: Jointly identify the areas for change that are agreed upon between family members and provider. Identify specific areas from self-assessment tools for focused intervention under each appropriate category. Number the priority areas for intervention in the column to the right accordingly. Identify the selected method of assistance that the family would like used to assist the change process and identify it by number in the appropriate phase targeted for change. When resolved, check off in the column to the far right.

Targeted Area for Family Intervention:	Priority	Methods of Assistance:	✓
Planning for Family Development Change		1. Behavior Modification	
		2. Contracting	
		3. Case management	
• Unfreezing phase		4. Collaboration	
• Moving phase		5. Consultation	
• Refreezing phase		6. Counseling	
		7. Environmental modification	
Planning for Family Structure Change		8. Family advocacy	
		9. Lifestyle modification	
• Unfreezing phase		10. Networking	
• Moving phase		11. Referral	
• Refreezing phase		12. Reminiscence Therapy	
		13. Role Modeling	
Planning for Family Function Change		14. Role supplementation	
		15. Teaching strategies	
		16. Values Clarification	
• Unfreezing phase			
• Moving phase			
• Refreezing phase			
Planning for Family Systems Change			
• Unfreezing phase			
• Moving phase			
• Refreezing phase			
Planning for Family Health Behaviors Change			
• Unfreezing phase			
• Moving phase			
• Refreezing phase			
—Self-actualization			
—Exercise			
—Nutrition			
—Communication			

INTERVENING TO FACILITATE FUNCTIONAL FAMILY COMMUNICATION

To facilitate functional family communication, you must first understand how functional family communication works. Functional family communication theory emphasizes the sending and receiving of both verbal and nonverbal messages. In this theory, communication with a high level of clarity and congruence between the sender and receiver promotes positive behavior within the family. Examples of functional family communication include reliable and valid communication between sender and recipient. Reliable communication is consistent in delivery and receipt just as valid communication is accurately understood between sender and receiver. You would expect in functional communication that when there is a lack of understanding, clarification is sought between recipient and sender. Current research on functional family communication (Olsen et al., 1999) indicates that communication that is lacking clarity (such as when it is disharmonious or disruptive) is likely to lead to problematic family behaviors. Conversely, you can visualize how functional communication and a dynamic group process between family members leads to family health. It may be helpful for you to review the model illustrating family communication found in Figure 20.2.

Remember that communication is both verbal and nonverbal, and your first step in facilitating functional family communication is to assess these areas of communication. It will help you begin facilitating communication by teaching family members that the majority of communication involves nonverbal cues, such as tone of voice, facial expression, and gestures. You will also want to help family members understand how their family communication

process has developed over time. Ask the family to draw in a genogram format to show how their communication has evolved from a historical perspective across the changing constellation of the family. An example of this family communication process diary appears in Figure 20.3.

Once you have all the possible communication lines drawn, you can ask family members to indicate either positive or negative dynamics next to the communication lines, according to their perspective. This can be accomplished as a one-time assessment or even on a daily basis. Remind family members that these are their perspectives only, based on their self-assessment, and so there is no right or wrong answer. After all the family members have illustrated their perception of family communication, encourage them to think about various family events that have been stressful or difficult to handle and that may have influenced those communication patterns.

Throughout your intervention to facilitate functional family communication, ask family members to practice using "I" statements that reflect ownership of one's perceptions versus "you" statements, which tend to project blame onto others. Examples of "I" statements include: "I feel angry when nobody helps me do the laundry," and "I feel discouraged when I come home from work and everyone is yelling." Examples of "you" statements include: "You are all too lazy to help with the laundry," or "All you contribute to the family is yelling and screaming." Remember that facilitating healthy family communication will take practice with the family members as well as encouraging healthy forgiveness of family member shortcomings.

INTERVENING TO FACILITATE FAMILY HEALTH AND WELLNESS

You will want to utilize multiple approaches when intervening with the family to facili-

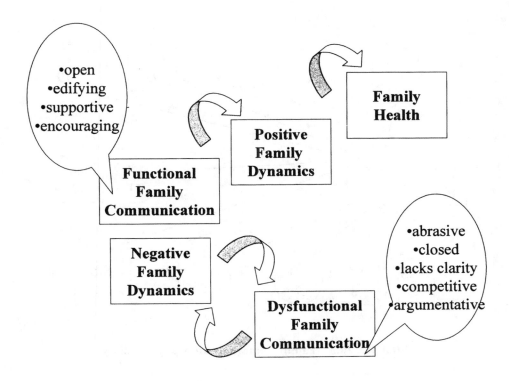

FIGURE 20.2   Family communication model.

tate family health and wellness. Suggested approaches are also provided for you in Table 20.5. These approaches to intervening with the family can be used to organize your methods of assistance broadly or specific to wellness issues of the family. For example, it may be helpful for you to break down your approaches into categories of common family concerns. For this reason, common areas for focused intervention within the family are provided in the remainder of this chapter.

- *Spirituality* involves the values, beliefs, moral codes for conduct, and ethical approaches held by the family. Help the family identify aspects of its spirituality because it differs between families. Culture and religion play an important role in family spirituality.

For some families spirituality involves church attendance, prayer, fasting, and reading scripture. For others, spirituality encompasses self-actualization, meditation, reading great books, and self-reflection. Ask each family member what their spiritual and religious beliefs are and provide support and encouragement for their healthy practices.

- *Exercise* involves both enjoyable physical activity and purposeful activity designed to reduce the risk of disease or to promote health. Assess the level of activity within the family and the amount of time the family exercises weekly. Suggest to families that they exercise together, which will increase family function by providing an opportunity for togetherness with a common

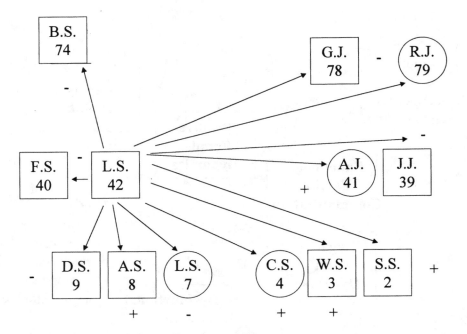

FIGURE 20.3   Family communication process diary.

positive goal. It can also reduce family stress and introduce new coping opportunities. Ask families to select physical activity or exercise programs that are appropriate for the developmental ages and capability of the family participants. For example, a family with six children under the age of 12 might want to structure a weekly activity plan that includes one parent walking with a different child each day and a family walk on the weekend. Families with adolescents might want to structure a weekly game of family baseball, swimming, tennis, football, basketball, or other sport. Encourage all family members to participate and invite those family members who have special activity-related talents to assume leadership in teaching and helping those with less skill. You will want to

familiarize yourself with other fitness issues found in chapter 11 of this book.

• *Nutrition* involves dietary choices and behaviors that facilitate the health status of family members. Your focus should not be limited to specific food choices of the family, but should include how the family does its food shopping, preparation, clean-up, and even its approaches to herbal and vitamin therapy. Ask family members to tell you their typical day's dietary intake. Although not all family members eat the same things throughout a given day, having the family provide a 24-hour food history for a typical day when the family is together is valuable in determining food choices that are influenced by family nutrition values and behaviors.

Also ask how food is used within the

context of the family for social interaction and as a method of coping with stress or to reward behavior. You will want to provide family members with information about healthful eating such as that provided in chapter 10, and encourage family members to identify shared values and behaviors associated with eating.

- *Stress management* involves an entire continuum of dealing with individual and family pressures as well as affording appropriate rest and personal space in which to renew one's abilities to deal with life's pressures. Regardless of developmental stage, family stress levels have implications for family health and function. For example, the baby that is under stress from hunger or a wet diaper will cry in an attempt to alleviate his or her stress. As family members grow and develop, they will learn other patterns of stress management that may be positive or negative. When one family member is distressed, other family members may feel and react to the stress themselves. Your role is to help the family identify its stress-management behaviors. Teach family members the benefit of identifying stress-management behaviors, because the way stress is handled tends to be passed from one generation to the next. Encourage family members not to label stress-management behaviors as good or bad, but state that some methods are healthier and that you are interested in helping them find and use more healthy approaches to stress management.
- *Sexuality* involves the healthy expression of intimacy between participants and should be fulfilling to the individual family member. It has been reported that healthy family behaviors in this area are evidenced by members

having a mutually exclusive and committed relationship where there is an exchange of affection, intimacy, and love (Hogan, 1985). You can facilitate the level of satisfaction within a couple's sexual relationship, including levels of healthy communication and loving support, by encouraging discussion of sexuality as a wellness function of the family. When concerns are voiced by family members, encourage partners to communicate their concerns to each other, by saying such things as "Tell your wife your feelings about that," or "Share your thoughts with your husband." You can also teach healthy sexual practices to other family members. For example, when working with a family that has teenagers, you will want to address the development of healthy sexual practices in a culturally sensitive way to assess whether the family has provided teaching and guidance about sexually transmitted disease, birth control issues, and safety of sexual practices.

- *Environment* involves both internal and external factors that either promote or detract from health. Ask the family to identify potential threats to family wellness in the following areas:
  - environmental toxicants like lead in house paints or dirt
  - occupational hazards such as exposure to extreme heat, sound, vibration, or radiation
  - recreational hazards and safety issues
  - home safety issues such as ventilation, rodents, temperature, and space
  - personal safety issues
  - potential deterioration of natural resources such as air, food, and water

Teach the family to problem-solve the

issues that emerge from their self-assessment. For example, you can encourage the family to discuss specific ways to reduce dangers. You can also provide the family with a list of specific steps to resolve potential threats to health and then ask them to decide which methods they might like to use.

Ultimately, intervening to facilitate health and wellness of the family will involve developing personalized interventions to meet the expressed needs of the family. An example of this personalized approach in jointly assessing, planning, and intervening to meet family health needs is provided for you in the family case study that follows.

SELECTED FAMILY CASE STUDY

Lynn and Autumn D. have been married for sixteen years. They live in a suburban community with their biological children, Dallas, age 9; Austin, age 8; Linae, age 7; Callie, age 4; Winston, age 3; and Sammy, age 2. Lynn (age 42) and Autumn (age 41) earn just over $50,000 per year and live in their parents' old home. Autumn supports the family as an attorney while Lynn has been either underemployed or unemployed for the last 10 years. The parents report significant role strain as both were raised in strict Catholic homes where each learned traditional values such as the role of father as provider and disciplinarian and the role of mother as homemaker and nurturant. Lynn serves as the primary caregiver while Autumn works outside the home.

Lynn is diabetic and has been recently diagnosed with hypertension. Autumn has a chronic history of anemia since childhood which has been unresponsive to iron therapy. Other sources of stress for the family include:

- *one child (Austin) is autistic and requires medication*

- *inability to fund recommended medical testing and educational interventions for Austin*
- *inability to fund dental interventions for all family members*
- *inability to pay balance of Autumn's educational loans*
- *lack of social support from neighbors, coworkers, or church members*
- *tensions among extended family members*
- *lack of consistent diet in the home*
- *lack of exercise or relaxation among family members*
- *lack of privacy for family members and frequent interrupted sleep due to Austin's intrusive behaviors*
- *frequent angry outbursts by Lynn that are directed at Autumn when laundry piles up or meals aren't prepared*

Autumn and Dallas have a good relationship, but appear to be carrying the load for meeting the needs of the family. Both are overweight. Autumn is concerned about Lynn's behavior, which has recently escalated to threats of suicide. Lynn has pressured Autumn to meet family demands over workplace demands, which has threatened Autumn's job. Autumn acknowledges that Lynn is frequently verbally and emotionally abusive, but does not consider divorce optional due to religious values. Lynn acknowledges that he is depressed, but tends to look to others to solve his problems.

Family Development *is identified to be at the expected level of a family with school-age children.*

Family Structure *is illustrated by the genogram found in Figure 20.1, which family systems data can further amplify.*

Family Function *is self-assessed by family members using the APGAR as moderately dysfunctional with a mean score of 5 when responses from Lynn, Autumn, and Dallas are combined.*

Family Health *is evaluated by two tools that collectively provide data on the cultural determinants that influence the family as well as the biological, psychosocial, and spiritual determinants of the family. The community practitioner interviews the family using the Family Cultural Heritage Assessment Tool (FAMCHAT) and identifies that* Lynn and Autumn come from two different ethnic backgrounds with differing communication patterns and food preferences, representing an additional stressor in the family. Lynn, Autumn, and Dallas each complete the FAMTOOL with respective scores of 19 (Lynn), 18 (Autumn), and 17 (Dallas), an average of 18 of the maximum potential total score of 36, or approximately 50%, which directly correlates with the APGAR score.

The community practitioner asks Lynn, Autumn, and Dallas to keep a 24-hour food diary and a family communication process diary. Based on family input from these multiple measures, the community practitioner uses the family empowerment work sheet to develop a plan to assist the family in meeting the following wellness needs:

- *Family Function Change*
  Intervention goal: To increase APGAR measurement by 30%.
  Requested methods of assistance:
  1. Collaboration
  2. Family advocacy
  3. Networking
- *Family Health Behaviors Change*
  Intervention goal: To increase FAMTOOL measurement by 30%.
  Requested methods of assistance:
  1. Behavior modification
  2. Networking
  3. Reminiscence therapy
- *Self-actualization*
  Intervention goal: To increase Lynn's sense of self-actualization.
  Requested methods of assistance:
  1. Consultation

2. Contracting
3. Values clarification
- *Exercise*
  Intervention goal: To increase family exercise and activity patterns with daily walks.
  Requested methods of assistance:
  1. Environmental modification
  2. Lifestyle modification
  3. Teaching
- *Nutrition*
  Intervention goal: To increase fruit and vegetable intake.
  Requested methods of assistance:
  1. Lifestyle modification
  2. Role supplementation
  3. Teaching
- *Communication*
  Intervention goal: To increase functional communication between family members identified in the communication diary.
  Requested methods of assistance:
  1. Counseling
  2. Referral
  3. Role modeling

SUMMARIZING FAMILY WELLNESS APPLICATION

You have been provided information on family theory and research, family development, family structure, family function, family systems, and family health. The bottom line and "take-home" point to remember in working with families is that addressing healthy behaviors from the family perspective can facilitate wellness across communities, cultures, and from generation to generation.

REFERENCES

Bowen, M. (1985). *Family therapy in clinical practice.* Northvale, NJ: Jason Aronson.

Campbell, D. W. (1991). Family paradigm theory and family rituals: Implications for child and family health. *Nurse Practitioner, 16,* 22–31.

Champion, J. D. (1998). Family violence and mental health. *Nursing Clinics of North America, 33*(1), 201–215.

Clark, C. C. (1998). Wellness self-care by healthy older adults. *Image: Journal of Nursing Scholarship, 30*(4), 351–355.

Comana, M. T., Brown, V. M., & Thomas, J. D. (1998). The effect of reminiscence therapy on family coping. *Journal of Family Nursing, 4*(2), 182–197.

Cox, R. P., & Davis, L. L. (1999). Family problem solving: Measuring the elusive concept. *Journal of Family Nursing, 5*(3), 332–360.

Davidson, J. U. (1984). Historical perspective of self-care agency among elderly Mennonites at the turn of the twentieth century. (Master thesis, Wichita State University, 1984). *Masters' Abstracts International, 26*(4), 418.

Davidson, J. U. (1989). Health embodiment: The relationship between self-care agency and health-promoting behaviors. (Doctoral dissertation, Texas Woman's University, 1988). *Dissertation Abstracts International, 49*(08-B), 3102.

Davidson, J. U., Regier, T., & Boos, S. C. (2001). *The KS Nurse, 76,* 10.

Denham, S. A. (1995). Family routines: A construct for considering family health. *Holistic Nursing Practice, 9*(4), 11–23.

Denham, S. A. (1999a). Pt. I: The definition and practice of family health. *Journal of Family Nursing, 5*(2), 133–159.

Denham, S. A. (1999b). Pt. II: Family health during and after death of a family member. *Journal of Family Nursing, 5*(2), 160–183.

Dixon, D. M. (1996). Unifying concepts in parents' experiences with health care providers. *Journal of Family Nursing, 2,* 111–132.

Duvall, E. M., & Miller, B. (1985). *Marriage and family development* (6th ed.). New York: Harper & Row.

Dzurec, L. C. (1995). Assessing fit: A key indicator of family health. *Journal of Nurse-Midwifery, 40*(3), 277–289.

Eddy, L. L., & Walker, A. J. (1999). The impact of children with chronic health problems on marriage. *Journal of Family Nursing, 5*(1), 10–32.

Erikson, E. (1986). *Childhood and society.* New York: Norton.

Faux, S. A., & Seideman, R. Y. (1996). Health care professionals and their relationships with families who have members with development disabilities. *Journal of Family Nursing, 2*(2), 217–238.

Gordon, M. (1994). *Nursing diagnosis: Process and application.* St. Louis, MO: Mosby.

Hartrick, G. (1997). Beyond a service model of care: Health promotion and the enhancement of family capacity. *Journal of Family Nursing, 3*(1), 57–69.

Hartrick, G., Lindsey, A. E., & Hills, M. (1994). Family nursing assessment: Meeting the challenge of health promotion. *Journal of Advanced Nursing, 20,* 85–91.

Hogan, R. (1985). *Human sexuality: A nursing perspective* (2nd ed.). Norwalk, CT: Appleton-Century-Crofts.

Hooper, J. I. (1996). The family receiving home care: Functional health pattern assessment. *Home Care Provider, 1*(5), 238–245.

Hulme, P. A. (1999). Family empowerment: A nursing intervention with suggested outcomes for families of children with a chronic health condition. *Journal of Family Nursing, 5*(1), 33–50.

Jones, S. L., & Dimond, M. (1982). Family theory and family therapy models: Comparative review with implications for nursing practice. *Family Theory and Therapy, 20*(10), 12–19.

Matsunaga, M. (1975, April). Nurse administrator must be chief initiator of change. *The American Nurse,* 4.

Loveland-Cherry, C. J. (1983). Family system patterns of cohesiveness and autonomy: Relationship to family members' health behavior. (Doctoral dissertation, Wayne State University, 1982). *Dissertation Abstracts International, 43*(11-B), 3537.

McCubbin, M. A., & McCubbin, H. I. (1993). Families coping with illness: The resiliency model of family stress, adjustment, and adaptation. In C. B. Danielson, B. Hamel-Bissell, & P. Winstead-Fry (Eds.), *Families, health and illness* (pp. 21–63). St. Louis, MO: Mosby.

Olsen, S. F., Marshall, E. S., Mandleco, B. L., Allred, K. W., Dyches, T. T., & Sansom, N. (1999). Support, communication, and hardiness in families with children with disabilities. *Journal of Family Nursing, 5,* 275–292.

Padula, C. A. (1997). Predictors of participation in health promotion activities by elderly couples. *Journal of Family Nursing, 3*(1), 88–106.

Pender, N. (1996). *Health promotion in nursing practice* (3rd ed.). Norwalk, CT: Appleton & Lange.

Plager, K. A. (1999). Understanding family legacy in family health concerns. *Journal of Family Nursing, 5*(1), 51–71.

Robinson, D. L. (1997). Family stress theory: Implications for family health. *Journal of the American Academy of Nurse Practitioner, 9*(1), 17–23.

Smilkstein, G. (1978). The family APGAR: A proposal for a family function test and its use by physicians. *Journal of Family Practice, 6,* 1231–1239.

Weeks, S. K., & O'Connor, P. C. (1994). Concept analysis of family + health = a new definition of family health. *Rehabilitation Nursing, 19*(4), 207–210.

Weeks, S. K., & O'Connor, P. C. (1997). The FAMTOOL family health assessment tool. *Rehabilitation Nursing, 22*(4), 188–191.

Wright, L. M., & Leahey, M. (2000). *Nurses and families: A guide to family assessment and intervention* (3rd ed.). Philadelphia: F. A. Davis.

PART V

Health Promotion in a Cultural Context

CHAPTER 21

Health Promotion with African American Women

Marva Mizell Price

T his chapter examines health promotion topics for African American women. The focus is applicable for nurses who provide care in private and public clinics and in community settings. While lifestyles concerns, health promotion, and strategies for nursing intervention are the emphasis of the discussion, other factors are included in the chapter that impact how African American women achieve and maintain their health through primary and secondary prevention.

In an era of technology and scientific advances, health care researchers devote increased attention to women's health issues. Research findings are being translated into improved clinical care. At the same time, women are being encouraged to gain insight on how their lifestyle choices affect their health.

One goal of *Healthy People 2010,* the health care agenda for the nation, is to eliminate health disparities among different segments of the population. These include differences that occur by gender, race, or ethnicity, education or income,

and disabilities (*Healthy People 2010,* [Online] 2000). An acknowledgement of the large gaps in health status between African American women and White women has stimulated research that is focused on collaborating with individuals and their communities to improve health outcomes. You will find that African American women who are healthy, well educated, and economically secure value health and health-promoting activities. Your hard work to provide culturally sensitive care will be appreciated.

In contrast, findings show that perception of self responsibility is not always easy for women who are less well-educated with limited social and economic resources. Nevertheless, with careful collaboration it can be equally satisfying and possible to work with women who need more of your time to acquire health knowledge and skills in self care. Remember that individuals, families, and communities differ in their readiness to move along the continuum toward holistic behaviors. Prepare to prioritize and set targets that are individualized and realistic for your client.

This chapter will help you understand personal attitudes, beliefs, and values that determine African American women's acceptance and ability to engage in health-promoting practices. Important background discussion is included on the impact of other factors that influence health such as education and economics. The overall intent of this chapter to help you identify a variety of parameters that correlate with improving the health status of African American women across socioeconomic levels.

CULTURAL PERSPECTIVES

African American refers to a people who are distinguished from other racial groups by their heritage of African ancestry. Among African Americans are individuals and families from various parts of the United States with different and even mixed ethnic heritages and varied hues of skin color. Some African Americans will prefer *African American* as their racial identity while others will prefer to be designated as *Black*, the terminology used in the era of the 1960s. *African American* and *Black* continue to be used interchangeably to denote nonwhites born in the United States whose ancestors include descendants of sub-Sahara Africa (Chisholm, 1996).

Not all African American women are similar, and so this chapter will not be a bible of health promotion strategies for all of them. The topics included are those considered of great significance to their well-being by many women of color from geographically diverse parts of the United States. Furthermore, the *Healthy People 2010* agenda emphasizes these areas to narrow the gap in health indicators between African American and White women.

African American women come from urban and rural settings across the United States and vary from one geographic area of the country to another and even within the same geographic locales. Many identify ethnically with one another through some commonly associated cultural distinctions such as heritage and customs. The ethnic bond for these women is a common heritage of African descent. The cultural distinctions associated with being African American are quite complex and are believed to be more sociocultural than scientific or genetic (Caldwell & Popenoe, 1995).

You probably agree that genetics predispose individuals to various diseases, but how a condition will manifest, as well as how an individual responds to move to a higher level of wellness is often mediated or affected by sociocultural and socioeconomic factors. Therefore, cultural beliefs and economic influences are also included in this chapter.

Anthropologists and public-health scholars have brought attention to the fact that biological differences among human beings are getting harder and harder to distinguish. You need only count the number of new categories for self-identifying categories of race in the census of 2000. Nearly two decades ago, population geneticist Richard Lewontin measured the degree of population difference in gene frequencies for 17 different traits, and found that only 6.3% of all variation could be accounted for at the level of major geographic race (Lewontin, 1982; Molnar, 1983). The visible characteristics of race alone were unreliable indicators of genotypic variation.

Likewise, women in your community who are grouped as African American are often widely divergent in beliefs, habits, reactions to various wellness activities, and adoption of healthful behaviors. Age, income, geographic region, cost of health care and health care coverage, and beliefs about the health care system influence our perceptions of wellness. Your interventions will need to incorporate beliefs and values into strategies aimed at changing unhealthy lifestyle behaviors (Feldman & Fulwood, 1999).

If the term African American were deleted from this chapter, it is hoped that you would still find this discussion on health promotion useful in your day-to-day environment and work with women from many different backgrounds, whether in a clinic or community setting.

Beliefs About Wellness

Early studies by nurses and other health care researches about gaps in health outcomes for African Americans traditionally focused on the effects of poverty. Very recently, studies have focused on the dynamics of African Americans' individual perceptions of illness and wellness. Frequency of poor health and how often women experience altered quality of life can be attributed to lower levels of health promotion activities.

To gain effective insight and promote culturally sensitive care, take time to talk to women themselves and other health professionals who have served in advocacy roles. A woman's belief about normal or abnormal health status determines her thinking and decisions to seek health care when she is not sick. Over generations, many African American families were oriented toward an external *health locus of control* (Dohrenwend & Dohrenwend, 1981). Health locus of control may be internal or external. Internal locus of control allows a woman to believe that her health outcomes are due to her own efforts and abilities of self care and that she has the ability to regain or maintain a state of wellness. Self care or preventive behaviors are behaviors

that a person might engage in to promote personal health or well-being.

On the other hand, external control places a state of health or illness under the predetermined control of others. State of health in external locus of control does not depend directly on the woman's or her family's health behavior. Whether she becomes sick or can influence health events is beyond her personal control. Illness may be due to chance, fate, or the spiritual power of God. Health professionals or even powerful family members may be felt to exert control over the individual's body. You may hear your client say, "All the women in our family died of cancer at a young age." This comment suggests coincidence and may be a multigenerational statement of perceived biological vulnerability. In addition, it can be a legacy and expectation of untimely death regardless of healthful self-care behaviors.

Comments of age-related multigenerational patterns may emerge when an illness has been diagnosed at a family member's particular state of the life cycle. A woman's belief about mastery over her health strongly affects her relationship with the health care system. Beliefs about control over health will predict certain health behaviors, particularly compliance with screening recommendations that you suggest for her. If you provide care to African American women who do not have strong belief in their ability to control their health circumstances, you are likely to find that her relationship with you and your health care setting will lack commitment. She will minimize the importance of her own ability or yours to maintain a level of wellness. When you work with her on recommendations, the recommendations will appear to be heard and understood, but never followed. Your client also may miss future follow-up appointments that are scheduled.

Family Influences and Social Support

Social support is that given to a person from the people in their social network. It is a means to provide assistance and encouragement to individuals in order that they may better cope with a situation or circumstance. Peers, friends, kinships, groups, and churches can provide social support. When provided by family members, their beliefs about mastery over one's health, family relationships and norms, and social networks strongly affect the nature of health promotion in nurse-client relationships (Stewart, 1993). There are some classic studies that help us understand how ethnic differences in social network and social support and age can make a difference in health status. Gottlieb and Green's work (1987) provided some of the early research on social support and social networks among African Americans. Their investigations found that middle-aged and older blacks tended to rely on an informal system of multiple family members and friends for social support.

Research has been conducted to examine associations between social ties and instrumental and emotional support among African American women in the use of cancer screening (Kang, Bloom, & Romano, 1994). These researchers found that women with more social ties were more likely to have had routine mammograms than were those with fewer social ties, even after controlling for health status, age, education, type of health insurance, and whether there's having a primary care source.

In many African American families, a woman's personal attitudes and values for healthy behaviors originate through her family experiences that are passed on from generation to generation. For example, a young child who is taken for her scheduled well-child visits and who sees her mother attack significance to the annual well-woman exam tends to value preventive health care as a young adult as well. These attitudes and beliefs serve to provide a sense of unity to family life. It facilitates continuity between past, present, and future experiences. African American women have been accustomed to placing family needs first and working toward healthier lifestyles last. In the past decade, research was conducted to show that African American women often value the health of their children and other dependent family members over their own health and may value personal health primarily as a dutiful honor to close family ties (Dignan et al., 1990).

You may be surprised to find that some of the women with whom you collaborate for healthier lifestyles already have some awareness of screening recommendations. Your first inclination is to ask why they have not followed them. Each woman's belief system can be compromised by the role that family and social networks play in her ability to adopt healthful behaviors. Show that you respect and care about her by listening and conveying acceptance of her day-to-day family and career responsibilities. Explore areas of social and community support. When there are family and friends who can have influence and involvement, explore ways to involve them in helping your client prioritize health-promotion strategies. Think about incorporating a few of the brief questions below to assess your client's social support:

- Tell me about your day-to-day responsibilities.
- What are your responsibilities for family members or friends?
- Whom do you turn to in your family and among your friends? Are there

places in your community that you can turn to when you are concerned about your health?

- What are some situations in which you are more likely to seek advice from others?

Convey a positive attitude toward your client. Find out what she believes. Discuss her perceptions about what constitutes wellness. Your next step will be to help her clarify what she and her support system understand. This will be a beginning step in building trust to engage your client as a partner in working toward a healthier lifestyle. You will encounter older women in your practice who adapt to healthy interventions more readily when there are close family and social ties in place. Encourage your client to follow through on positive health advice. Promote a positive attitude towards accepting your recommendations, keeping appointment schedules, and receiving health-promotion screenings.

The Role of Spirituality

Spirituality is an individual's proper relationship to God or the religious practices by which she may attain that relationship (Stolley & Koenig, 1997). Knowledge of the effects of religious beliefs on African American health can help you provide care that is sensitive to their beliefs. Without such awareness, you might interpret spiritual and religious influences as counterproductive to your health-promotion strategies.

Spirituality or the religion in which spirituality is expressed is very important to the support system in everyday living for many African Americans. This is especially true for older African Americans. Spirituality provides support in daily coping, increases

self-worth, and is especially vital in periods of distress and illness (Williams, 1994).

Historically, the church has been a catalyst for social, economic, and political change in the African American community. It is the central institution in the African American community, serving religious needs and providing contacts for social support. Membership in a congregation brings people together (Koenig, 1999). In fact, the church can be a second family for the individual. A growing number of church congregations have health screening programs for chronic diseases like hypertension (often referred to by consumers as pressure or high blood) and diabetes mellitus (often referred to by consumers as sugar). Concern and mutual respect are a part of the social support system of the church, and the social bond can become an informal health promotion network.

Seventy-five percent of all older African Americans have church affiliation and at least half attend religious services at least once a week (Koenig, 1999; Stolley & Koenig, 1997). This is particularly important for older African American women, who tend to center their daily lives around private prayer sessions (Koenig, 1999). Differences in the importance of prayer have been found with decreased religious involvement for divorced and widowed African American women (Chatters & Taylor, 1989; Stolley & Koenig, 1997; Taylor & Chatters, 1991). However, even women who do not have close ties with formal religious activities will seek emotional support through spirituality during stressful events and illness. Within the last decade, nurses and public health researchers have extended themselves into communities to work hand in hand with religious and civic organizations to incorporate health-promotion activities into the group's outreach plans.

SOCIOECONOMIC INFLUENCES AS A DETERMINANT OF HEALTH PROMOTION

Inequalities in income and education underlie many health disparities in the United States. Close correlation exists between an African American woman's financial resources and her readiness to consider health promotion behaviors (*Healthy People 2010*, 2000; Sanders-Phillips, 1997). The effect of socioeconomics on African American health care has been the subject of political campaigns and citizen advocates. Furthermore, disparities in health care for African Americans have been the focus of several scientifically conducted studies. The inadequacies in health status are multifaceted, but frequently are associated with generations of poverty, inadequate access to quality health care, health care policy, and lifestyle factors.

African Americans are the largest minority group in the United States, comprising 12.6% of the population (U.S. Census Bureau [On-line], 2000). A little more than half of African Americans live in urban areas, with the remainder in rural communities (U.S. Census Bureau). A large number of the urban dwellers live in central cities with undesirable conditions of dense housing, low income and unemployment, exposure to drugs in the community, periodic street violence, and generally high levels of stress. American cities with the largest African American population are Detroit, Washington, DC, New Orleans, Baltimore, Memphis, and Philadelphia (Boston University Library [On-line], 2000). However, you will find African American families in nearly every urban or rural community.

The median age of African Americans is 30. The average size of the African American family is larger than the general population with an average of three to four members per household. In addition, female-headed households have increased over the past 30 years. The average life expectancy for African American women is 73.4 years compared with 78.7 years for their White counterparts (U.S. Census Bureau; Feldman & Fulwood, 1999).

While 8 out of 10 African Americans have completed high school and many have attended some community or technical college, only about 13% of African Americans are college graduates (Boston University Library, 2000). Regardless of education, men in the United States on average earn more than women at every educational level (U.S. Census Bureau). Women are employed in nearly every profession; however, given educational attainment there are few African American females at the top of organizations and corporations.

There are distinct demographic differences in poverty by race, ethnicity, and household composition as well as geographical variation in poverty across the United States. Lower socioeconomic groups continue to lag behind (*Healthy People 2010*, 2000). Although the annual income for African Americans has risen, approximately 30% of African American families still live below the poverty level (U.S. Census Bureau). Income inequality has increased over the past three decades, and 50% of female-headed households are below poverty level (U.S. Census Bureau). African Americans with low incomes, including many women who are employed with minimal or no insurance coverage, often fall through the cracks without adequate insurance benefits for health maintenance and health promotion.

A significant portion of federal health care funding is divided into categories for specific age groups and health needs. For example, low-income pregnant women qualify for prenatal care and limited health screenings through federal dollars allocated to states. Preventive care for reproductive health services is provided through federal- and state-funded family planning and rural health clinics. Low-income women over 50 years of age receive cancer prevention care through federal grant funds to state public health and rural health clinics for breast and cervical cancer prevention. Women who are 65 and older are guaranteed breast and cervical cancer screening services in private physicians' offices through Medicare. Medicare provides health insurance and preventive health benefits to people who are 65 years and older and to others who are eligible for Social Security benefits. An increasing number of communities are working with creative managed care and Medicaid funding through public and private collaborations. The federal and state governments finance Medicaid funding, which provides health care benefits to poor and medically needy persons.

Currently, private physicians' offices may accept or reject patients covered by Medicaid Managed Care funds. This is an alternative health care delivery and financing system that integrates the financial processes with service delivery. Contracts are made with employers and insurers to provide a package of services. Your clients who participated in Medicaid Managed Care or who are members of managed care organizations will have access to packages that include health promotion services. These include individualized health education profiles, immunizations, HIV education and screening, eye care, basic nutrition services, and breast and cervical cancer screening. If you are employed in private health care clinics, familiarize yourself with a variety of private insurance plans and acquaint yourself with which health-promotion interventions are reimbursable.

HEALTH AND LIFESTYLE CHALLENGES AND CONCERNS

There are certain health problems in African American females where health promotion has been shown to make a positive impact. The topics that are discussed in this section are a threat to health. Listed in random order they are: obesity, decreased physical activity and fitness, hypertension, diabetes, stress, tobacco use, inadequate breast and cervical screening, osteoarthritis, lupus, menopause—particularly as it relates to cardiovascular and bone health—and exposure to the HIV virus (*Healthy People 2010*, 2000). This list is not all-inclusive of the many health issues that are important to the whole person. However, these issues are among the top concerns for an agenda aimed at making a positive impact on the health of African Americans. The *Healthy People 2010* leading indicators prioritize these issues as crucial for prevention-oriented interventions for African Americans, and these health problems can be addressed by nurses in clinics and in their outreach in community settings (*Healthy People 2010 Objectives* [Online], 1998).

NUTRITION AND OBESITY

Obesity, defined as excessive body storage of energy in the form of fat, has adverse effects on other chronic diseases and certain cancers, which contribute to increased morbidity and mortality. Obesity is defined as *body mass index* (BMI) above the desirable index. BMI is the ratio of weight to height as seen in the formula in Box 21.1.

BMI correlates to body fat content in adults. Being overweight is a significant health issue for most industrialized societies and more important for African American women than any other ethnic group

---

Box 21.1   BMI Calculation (Report of the U.S. Preventive Services Task Force)

- Divide your client's weight in kilograms by the square of her height in meters
- kg/m^2
- Healthy BMI = 27.3 or less

---

in the United States. A strong relationship exists between high BMI and chronic health conditions like diabetes, hypertension, and high serum lipids (Sowers, 1998).

Studies of obesity in African American women across educational levels find that obesity is prevalent across age groups and predominant after 18 years of age. The weight gain is maintained through adulthood. Individual decisions about weight management and success of the undertaking are complex and thought to be culturally influenced. For example, there may be special cultural constraints and attitudes about food selection and preparation methods that negatively influence behavior change. These include ambivalence about the health benefits of weight reduction and dietary change, a relatively tolerant attitude toward moderate obesity, positive value placed on certain high-fat and high-sodium foods, and a failure to identify with maintenance of cardiovascular health. Other contributing factors include inadequate social support and a lack of daily coping methods, which can lead to unhealthy eating patterns (Holmes et al., 1998).

Although African American women may be conscious of being overweight, they are less likely to be preoccupied with their weight or feel a strong social pressure to lose weight, even when weight reduction is attempted (Maillet, D'Eramo, & Spollett, 1996). Fuller body figures are viewed positively and are largely acceptable among many African American families. Obsession with thinness and stigmatization of obesity

pose little societal pressure to African American women.

Another important factor in being overweight for African American women is the lack of adequate exercise and leisure physical activity. Increased weight can be the result of an unbalanced energy equation (i.e., a higher level of food intake and lower level of energy output) (Stolley & Fitzgibbon, 1997). Research findings support inclusion of cultural frameworks in health promotion activities aimed at weight reduction (Rosenberg, Palmer, Adams-Campbell, & Rao, 1999).

African American women need culturally relevant interventions that address obesity prevention across income levels. You will need to incorporate lifestyle changes that support a low-fat, low cholesterol, high-fiber diet while keeping in mind how to incorporate cultural preferences for foods. Don't forget to emphasize the importance of an intake of 8 or more 8 oz. glasses of water each day. A large study of dietary intake of African American residents in a southern community found that their diets contained beneficial quantities of fruits and vegetables that included broccoli, cabbage, collards, and citrus juices and fruits. Find out what your client's food preferences are and the amount of her daily intake. If she includes fruits and vegetables, praise her for including these in her diet, as they contain nutrients (ascorbic acid, B-carotenes, and phytochemicals), which are known to have a direct benefit on preventing chronic diseases (McClelland, Demark-Wahnefried, Mustian, Cowan, & Campbell, 1998). Try incorporating the components below when developing an intense weight management plan for your client (Stolley & Fitzgibbon, 1997).

- Plan for long-term interventions
- Family or peer participation
- Conduct program in an easily accessible clinic setting with hassle-free parking or a safe and familiar community location
- Incorporate culturally appropriate music, dance, and media when the individual prefers these
- Acknowledgement and knowledge of neighborhood food stores in which families shop
- Acknowledgment and inclusion of foods commonly prepared and eaten by the individual and her family
- Attention to the challenges of adopting a low-fat dietary plan within a strict financial budget
- Follow-up booster sessions to support maintenance of dietary changes
- Inclusion of intensive exercise components
- Integrate low-fat food preparation activities in the weight maintenance program

We must also remember that the struggle with excess weight should not overshadow those African American women who are not overweight but who are at high risk instead because of preoccupation with their weight. African American females have been largely excluded from studies of eating disorders due to the assumption that the African American community's acceptance of women with fuller shapes protects its women from eating problems. However, recent studies are beginning to show that race, class, and exposure to a dominant culture that denigrates African American features and physiques have an impact on body image among African American women and may play a role in the development of eating problems (Williamson, 1998). Problem eating behaviors such as anorexia, bulimia, and binge-eating should be remembered when assessing abnormal eating behaviors.

Physical Activity and Fitness

The term physical activity is used in this chapter to indicate any type of exertion of sufficient duration, frequency, and intensity to be associated with a potential health benefits. Women in general are involved in physical activity less often than men.

A limited amount of research (Duey et al., 1998; Ward et al., 1997) suggests that for those African American women who are overweight, the origin of the weight problem, though not well understood, may lie in childhood and adolescence. An area of concern is a lower level of aerobic fitness for many African American girls compared to girls of other ethnic backgrounds. Girls who were studied were less likely to engage in vigorous weight-bearing or aerobic activities such as jogging or running, aerobic dance, swimming and competitive sports, walking, and bicycling. Sedentary behavior may be an important contributing factor in the development of obesity that starts in adolescence and increases in adulthood. In addition, physical inactivity can be the beginning of unfavorable changes in serum cholesterol levels.

Nursing theorists have studied the relationship of ethnic background and socioeconomic status to physical activity for African American women (Felton, Parson, & Bartoces, 1997). Findings show that nurses can motivate women to exercise.

Help women become knowledgeable about the long-term health problems associated with inactivity and the benefits of physical activity.

Work with your client for modification in her environment to overcome her everyday barriers to physical activity. A list of barriers to regular physical activity for many African American women resulted from research conducted by nurse researchers Nies, Vollman, and Cook (1999). See Box 21.2 to learn about barriers to regular physical activity.

Physical activity is not an easily modified behavior. However, in your client-nurse relationship you will have the opportunity to develop and evaluate individualized interventions for African American girls and women. These might include modification of diet along with increased regular physical activity. Assess how your client can integrate practical, convenient, and enjoyable forms of physical activity into her schedule. Does your client work traditional hours? An evening or night work schedule can make a regular exercise regimen difficult to arrange. Are there church or other community-based or work-based programs that are available to her? Talk with your client and find out from others who are involved in community outreach about the community resources that are available for informal sports such as softball, basketball, tennis, aerobic dance, and other organized exercise programs or gyms. What are her social supports? Social support by family or friends can provide a supportive social structure to facilitate exercise. Does she have access to a safe place that is conducive to exercise? If not, help her locate one or even assist her in finding other women who experience similar barriers to regular exercise. With your help, they may be able to organize an exercise program tailored to their specific needs.

Assess these important areas before developing an exercise regimen with your client. The following questions may be helpful in your preassessment for an exercise regimen:

- Does your client work traditional hours?
- Are there church or other community-based or work-based programs that are available to her?
- What are her social supports?
- Does she have access to a safe, conducive place for exercise?

Women with sedentary lifestyles will benefit from a prescribed regimen of physical activities, which will improve their overall health status. Aerobic exercise such as walking or dancing for 30 minutes duration 3 days a week raises the heart rate to improve

---

Box 21.2　Barriers to Regular Physical Activity

- Lack of childcare
- No person to exercise with
- Competing responsibilities
- Lack of space in the home
- Inability to use exercise facilities at work
- Lack of motivation
- Fatigue
- Unsafe neighborhood

overall cardiovascular and physical fitness. Other forms of aerobic exercise like softball, basketball, tennis, and even walking a pet should be encouraged once an individual has integrated a plan for physical activity in her lifestyle.

Older African American women can benefit from your helping them set goals for regular physical activity. Some may be at risk for developing disabling diseases. These individuals will find it hardest to change their sedentary lifestyles because they may have the least tolerance for starting with 30 minutes of aerobic activity three times a week. Discuss the benefits of physical activity. It can improve their strength, endurance, flexibility, and balance and prevent the onset of further disabilities. Also discuss the benefits of exercise on chronic diseases. Exercise reduces the severity of hypertension, diabetes, and osteoarthritis (Carlson et al., 1999). It may also be helpful to tell the women about little ways to increase exercise in their daily routine like parking farther away or taking the stairs instead of the elevator.

Assess their activity level. Your goals for your older clients might include teaching them about flexibility, weights, and endurance exercises. Find out about senior programs and community recreational facilities that offer individualized or group instruction in resistance training with weights, stationary bicycles, aerobics, and flexibility. Help your senior clients set goals to start their exercise regimen at an appropriate pace depending on the individual's baseline ability. Low-intensity exercise will help your older clients improve muscle strength in upper and lower extremities. Some of your clients will only be able to perform activities of daily living (ADL) as their baseline. Praise them, too, because ADLs will prevent a decline in their physical ability. Others will be able to engage in spontaneous and moderate physical activity

at a steadily increasing pace to improve their gait speed and stair-climbing power.

Hypertension

The number one health problem for African Americans is hypertension (*Healthy People 2010*, 2000). Some of the highest rates of cardiovascular disease are found in African American women and are caused by hypertension. Cardiovascular disease is the leading cause of death among African American women, even at young ages, and is highest in the southeastern United States (Gillum, 1996). Cardiovascular disease takes more lives than the next 14 leading causes of death combined. Compared with White American women, African American women have a higher incidence of hypertension that occurs at an earlier age and that if not reversed continues for a lifetime. The increased incidence of hypertension begins in the childbearing years. Very little difference has been found between White and African American blood pressure in childhood and adolescence. It has been estimated that a reduction in systolic blood pressure of 9 mm Hg and one of 5 mm Hg in diastolic blood pressure could result in a 21% decrease in deaths from cardiovascular heart disease (Potts & Thomas, 1999). The criterion for Hypertension is listed in Box 21.3.

Box 21.4 displays the Healthy People 2010 objectives for hypertension prevention and control in African American women.

The *stroke belt* consists of states in the southeastern United States with the highest number of residents with hypertension, and a death rate from strokes greater the national average (Gillum, 1996; Hall et al., 1997). These states are Alabama, Arkansas, Florida, Georgia, Kentucky, Louisiana,

---

Box 21.3 Criteria for Hypertension

Systolic blood pressure $\geq$ 140 mm Hg
  or diastolic blood pressure $\geq$ 90 mm Hg three consecutive times

(Joint National Committee on Prevention, Detection, Evaluation, and Treatment of Hypertension VI, 1997)

Box 21.4 *Healthy People 2010 Objectives* for Hypertension Prevention and Control in African American Women

- Increase to $\geq$ 50% the proportion of persons with high blood pressure whose blood pressure is under control.
- Increase to $\geq$ 90% the proportion of persons with high blood pressure who are taking action to control their blood pressure by taking medication, dieting to lose weight, reducing salt intake, and exercising.
- Reduce overweight to $\leq$ 30% in Black women aged 20 years and older and 15% among persons aged 12 to 19 years.
- Increase to $\geq$ 30% the proportion of people aged 6 years and older who engage regularly in light to moderate physical activity for $\geq$ 30 minutes per day.
- Decrease salt and sodium intake so that $\geq$ 65% of home meal preparers prepare foods without adding salt, $\geq$ 80% of people avoid using salt at table, and $\geq$ 40% of adults regularly purchase foods modified or lower in sodium.
- Increase to $\geq$ 90% the proportion of adults who have had their blood pressure measured within the preceding 2 years and can state whether their blood pressure was normal or high.
- Increase to $\geq$ 50% the proportion of employers with 50 employees that offer high-blood-pressure education and control activities to their employees.

From Department of Health and Human Services. *Healthy People 2000: National Health Promotion and Disease Prevention Objectives.* Washington, DC: Public Health Service, 1991.

Maryland, Mississippi, North Carolina, South Carolina, Tennessee, Virginia, West Virginia, and the District of Columbia. South Carolina has the highest number of stroke deaths in the United States (Hall et al., 1997), but hypertension is not confined to these states. Stroke, often associated with hypertension, is the third leading cause of death among African American women nationwide.

Poor health outcomes from cardiovascular disease are related to genetics, environment, lifestyle, and access and use of health care (Dennis, 1999; Gillum, 1996). Studies about hypertension in African American women have been associated with the following list of lifestyle factors:

- being overweight
- abdominal obesity (Dennis, 1999; Gillum, 1996)
- inactivity
- increasing age
- eating foods high in saturated fats and cholesterol
- behavioral factors

- stress
- tobacco use

Family History

A woman's family history for hypertension is important and can be influenced by her family genetics and generations of family lifestyle habits. It will be important for you to ask your client about her family history. The Working Group on Research in Coronary Heart Disease in Blacks (1994) found that a family history of hypertension is a major risk factor for another family member's being four times more likely to be diagnosed with it. Elevated blood pressure in a mother has been found to be related to an elevated blood pressure in her daughter (Morrison, Payne, Barton, Khoury, & Crawford, 1994; Gillum, 1996). These findings are suggestive that deleterious lifestyle habits may be present in a family across generations that are high risk for increasing the blood pressure. Over time, this has the appearance of a genetic link. *Healthy People 2010* points out that current biological and genetic characteristics of African Americans do not explain the health disparities compared to Whites in the United States. If your client's family history includes family members who were diagnosed with hypertension, the health promotion contract for your client will include health advice about yearly blood pressure measurement, even if her current blood pressure reading is within the normal range (less than 140/90). Diet and exercise can normalize early blood pressure elevation.

Physical Activity

Hypertension is seen frequently in African American women with low levels of physical fitness. Moderate physical activity that raises the heart rate for 20 to 30 minutes three or more times a week has been shown to protect against hypertension and cardio-vascular disease (National Institutes for Health [NIH] Consensus Development Panel on Physical Activity and Cardiovascular Health, 1996). African American women who have been diagnosed with mild hypertension have been able to reverse the disease by beginning a regimen of walking three times a week. For individuals who lead sedentary lifestyles, walking is an easier form of exercise to begin.

Weight Gain

In the Southeast, nearly three fourths of African American women are overweight (Hall et al., 1997). Weight gain contributes to an increase in blood pressure for African American women that occurs in young adulthood and continues with aging. Weight gain in young adulthood is one of the best predictors for risk of an African American woman's developing hypertension later in life. Refer to the discussion of nutrition and obesity in this chapter.

Food Choices

Many African American women often have misperceptions about the serious effect on their blood pressure of the excess intake of certain foods. Dennis (1999) points out the relationship between African American women's cultural attitudes and their food purchases. Investigators have found that African Americans of lower socioeconomic status consume larger quantities of salt than those at higher income levels or all other ethnic groups (Flack & Hamaty, 1999). Despite widespread concerns about fat and salt consumption, lower-income African American women have a harder time selecting food with lower salt and fat content.

Excess dietary salt and a lack of potassium in the diet has been associated with hypertension in African Americans due to a greater dietary sodium/potassium ratio. Long-term high salt intake causes vascular wall damage and kidney damage. Low potassium intake contributes to constriction of the blood vessels. This complex chain of events increases your client's systolic blood pressure, leads to more severe forms of hypertension as she ages, and increases the likelihood of further cardiac damage, permanent changes in the vessels of the eyes, and irreversible kidney damage that leads to end-stage renal disease.

Stress

Middle- and upper-income African American clients will have a higher level of self-esteem, resilience, and internal and external resources to cope with stress. Resilience is the capacity of those who are exposed to identifiable risk factors to overcome those risks and avoid negative outcomes. The lives of these same African American clients are typical of the majority of American families with two parents, job security, and economic stability. They possess the ability to engage readily in a collaborative nurse-client relationship for stress-reduction techniques. On the other hand, you will find it helpful to understand the sources of stress for your clients with fewer financial resources. Potential stressors of a socioeconomic and environmental nature are listed below.

- low educational attainment
- high levels of either unemployment or low paying occupations
- stressful work environment
- low family income
- undesirable living conditions

African Americans of lower socioeconomic status are twice as likely as the White population to be unemployed or underemployed in jobs that do not reflect their education or skill level. Often they struggle in frustration for upwardly mobile employ-

ment, which can lead to insecurity and low self-esteem. Furthermore, it can lead your client to feel like a victim with little ability to determine her own destiny (Rodriguez, Allen, Frongillo, & Chandra, 1998; Chisholm, 1996).

The strength displayed by many African American women, which is perceived as a positive characteristic, can also lead to stress (Chisholm, 1996). African American women traditionally have worked outside the home in demanding jobs, have been the sole wage earner even in times of low employment for spouses, have experienced high levels of single parenthood and cared for children and extended family, all while relying on themselves for psychological support. When she cannot provide adequately for herself and family, the African American woman may feel overwhelmed and weak, perceiving that these feelings make her vulnerable. This woman will think of herself as having failed to live up to the strength of previous generations of women in her family. It will be difficult for her to tell you that she can not handle her responsibilities. Offer a compassionate ear and listen nonjudgmentally.

Research has shown that stressful events cause elevation in blood pressure by a direct physiologic effect related to suppressed anger and hostility. Frequent exposure to anxiety and tension and long-term suppression of the strain among African American women has been shown to cause a higher resting blood pressure (Anderson, McNeilly, & Myers, 1991). She may think that stress is part of life's burden that cannot be changed; apathy develops. Her exposure to stressful situations over time might lead to negative, self-defeating behaviors as her way of coping. Consequently, long-standing worry and stress may emerge in mood disorders, unhealthy eating patterns, or abuse of tobacco, alcohol, or drugs.

Listen to your client; provide empathy while trying to understand her circumstances. Introduce lifestyle changes at a pace that your client feels she can integrate successfully. Provide opportunities for follow-up and evaluation. Explore her receptiveness to a referral to an understanding counselor, one who is culturally sensitive, open, and responsive to the counteractive coping issues that have emerged.

Tobacco Use

In your assessment and planning for a healthier blood pressure level, ask your client about tobacco use, and remember to ask about smokeless tobacco, too. African American females are least likely to use cigarettes among all other racial groups. However, sustained smoking cessation is more challenging for African American women. Tobacco use, including cigarette smoking and smokeless or spit tobacco, can contribute to elevated blood pressure. Smokeless tobacco use is seen more frequently among older women in the southeastern states.

You communicated to your client that her use of tobacco could affect her blood pressure, and now you are wondering how to determine if your client is serious about making a change in her behavior. The stages of change model and health-promoting lifestyle profile are two theories that can guide your plan and interventions. Nurse researchers have utilized health promotion theories to determine factors important to smoking cessation for African American females (Tessaro et al, 1997; McCleary-Jones, 1996). Tessaro et al. (1997) used the stages of change model to determine readiness for successful behavior changes of a clinic's low-income African American population. The components of this model are shown in Box 21.5.

African American tobacco smokers have a stronger desire to quit than other ethnic groups and are more likely to have made serious attempts to quit (Tessaro et al., 1997). A quit attempt in the past was shown to predict interest in changing smoking behavior. Moreover, risk perception was important to the cessation process, meaning that when an individual perceived that smoking might damage his or her health, there was more motivation to stop tobacco use.

Consider using the health-promoting lifestyle profile for your client assessments where your intent is to integrate their tobacco cessation plan in an overall holistic health-promotion model. This model incorporates self-actualization, health responsibility, exercise, nutrition, interpersonal support, and stress management (Walker, Sechrist, & Pender, 1987; Pender, 1982). This model has been used with African American clients who are 40 years of age and younger, of lower socioeconomic and social class and lower education level. It can determine how your client's self-initiated action interacts with other factors for readiness to change her behavior (McCleary-Jones, 1996).

A health-promotion plan should include a discussion about each of your client's lifestyle risk factors and how they contribute to hypertension. Depending on her risk factors, you and your client can decide which of the antihypertensive behaviors listed in Box 21.6 to include in a health promotion contract. You can provide guidance to help her prioritize one or two areas to start first. Practical approaches, possibly including self-help printed materials, motivational telephone follow-up, and referral for a hypertension work-up can initiate behavioral change for a healthy heart.

Diabetes Mellitus

Diabetes is one of the most serious health problems in the African American popula-

---

Box 21.5   Stages of Change Model

- *Precontemplation:* considering the possibility of change
- *Contemplation:* thinking about change
- *Preparation:* readiness to make a decision
- *Action:* undertaking change
- *Maintenance:* maintaining positive change

Box 21.6   Antihypertensive Activities

- Lower intake of foods containing salt and fats
- Decrease salt and fat intake
- Increase intake of foods containing potassium
- Increase physical activity to reduce weight and stress
- Adopt leisure-time activities
- Stop tobacco use

---

tion, surpassed only by cardiovascular disease and cancer. Diabetes is a chronic disorder characterized by abnormalities in insulin secretion and action. African Americans are among the ethnic groups at higher risk for non-insulin-dependent diabetes (Type 2 or NIDDM). Approximately two thirds of persons with diabetes have hypertension. When diabetes and hypertension coexist, complications occur more frequently, as early as the middle years and are more severe (Flack & Hamaty, 1999). Diabetic complications may include cardiovascular-related complications, nerve damage, blindness, renal complications, and lower limb amputation. End-stage renal disease has been documented to have a three-fold occurrence in African Americans with diabetes.

Genetics, obesity, and low levels of physical activity are strongly linked to diabetes. However, obesity has been shown a significant risk factor for the disease. In overweight adults aged 20 to 75, the risk of diabetes is nearly three times greater than

for those of similar ages who are not overweight. Dietary management and exercise are key to self-management, in addition to medications. Stress regular exercise as a starting point in improving diabetes management. For your sedentary client, mutually set a goal of walking for exercise 10 to 30 minutes a day once a week, until she can build up to 20 to 30 minutes three times a week. Researchers in this area have shown that diabetes is less common in individuals who exercise regularly because exercise lowers glucose levels and increases insulin sensitivity.

Your role in health promotion might include reaching out into the community for community education activities. Show sensitivity to the role of culture in diabetes management. African American churches are a valuable link between their members and the community. Become acquainted with churches in your area where you might provide resources for diabetes education. Include information on detection, sources of care, and the importance of dietary management and exercise. The American Diabetic Association provides a nice variety of culturally sensitive materials, including pamphlets, flyers, and videos that are readily available for consumer use.

Breast Health

African American women believe that breast cancer is the greatest threat to their health, although statistics show that heart disease causes more deaths (Boston University Library, 2000). Breast cancer is the leading cause of cancer deaths for African American women. Cancer deaths declined overall for Americans over the past few years without a decline among African Americans, despite advances in detection and treatment (American Cancer Society [ACS] [On-line], 2000). The number of African American women who get breast cancer is lower than that of White women, but African American women under the age of 40 get breast cancer more often. It occurs more often in women in the United States of all ethnic groups over 50 years of age, and likewise in African American women occurs at an older age. However, an increasing number of African American women are being diagnosed with breast cancer in their 30s and 40s. These cancers often are larger when found and are more aggressive. Among African American women, the use of screening procedures is low (Burns et al., 1996). Although breast cancer often is diagnosed in advanced stages, the outcome is worse at each stage of diagnosis. Recent findings show that therapies for cancer treatment and life extension are used less frequently in African American women (Lambert, Newton, & de-Meneses, 1998; Lannin et al., 1998). Figure 21.1 shows factors that influence breast cancer screening in African American women.

African American women, especially older ones, who do not seek regular mammography, have more barriers to preventive health screening than other women (Lambert, Newton, & deMeneses, 1998; Underwood, 1999). Box 21.7 shows factors that influence breast cancer screening in African American women.

Nonparticipation in screening can be linked to inadequate awareness and knowledge about breast examinations, cultural beliefs, and attitudes about breast cancer (Douglas, Bartolucci, Waterboro, & Sirles, 1995), competing family priorities, and inadequate access to low-cost health care and mammograms when a woman does not have adequate health care benefits.

Women who do not perform regular breast self-exam (BSE) are less able to decide if something they find is new or different. Emphasize to them that all areas of concern should be reported to you or another health care provider. The following is a list of breast symptoms that need timely attention:

- Changes in the size or shape of the breast or areola
- Skin changes such as pitting, dimpling, or redness
- Nipple redness, irritation, new inversion of the nipple
- Changes in the vein pattern of breast tissue
- A lump, irregularity, or thickness in the breast or underarm tissue
- Unexplained breast pain

Address your client's personal concerns. You may have to discuss these symptoms in repeated sessions to impress on her their importance. These women may think that CBE and mammography are unnecessary in the absence of symptoms. There are also women who will accept a Papanicolaou

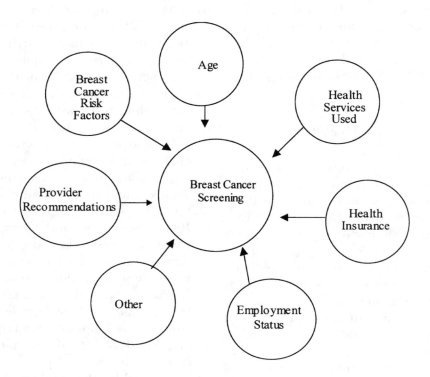

FIGURE 21.1   Factors influencing breast cancer screening.

Note: From "Breast cancer screening among African American women: Addressing the needs of African American women with known and no know risk factors," by S. M. Underwood, 1999, *Journal of the National Black Nurses Association, 10*(1), pp. 46–55. Reprinted with permission.

Box 21.7   Personal Barriers for Breast Screening

- Unfamiliarity with breast changes and discomfort with performing BSE
- Embarrassment to disrobe for exams or mammograms
- Lack of information about mammography and early detection
- Lack of knowledge about susceptibility
- Lack of knowledge about the benefit of early detection and improved survivorship of breast cancer
- Misinformation about how the costs of breast screening, especially mammograms can be covered
- Prioritization of other family needs

(Pap)—the most widely recommended test to check for abnormal cervical cells—but do not initiate a CBE or mammogram (Mayer-Oakes et al., 1996). Further, they may feel that paying too much attention to the breasts might bring on breast cancer. Try the tips below to increase the number of women in your clinical setting who receive a full array of breast services.

- Discuss information about the importance of BSE.
- Discuss with your client that the CBE is done at least annually.
- During an annual preventive exam, episodic or follow-up visit for chronic disease, look through the record to see if your client is due for a CBE, mammogram or nutritional consult.
- Arrange a convenient time for a CBE, mammogram or nutritional consult before she leaves the clinic if it cannot be done while she is there.
- Develop effective reminder systems in your setting, either through direct contact to women or through effective chart reminders

Your role is to offer information, clarify misconceptions, and help guide clients through proper decisions. Women who face a higher than average risk for breast cancer may ask your advice about whether they should begin screening before age 40. Help them seek expert medical guidance on the frequency of screening. There is no consensus among breast-care specialists on the age at which mammograms should be discontinued. There is insufficient data on women over the age of 70, which is not to say they should not have mammograms. Cases of breast cancer increase with advancing age. As long as a woman is healthy and can benefit from early detection, you should advise screening for her.

Limited research on breast cancer diagnosis and survival in African American women suggests that dietary fat and patterns of weight gain may be important risk factors. Environmental toxins may also contribute. Future research will shed more light.

You can play a very important role in informing your clients about secondary prevention measures. Teach your African American clients the importance of the annual CBE and the monthly breast self-examination (BSE) for early detection of breast changes. ACS guidelines for the mammogram are in Box 21.8, and important information to help reassure your client is in Box 21.9.

Failure to discuss mammograms, inadequate explanations, and inattentiveness to a woman's concerns when her health care provider communicates with her contribute to the low screening rate for breast and cervical cancer among African American women. Remember to discuss breast health promotion including nutritional changes they can make. If you fail to, they often assume it must not be important.

For the client with visual impairment, decreased tactile sensitivity in her finger pads from diabetic complications, or physical limitation in her extremities because of arthritis, check the adequacy of her BSE. If she has shoulder arthritis, determine whether she can raise the opposite arm during the self-breast exam to provide sufficient flattening of the breast mound. Demonstrate BSE techniques and have her repeat the demonstration; encourage her to perform the best BSE that she can with limited shoulder mobility. However, for women with disabilities, her health care provider will need to provide increased vigilance with more frequent clinical breast exam. When a woman can not perform an adequate breast self-exam, make a notation

---

Box 21.8   American Cancer Society BSE Guidelines

- Age 20–39: Monthly breast self-examination right after the period; clinical breast examination (CBE) every 3 years by a doctor or nurse
- Age 40+: Monthly breast self-examination; annual clinical breast examination close to the time of the mammogram; annual mammogram (American Cancer Society, 2000).

Box 21.9   Important Information about Breast Screening

- Women detect 8 out of 10 breast cancers between visits to their health care providers.
- Women who routinely perform BSE can usually detect an unusual mass in their breasts much sooner than women who do not practice breast self-exams.
- Learning the technique for breast self-examination is easy, although the exam is done carefully 1 week after completion of the menses.
- For women who no longer have a period, instruct them to pick a convenient easy-to-remember time like the first day of the month.

---

in her clinic record problem list as a reminder for more frequent CBEs.

Cervical Health

Cervical cancer is a preventable disease, but it continues to be a significant disease for African American women. This cancer is the third leading cause of gynecologic cancer deaths nationally for older African American women (ACS, 2000). African American women are less likely to be diagnosed with cervical cancer while it is still confined to the cervix (Dignan, Michielutte, Wells, & Bahnson, 1994). Regular cervical cancer screening among many of these women may be poorly accepted and underutilized despite the Pap test's effectiveness in drastically reducing cervical cancer deaths.

The cervical cancer problem is highest among women who lack access to quality preventive care or who avoid cervical cancer screening for cultural or other reasons because they do not perceive themselves to be at risk. Barriers that appear more significant for African American women who are 50 and older include:

- Lack of knowledge about the importance of the Pap test
- Not knowing how and where to get a Pap test
- Costs (Powell-Griner, Bolen, & Bland, 1999)
- Long waits to see a health care provider or no usual source of care
- Lack of physician's recommendation
- Unpleasantness of the gynecologic exam
- Social and cultural attitudes about cancer
- Fear of finding cancer
- Emotional discomfort and embarrassment associated with the exam (Jennings, 1996; Sawyer, 1990).

The Pap test is a simple procedure that is performed by a health care professional as part of the annual pelvic exam. The ACS recommends this test for all women who have reached age 18 or who have ever been sexually active. After three consecutive annual exams with normal findings, the Pap test may be performed less frequently at the discretion of the physician (ACS, 2001). Important factors in the prevention of cervical cancer are:

- Monogamous sexual relationships
- Delay of first sexual intercourse until a later age
- Protection from human papillomavirus (HPV) infections, a tumor-producing virus with more than 70 identified strains that produce genital warts, cervical cell changes and cancer (Daley, 1997; MMWR, 1998; Koutsky, 1997)
- Avoidance of tobacco (tobacco chemicals accelerate HPV infections) (Nischan, Ebeling, & Schindler, 1988)
- Eating a balanced diet with adequate fruits and vegetables for a strong immune system
- Regular Pap tests (American Cancer Society, 2001; National Cancer Institute, 2001).

Health promotion interventions will change knowledge and attitudes among clients who are reluctant to get pelvic exams and Pap tests. You play a vital role in helping women address their concerns about cervical cancer screening, understanding the current screening practices, and obtaining access to preventive care. Older African American women often do not think of cancer screening as part of their routine preventive health care. They are less likely to initiate discussions about Pap tests or mammograms. They depend on their health care provider to discuss which health care behaviors they need to follow (Mouton, 1997).

Osteoarthritis

Osteoarthritis is a nonfatal, degenerative form of arthritis that causes physical impairment and joint pain in older African American women. More women are affected in the southeastern United States (Mouton, 1997). This condition affects the daily functional health and quality of life by narrowing the weight-bearing joint spaces. The spine, shoulders, elbow, hips, knees, and fingers are the usual sites of degeneration; the knees are affected more frequently in African American women. Obesity is associated with joint degeneration. In women with osteoarthritis, the health promotion contract should include measures for weight reduction, slow-paced ambulation, and continued mobility. Consider recommending senior center programs or recreation centers that have programs for older clients, with light activity to support functional activity. Nutritional recommendations include maximizing whole foods and minimizing refined, packaged goods, and drinking 8–10 glasses of water per day.

Systemic Lupus Erythematosus (Lupus)

Lupus is a very complex chronic autoimmune and inflammatory condition that unpredictably attacks the healthy tissues of one or multiple organs of the body (Kahl, 1996). The trigger for the disease differs from one person to another, and lupus is found predominately in women in the childbearing years. The highest rates of lupus are seen in African American women (Boston University Library, 2000). There are periods of remission with acute and chronic relapses. Fatigue, fever, and weight loss are the chief complaints of many of those affected with lupus. However, other organs that might be affected are the skin, eyes, joints, lungs, kidneys, brain and liver, and the immune system.

Lupus in not well understood by the public. Several misconceptions exist about lupus, that it is always fatal, contagious, strongly genetic, or a form of AIDS. None of these is true. Your client with lupus needs psychosocial and educational interventions. Women with lupus often look quite well despite overwhelming fatigue and joint pain. Their healthy appearance can lead to unrealistic expectations and a lack of understanding from family, friends, and coworkers.

Focus on stress management and relaxation, and direct your client to organizations that can provide emotional support and educational materials. The Arthritis Foundation and the Lupus Foundation of America are excellent sources of support and information. Information about their services can be found on the World Wide Web or in the business section of your phone directory.

Menopause

Menopause is a phase in a woman's life that can be viewed from physiologic, emotional and cultural perspectives. Preventative actions for African American women in perimenopausal and menopausal phases of their lives include information on how to reduce conditions associated with a decrease in estrogen. Some research has supported the reduction of hot flashes, maintenance of mental alertness, possible prevention of osteoporosis and protection against urinary incontinence from hormone replacement therapy or HRT (Maki,

Zonderman, & Resnick, 2001). HRT is used daily in the form of a table or patch to replace dwindling natural hormones. African American women are least likely to accept HRT (Rosenberg, Palmer, Rao, & Adams-Campbell, 1998).

Drawbacks to HRT include increased breast cancer risk after long-term use and possible risk of gallbladder surgery (Clemons & Goss, 2001; Uhler, Marks, & Judd, 2000). Women with a history of any blood-clotting, breast cancer, liver impairment or unexplained vaginal bleeding are unsuited to HRT (Hoibraaten, Qvigstad, Arnesen, Larsen, Wickstom, & Sandset, 2000).

For women who choose not to take HRT, collaborative nutritional, herbal and exercise programs can be developed. For example, clients may decide to eat 4 ounces of tofu, drink a glass of soymilk, or eat a serving of chick peas, lentils, flax seed, clover or alfalfa sprouts daily to provide phytoestrogens. Evidence for the beneficial effects of phytoestrogens on menopausal symptoms is growing (Glazier & Bowman, 2001).

Herbs such as black cohosh, dong quai, red clover, sage and other herbs have been used in China and other countries for thousands of years by women to reduce their menopausal symptoms (Clark, 2000; Nestel, Pomeroy, & Kay, 1999). Kegel exercises can be used to reduce incontinence. Foods high in B-vitamins (sunflower seeds, wheat germ, brown rice, soybeans, white beans, chicken, mackerel, salmon, tuna, bananas, walnuts, peanuts, sweet potatoes, and cooked cabbage) can be eaten to ward off mood swings and feelings of depression (Benton & Donohoe, 1999). Walking, swimming or weight training (resistance) can provide the kind of movement that enhances muscular and bone strength (Bemben, Fetters, Bemben, Nabavi, & Koh, 2000). Your role is twofold: (1) provide an environment where clients can speak openly about their concerns and fears as well as the benefits of natural remedies and HRT, (2) assist women to develop a menopausal plan that works for them.

Prevention of Human Immunodeficiency Virus Infection

Evaluate your comfort level for discussing HIV and safe sex as part of promoting high-level wellness. HIV and AIDS are serious threats to the health of women. In the United States AIDS is the fourth leading cause of death among women aged 25 to 44 (Center for Disease Control and Prevention [CDC], 2000). Your clients need to know that HIV has slowly increased among African American women, the fastest growing segment of the HIV-infected population, making it the leading cause of death for African Americans aged 25 to 44 (CDC, 2000). A comprehensive review of nursing research shows that prevention remains the most effective strategy for sexually active women against contracting HIV (Mallory & Fife, 1999).

African American women are more likely to contract HIV through sexual contact with partners infected with HIV. For a smaller number of women, intravenous drug use is the source of their infection. Latex male or female condoms and latex dental dams (an oral barrier) for sexually active male and female partners are effective strategies against the transmission of HIV. The effectiveness depends on consistent and proper use.

Nurses can help sexually active women of all ages (who least expect that their partner may have been infected with HIV) identify sexual behaviors (unprotected vaginal, oral, and anal sex) and interpersonal and gender-related obstacles that increase their likelihood of contracting the virus. Identify community resources to educate African American women about their chances of contracting the disease, measures to take to protect themselves against it, and where to get HIV testing. Equally important for women to understand is that they can be unknowingly infected with HIV and transmit it to an unborn fetus during pregnancy.

Power and control in partner relationships are not talked about often. However, they are essential to understanding women's vulnerability to HIV (Dancy, 1996; Mallory & Fife, 1999; Wingood & DiClemente, 1998). Many women do not have practical skills to turn their abstract knowledge into HIV prevention. For example, a woman may not know how to ask about a partner's sexual practices and past or current sexual partners and their practices. Your client may not be able to demand that a partner use a condom or other latex device, although she knows that being assertive could lessen her chance of contracting HIV. Prevention strategies must include resources for teaching negotiation skills and assertiveness combined with the facts about HIV transmission. Find out about these resources in your community.

SUMMARY

The African American community acknowledges an alarming health crisis and urgency for health promotion for women of all ages. Their well-being and quality of life are threatened and often assaulted by socioeconomic, environmental, and political forces beyond their control and by personal choices within their control. A vital part of primary and secondary prevention lies in outreach to women to offer them a plan for lifestyle changes that can improve and extend life. Much work needs to be done and you are an invaluable link to interventions that chart a path toward wellness for a resilient but vulnerable society of women. Each goal reached is exhilarating and is evidence of what carefully planned health promotion strategies can produce.

REFERENCES

American Cancer Society. (2001). *Cancer Prevention and Detection: Facts and Figures.* Atlanta, GA: American Cancer Society. [On-line]. Available: http://www3.cancer.org/cancerinfo.

Anderson, N. B., McNeilly, M., & Myers, H. F. (1991). Autonomic reactivity and hypertension in Blacks: A review and proposed model. *Ethnicity and Disease, 1*(2), 154–170.

Bemben, D. A., Fetters, N. L., Bemben, M. G., Nabavi, N., & Koh, E. T. *Medicine and Science in Sports Exercise, 32*(11), 1949–1957.

Benton, D., & Donohue, R. T. (1999). The effects of nutrients on mood. *Public Health Nutrition, 2*(3A), 403–409.

Boston University Library Health Statistics. 2000. [On-line]. Available: http://med-lib-www.bu.edu/library/stats.html.

Burns, R. B., McCarthy, E. P., Freund, K. M., Marwill, S. L., Shwartz, M., Ash, A., & Moskowitz, M. A. (1996). Black women receive less mammography even with similar use of primary care. *Annals of Internal Medicine, 125*(3), 173–182.

Caldwell, S. H., & Popenoe, R. (1995). Perceptions and misperceptions of skin color. *Annals of Internal Medicine, 122*(8), 614–621.

Center for Disease Control and Prevention (2001). *HIV/AIDS among African Americans.* Atlanta, GA: Center for Disease Control and Prevention. [On-line]. Available: http://www.cdc.gov/hiv/search.htm.

Chatters, L. M., & Taylor (1989). Age differences in religious participation among Black adults. *Journal of Gerontology, 44,* S183–189.

Chisholm, J. F. (1996). Mental health issues in African-American women. *New York Academy of Sciences, 789,* 161–179.

Clark, C. C. (2000). *Integrating Complementary Procedures Into Practice.* New York: Springer Publishing.

Clemons, M., & Goss, P. (2001). Estrogen and the risk of breast cancer. [erratum appears in New England Journal of Medicine 2001 June 7; 344(23):1804]. *New England Journal of Medicine, 344*(4), 276–285.

Daley, E. M. (1997). Clinical update on the role of HPV and cervical cancer. *Cancer Nursing, 21*(1), 31–35.

Dancy, B. (1996). What African-American women know, do, and feel about AIDS: A function of age and education. *AIDS Education and Prevention, 8*(1), 26–36.

Dennis, G. C. (1999). Cardiovascular disease in African-American women: A dilemma of culture. *Journal of the National Medical Association, 91*(6), 331–312.

D'Epiro, N. W., Col, N. F., Legato, M., & Schiff, I. (1988). HRT: New data, continuing controversies. *Patient Care Nurse Practitioner* (December), 18–34.

Dignan, M., Michielutte, R., Sharp, P., Bahnson, J., Young, L., & Beal, P. (1990). The role of focus groups in health education for cervical cancer among minority women. *Journal of Community Health, 15,* 369–375.

Dignan, M., Michielutte, R., Wells, H., & Bahnson, J. (1994). The Forsyth county cervical cancer prevention project–1: Cervical cancer screening for Black women. *Health Education Research, 9*(4), 411–420.

Dohrenwend, B.S., & Dohrenwend, B. P. (Eds.). (1981). *Stressful life events and their contexts.* New York: Prodist.

Douglas, M., Bartolucci, A., Waterboro, J., & Sirles, A. (1995). Breast cancer early detection: Differences between African American and White women's health beliefs and detection practices. *Oncology Nursing Forum, 22*(5), 835–837.

Duey, W. J., O'Brien, W. L., Crutchfield, A. B., Brown, L. A., Willford, H. N., & Sharff-Olson, M. (1998). Effects of exercise training on aerobic fitness in African-American females. *Ethnicity and Disease, 8*(3), 306–311.

Feldman, R. H., & Fulwood, R. (1999). The three leading causes of death in African

Americans: Barriers to reducing excess disparity and to improving health behaviors. *Journal of Health Care for the Poor and Underserved, 10*(1), 45–71.

Felton, G. M., Parson, M. A., & Bartoces, M. G. (1997). Demographic factors: Interaction effects on health-promoting behavior and health related factors. *Public Health Nursing, 14*(6), 361–367.

Flack, J. M., & Hamaty, M. (1999). Difficult-to-treat hypertensive populations: Focus on African-Americans and people with type 2 diabetes. *Journal of Hypertension, 17*(Suppl. 1), S19–S24.

Gillum, R. F. (1996). Epidemiology of hypertension in African American women. *American Heart Journal, 131*(2), 385–395.

Glazier, M. G., & Bowman, M. A. (2001). A review of the evidence for the use of phytoestrogens as a replacement for traditional estrogen replacement therapy. *Archives of Internal Medicine, 161*(9), 1161–1172.

Gottlieb, N. H., & Green, L. W. (1987). Ethnicity and lifestyle health risk: Some possible mechanisms. *American Journal of Health Promotion,* 37–45, 51.

Hall, W. D., Ferrario, C. M., Moore, M. A., Hall, J. E., Flack, J. M., Cooper, W., Simmons, J. D., Egan, B. M., Lackland, D. T., Perry, M., & Roccella, E. J. (1997). Hypertension-related morbidity and mortality in the southeastern United States. *The American Journal of the Medical Sciences, 313*(4), 195–209.

Healthy People 2010. (2000). [On-line]. Available: http://www.health.gov/healthypeople.

Healthy People 2010 Objectives: Draft for Public Comment. (1998). [On-line]. Available: http://web.health.gov/healthypeople/2010 Draft.

Hoibraaten, E., Qvigstad, E., Arnesen, H., Larsen, S., Wickstrom, E., & Sandset, P. M. (2000). Increased risk of recurrent venous thromboembolism during hormone replacement therapy. *Thromb Halmost, 84*(6), 961–967.

Jennings, K. M. (1996). Getting Black women to screen for cancer: Incorporating health beliefs into practice. *Journal of the American Academy of Nurse Practitioners, 8*(2), 53–59.

Joint National Committee on Prevention, Detection, Evaluation, and Treatment of Hypertension and the National high Blood Pressure Education Program Coordinating Committee. (1997). The sixth report of the joint national committee on prevention, detection, evaluation, and treatment of high blood pressure. *Archives of Internal Medicine, 157*(21), 2413–2446.

Kahl, L. E. (1996). Systemic lupus erythematous. In J. Noble (Ed.), *Textbook of primary care medicine* (pp. 1130–1139). St. Louis, MO: Mosby.

Kang, S. H., Bloom, J. R., & Romano, P. S. (1994). Cancer screening among African-American women: Their use of tests and social support. *American Journal of Public Health, 84*(1), 101–103.

Koenig, H. G. (1999). *The healing power of faith.* New York: Simon & Schuster.

Koutsky, L. (1997). Epidemiology of genital human papillomavirus infection. *American Journal of Medicine, 102*(5A), 3–8.

Lambert, S., Newton, M., & deMeneses, M. (1998). Barriers to mammography in older, low-income African American women. *The Journal of Multicultural Nursing and Health, 4*(2), 17–19.

Lannin, D. R., Mathews, H. F., Mitchell, J., Swanson, M. S., Swanson, F. H., & Edwards, M. S. (1998). Influence of socioeconomic and cultural factors on racial differences in late-stage presentation of breast cancer. *Journal of the American Medical Association, 279*(22), 1801–1807.

Levins, J. S., & Taylor, R. J. (1997). Age differences in patterns and correlates of the frequency of prayer. *The Gerontologist, 37*(1), 75–88.

Lewontin, R. D. (1982). Human diversity. In H. Nelson (Ed.), *Introduction to physical anthropology* (p. 203). St. Paul, MN: West.

Maillet, N. A., D'Eramo, G., & Spollett, G. (1996). Using focus groups to characterize the health beliefs and practices of Black women with non-insulin-dependent diabetes. *The Diabetes Educator, 22*(1), 39–46.

Maki, P., Zonderman, A., & Resnick, S. (2001). Enhanced verbal memory in nondemented elderly women receiving hormone-replacement therapy. *American Journal of Psychiatry, 158*(2), 227–233.

Mallory, C., & Fife, B. L. (1999). Women and the prevention of HIV infection: An integrative review of the literature. *Journal of the Association of Nurses in AIDS Care, 10*(1), 51–63.

Mayer-Oakes, S. A., Atchison, K. A., Matthias, R. E., DeJong, F. J., Lubben, J., & Schweitzer, S. O. (1996). Mammography use in older women with regular physicians: What are the predictors? *American Journal of Preventive Medicine, 12*(1), 44–50.

McCleary-Jones, V. (1996). Health promotion practices of smoking and non-smoking Black women. *The ABNF Journal, 7*(1), 7–10.

McClelland, J. W., Demark-Wahnefried, W., Mustian, R. D., Cowan, A. T., & Campbell, M. K. (1998). Fruit and vegetable consumption of rural African Americans: Baseline survey results of the Black Churches United for Better Health 5-a-day project. *Nutrition and Cancer, 30*(2), 148–157.

Molnar, S. (1983). *Human variations: Races, types, and ethnic groups.* Upper Saddle Field, NJ: Prentice-Hall.

Morbidity and Mortality Weekly Reports. (1998, January 23). Human Papillomavirus infection. *MMWR, 47,* 88–98.

Morrison, J. A., Payne, G., Barton, B. A., Khoury, P. R., & Crawford, P. (1994). Mother-daughter correlations of obesity and cardiovascular disease risk factors in Black and White households: The NHLBI Growth and Health Study. *American Journal of Public Health, 84*(11), 1761–1767.

Mouton, C. P. (1997). Special health considerations in African-American elders. *American Family Physician, 55*(4), 1243–1253.

Nagata, C., Takatsuta, N., Kawakami, N., & Shimizu, H. (2001). Soy product intake and hot flashes in Japanese women: Results from a community-based prospective study. *American Journal of Epidemiology, 153*(8), 790–793.

National Cancer Institute. (2001). Bethesda, MD: Author. [On-line]. http://cancernet.nci.nih.gov/wyntk_pubs/cervix.htm#5).

Nestel, P., Pomeroy, S., & Kay, S. (1999). Isoflavones from red clover improve systemic arterial compliance but not plasma lipids in menopausal women. *Journal of Clinical Endocrinology and Metabolism, 84,* 895–898.

Nischan, P., Ebeling, K., & Schindler, C. (1988). Smoking and invasive cervical cancer risk. *American Journal of Epidemiology, 128*(1), 74–77.

Nies, M. A., Vollman, M., & Cook, T. (1999). African American women's experiences with physical activity in their daily lives. *Public Health Nursing, 16*(1), 23–31.

NIH Consensus Development Panel on Physical Activity and Cardiovascular Health. (1996). Physical activity and cardiovascular health. *Journal of the American Medical Association, 276*(3), 241–246.

Pender, N. (1982). *Health promotion in nursing practice.* Norwalk, CT: Appleton & Lange.

Potts, J. L., & Thomas, J. (1999). Traditional coronary risk factors in African Americans. *The American Journal of the Medical Sciences, 317*(3), 189–192.

Powell-Griner, E., Bolen, J., & Bland, S. (1999). Health care coverage and use of preventive services among the near elderly in the United States. *American Journal of Public Health, 89*(6), 882–886.

Rodriguez, E., Allen, J. A., Frongillo, E. A., & Chindra, P. (1998). Unemployment, depression, and health: A look at the African-American community. *Journal of Epidemiology and Community Health, 53*(6), 335–342.

Rosenberg, J. R., Palmer, J. R., Adams-Campbell, L. L., & Rao, R. S. (1999). Obesity and hypertension among college educated Black women in the United States. *Journal of Human Hypertension, 13*(4), 237–241.

Rosenberg, L., Palmer, J. R., Rao, R. S., & Adams-Campbell, L. L. (1998). Correlates of postmenopausal female hormone use among Black women in the United States. *Obstetrics and Gynecology, 91*(3), 454–458.

Sanders-Phillips, K. (1997). Correlates of health promotion behaviors in low-income Black women and Latinas. *American Journal of Preventive Medicine, 12*(6), 450–458.

Sawyer, J., Earp, J., Fletcher, R., Daye, F., & Wynn, T. (1990). Pap tests of rural Black women. *Journal of General Internal Medicine,* 5(2), 115–119.

Sowers, J. R. (1998). Obesity and cardiovascular disease. *Clinical Chemistry, 44*(8), 1821–1825.

Stewart, M. J. (1993). *Integrating social support in nursing.* Newbury Park, CA: Sage.

Stolley, M. R., & Fitzgibbon, M. L. (1997). Effects of an obesity prevention program on the eating behavior of African American mothers and daughters. *Health Education Behavior, 24*(2), 152–164.

Stolley, J. M., & Koenig, H. (1997). Religion/spirituality and health among elderly African Americans and Hispanics. *Journal of Psychosocial Nursing, 35*(11), 32–38.

Taylor, R. J., & Chatters, L. M. (1991). Nonorganizational religious participation among elderly Black adults. *Journal of Gerontology, 46*(2), S103–111.

Tessaro, I., Lyna, P. R., Rimer, B., Heisler, J., Woods-Powell, C. T., Yarnall, K. S., & Barber, L. T. (1997). Readiness to change smoking behavior in a community health center population. *Journal of Community Health, 22*(1), 15–31.

Uhler, M. L., Marks, J. W., & Judd, H. L. (2000). Estrogen replacement therapy and gallbladder disease in postmenopausal women. *Menopause, 7*(3), 162–167.

Underwood, S. M. (1999). Breast cancer screening among African American women: Addressing the needs of African American women with known and no known risk factors. *Journal of the National Black Nurses Association, 10*(1), 46–55.

U.S. Census Bureau. (2000). [On-line]. Available: http://www.census.gov

U.S. Preventive Services Task Force. (1996). *Guide to clinical preventive services* (2nd ed.). Baltimore: Williams & Wilkins.

Walker, S. N., Sechrist, K. R., & Pender, N. J. (1987). The health-promoting lifestyle profile: Development and psychometric characteristics. *Nursing Research, 36*(2), 76–81.

Ward, D. S., Trost, S. G., Felton, G., Saunders, R., Parsons, M. A., Dowda, M.. & Pate, R. R. (1997). Physical activity and physical fitness in African-American girls with and without obesity. *Obesity Research, 5*(6), 572–577.

Wingood, G. M., & DiClemente, R. J. (1998). Gender-related correlates and predictors of consistent condom use among young adult African-American women: A prospective analysis. *International Journal of STD and AIDS, 9*(3), 139–145.

Working Group on Research in Coronary Heart Disease in Blacks. (1994). Report of the Working Group on Research in Coronary Heart Disease in Blacks. *National Heart, Lung, and Blood Institute.* Bethesda, MD.

Williams, D. R. (1994). Measurement of religion. In J. S. Levin (Ed.), *Religion, aging, and health.* Thousand Oaks, CA: Sage.

Williamson, L. (1998). Eating disorders and the cultural forces behind the drive for thinness: Are African American women really protected? *Social Work in Health Care, 28*(1), 61–73.

CHAPTER 22

Establishing a Lay Health Promotion Program in a Hispanic Community

Sandra K. Hopper

The Pew Health Professions Commission (1994) defines lay health promoters (LHPs) broadly as "individuals who connect health care consumers and providers, promoting health among groups who have traditionally lacked access to adequate care." Financial reforms in health care and pressures on the health care delivery system to be more culturally relevant are expanding opportunities for lay health promoters. Managed care programs, focusing on acute and episodic care, have done little to expand treatment for the indigent, the homeless, and the uninsured so preventive efforts become critical. Considerable evidence exists that it is this area of prevention in which lay health promoters functioning in partnership with community health teams have been able to demonstrate the greatest impact on health outcomes (Love, Gardner, & Legion, 1997). The use of LHPs increases access to primary and preventive health care services because their responsibilities include advocacy, outreach, health promotion, and disease prevention. The project described in

this chapter reflects the changing face of community health care and community health programs that serve the individuals who are most critically in need of services. Projects like this expose nursing students to vulnerable populations. This term is often used to define groups whose needs are not fully addressed by traditional service providers. This can include, but is not limited to, those who are physically or mentally disabled, blind, deaf, hard of hearing, who have cognitive disorders or mobility limitations, who are limited in or non-English-speaking, are geographically or culturally isolated, medically or chemically dependent, homeless, frail or elderly, and the children. In this chapter you will learn how to develop a lay health promoter program and examine a case study of one that has been implemented.

HISTORICAL DEVELOPMENT

With their roots in developing countries, lay health promoters are widely utilized in

Latin America, Asia, and Africa in rural areas that lack formal health care providers. The use of lay workers began in the United States during the 1950s and 1960s to support public health programs (Hoff, 1969). The Federal Migrant Act of 1962 and the Economic Opportunity Act of 1964 mandated outreach services in poverty neighborhoods and migrant labor camps. Following the World Health Organization's Declaration of Alma-Ata in 1978 promoting LHPs as primary health care providers, interest in lay health promoter programs has increased (Skeet, 1985).

NATURE OF THE WORK

Lay health promoter programs have been shown to improve communication between community members and health care providers; to bridge cultural gaps; to improve the delivery of health services to vulnerable populations such as low-income, ethnic, and rural and neighborhood groups; and to assist communities in problem-solving, increasing both individual and community empowerment (United States Department of Health and Human Services [DHHS], 1994; Barnes & Fairbanks, 1997; Giblin, 1989; Hoff, 1969; Leutz, 1976; Wallerstein, 1992).

There is no single accepted definition for a lay health promoter. According to the Centers for Disease Control and Prevention (CDC, 1998) the term lay health promoter denotes trusted and respected community members who provide informal community-based health-related services and who establish vital cultural and technical links between health care professionals and persons in the community. While the CDC listed 26 terms that may be used to identify this type of community worker, the National Community Health Advisor Study (National Center, 1998) identified 66 distinct yet similar titles. Some of these include community health worker, health facilitator, home visitor, indigenous paraprofessional, lay volunteer, outreach worker, peer counselor, and promotora.

STEPS TO IMPLEMENTING A LAY HEALTH-PROMOTER PROGRAM

In the following section, specific steps are outlined to assist the reader in implementing a lay health-promoter program. Also included are some lessons learned by those who have gone before you in the hope of facilitating your program development journey. The terms lay health promoter and the Spanish *promotora* will be used interchangeably.

Step 1: Assess Whether a Lay Health-Promoter Program Would Be Viable and Valuable to Your Community

Many communities are conducting broad health assessments either of a need- or capacity-based nature that reveals the kinds of services a lay health promoter program could provide. If this information is not available, look to existing agencies providing services to vulnerable populations— free clinics, public health departments, and hospital emergency departments—for statistics to determine problematic areas with health (mortality and morbidity) and access to services. Discuss with health care providers and members of the targeted population their perceptions of needs. This can be accomplished through key informant interviews and focus groups. Once the value is established, match the issue with a population from which to recruit the workers, tap into the rich resources of faith communities, community associations, clubs, etc. Team-building, unique learning opportunities, meeting real needs in the community, and bridge-building are some of the many rewards and dividends achieved through a well-planned and implemented community service project

Step 2: Meet with the Identified Community and Collaborate to Find a Place for the Program to Be Housed

Factors to consider when selecting program space are location to the targeted population; openness to program partnership in the form of an in-kind (rent-free) contribution; adequate physical space (size and equipment); and trust and respect of the targeted population. It could be housed in community organizations such as churches, tenants' organizations, or nonprofit entities that serve the targeted population.

Step 3: Obtain Community Support

Establishing trust and a level of confidence within the targeted population are critical to obtaining support. Discover the trusted key players in the health and human service arena who will provide entrée to the people you want to reach. Meet with them to inform them of the program objectives and invite them to participate in the planning process. The greater the community buy-in, the greater the chances of program success. Don't forget to include businesses as part of the community support network—they will grow to recognize the benefits the program offers the community.

Step 4: Design the Program

An optimal program schedule for the recommended 40 hours' instruction (includ-

ing graduation) is either a 2-hour class twice a week a 4-hour class once a week for 10 weeks. Topics are presented in each session to include general didactic information and prevention or assessment skills. Provision of child care and lunch if the class is over a mealtime decreases the barriers to participation. Choose your volunteer guest speakers carefully from area health care providers, health care students, or graduate lay-health promoters. Some speakers may not be able to connect with the audience to ensure that the lessons are adequately taught. The stethoscope, blood pressure cuff, and thermometer are important parts of the training and should be provided. They help the lay health-promoter gain access and credibility. They are also symbols of pride and evidence of what the lay health promoter has achieved. Ask the *promotora* student to make health contacts in her neighborhood to share what she has learned. They can report on their contacts during class where they can discuss what happened. This involves the *promotoras* in their communities from the start; it offers an opportunity for feedback from the staff and group, and builds lay health-promoter confidence. Graduation is very important. Let the group plan the graduation ceremony. Choose a speaker who is relevant to the group. Hand out certificates, serve refreshments, and invite guests. Allow the graduates to invite as many guests as they want. Make graduation dependent upon attendance at a specific number of classes— 80% attendance rate of the total classes offered is reasonable.

Step 5: Design the Program Evaluation

Evaluation consists of constantly asking meaningful questions, gathering information, summarizing responses, reporting information, and fine-tuning plans. Both process and outcome data lend programs greater credibility for their activity reports and funding proposals. Process evaluation is aimed at understanding the internal dynamics of program operations and identifying areas for improvement. Process evaluations are concerned with what was done, when it was done, who did it and to whom, how often it was useful, and how well it was done. Outcome evaluation is aimed at determining program effects on short-term, intermediate, and long-term objectives such as changes in health status or disease prevalence. An outcome evaluation might ask whether a program has changed participants' behaviors or attitudes such as changes in health status or disease prevalence.

from state or federal agencies and pharmaceutical companies. Funds must be raised for meals, graduation ceremonies, curriculum materials, salaries (recommend director, health educator, and childcare coordinator), and equipment (thermometers, stethoscopes, and blood pressure cuffs). Optional costs can include premium awards and travel for the health educator to do follow-up work with the program graduates. Pursue funding from local sources such as hospitals, churches, local and state foundations, and businesses. Local social service agencies and housing authorities may also be interested in supporting the initiative. Once the program is up and running, the program evaluation will provide valuable data to make the case for funding from the business community and others.

Step 6: Prepare a Budget and Obtain Funding

A lay health promoter program is a low-tech approach that can be started on a minimal budget, but it is vital that the budget provide the necessary infrastructure vital to the program's success. It is necessary to have a health educator or a nurse who has experience working in the community involved in coordinating the program. If the program is to be taught in a language other than English, this person must be bilingual. It is also useful to partner with a college or university that can provide a range of volunteer services and resources. Pamphlets and other handout materials are available from nonprofit health agencies such as the American Red Cross and the American Heart Association. These organizations are grateful to have LHPs distribute materials. Other materials can be purchased at low prices or obtained for free

Step 7: Implement and Maintain Your Lay Health-Promoter Program

Sensitivity to cultural differences and a degree of flexibility must be applied in recruitment, training, and supervision. Spread the word about LHP program class availability. In the beginning you may need to use all of your available channels to spread the word. Give talks at community meetings and announcements at churches. Cultivate a relationship with the local newspaper. Word of mouth is a great way to inform the community.

Step 8: Develop and Implement Mechanisms to Keep Program Graduates Involved and Connected

Given the volunteer nature of the work and the women's work and home responsibilities, it is important to try to develop ways to keep LHP graduates linked to the program.

This has been accomplished in some programs by means of a newsletter, continuing education workshops, and regularly scheduled meetings.

CASE STUDY

Assessment of Viability and Value

With expanding employment needs and church-sponsored resettlement activities, the Shenandoah Valley area of Virginia has seen a significant influx of immigrants. Hispanics are the largest immigrant population in the area with 1,277 according to a 1995 population survey. However, the Virginia Council of Churches Refugee Resettlement Program (VCCRRP) conservatively estimates that the number of Hispanics had grown to approximately 2,500 by 1996. Additionally, the VCCRRP had informed the local health department to expect six to eight Cuban refugees per month beginning in July 1998, with expectations that this would continue over the following year. Although Hispanics originally came to the Shenandoah Valley several decades ago as migrant laborers in the apple industry, the poultry processing industry has facilitated a more permanent settlement.

Hispanics rent apartments or houses, rent or buy trailers, bring their families, and send their children to school. Many still see themselves as temporary residents, yet some have lived here for 5 to 10 years or more. Hispanics come from various Spanish-speaking countries—Mexico, El Salvador, Guatemala, and other Latin American countries. According to the Report of Subcommittee on Immigrants (Zarrugh, 1997), unless Hispanics come as refugees they generally do not receive any formal community support services to help them settle except when the Catholic church provides assistance with immigration once they are there.

When Hispanics use health care services, they are more likely to use emergency rooms than to see a primary care physician (Furino & Munoz, 1991). Information on the utilization of Rockingham Memorial Hospital's Emergency Department (ED) in Harrisonburg-Rockingham County (H-R) for 1997–1998 reflects a similar pattern. Whereas the estimated Hispanic population for H-R is 1.4% of the total population, Hispanics accounted for a disproportionate rate of ED visits (2.5%) and number of patients (2.6%). Between August 1997 and July 1998, 647 Hispanic patients had 941 ED visits. Utilizing diagnostic codes for a minimum of five visits, the visits fall into four major categories. In rank order, these include infection, injury, gastrointestinal problems, and mental health–related concerns. The most recent available statistics from the H-R health department show 4,260 total contacts for fiscal year 1996–1997 for clients of Hispanic origin (Mexico, Puerto Rico, Central and South America, Cuba, and other). These contacts were predominately for child health, family planning, immunization, maternity, Women, Infants and Children Program (WIC), and tuberculosis. Many Hispanics test positive for TB and are followed for medication regimen. In 1998 there were 140 high-risk TB cases open with Hispanics representing 65.7% of the total, and this does not include those clients who test positive but refuse medication. Based on the 1994–1997 trends of Hispanic contacts, a 5-year straight line projection shows that these contacts will increase to more than 8,000 in years 2001–2002, a twofold increase over 1996–1998. Given that local Hispanics are slow to use services, it can be assumed that many who experience illnesses do not seek any care. Barriers leading to inadequate access and utilization of health care services

---

Box 22.1   Checklist for Implementing a Lay Health Promoter Program

Step 1: Make a decision to have a lay health promoter program.

❏ Use existing sources to identify the major health care needs of the community. Gather information about:
   ✓ Major causes of morbidity and mortality from the state or local health department
   ✓ Community demographics

Community forums where community residents discuss their health care needs may also be helpful or conduct focus groups.

❏ Determine the health information needs of your population:
   ✓ Talk to physicians and health care providers.
   ✓ Give your clients a health knowledge survey.
❏ Based on the information gathered, formulate a statement of health knowledge and skills needed for the target population and community.
❏ Make a go/no-go decision about the appropriateness of a lay health promoter program for your population by asking the following questions:
   ✓ Do we have a population that would benefit from increased health knowledge and if so, in what areas?
   ✓ Are the major causes of morbidity and mortality such that preventive maintenance and follow-up will benefit the population?
   ✓ Would a program such as the lay health promoter be accepted in the community?

Step 2: Determine where the program will be housed.

❏ Secure a "home base" in an organization that is trusted by the targeted population.
❏ Classroom and storage spaces are important.

Step 3: Obtain community support.

❏ Determine initial budget needs.
❏ Identify prospects for cash and in-kind contributions.
❏ Take the time to meet with health care providers in your community and explain the program to them. Ask for their ideas about how the lay health promoters can be of value to the community.
❏ Inform churches and (tenant) organizations of the program.
❏ Provide information to the local newspaper for a human-interest story.

Step 4: Design your lay health promoter program.

❏ Determine the topics for the curriculum.

Box 22.1 *(continued)*

❑ Develop a schedule for classes.
❑ Gather necessary materials and supplies.
❑ Find a classroom.
❑ Post flyers, talk to clients, present idea at churches and housing meetings.
❑ Arrange for child-care providers, including a coordinator.
❑ Make arrangements for lunches.
❑ Obtain any necessary audio-visual materials.

Step 5: Design the program evaluation.
Formative Evaluation

❑ Use client focus groups, interviews with community members, and community input meetings to assist in designing the program. Make sure that materials are at an acceptable reading level and are culturally sensitive.

Program Monitoring

❑ Design a computerized database to track health encounters reported by the health care promoter.
❑ Determine what service outcomes (e.g., increased clinic visits, referrals to physicians) can be expected from lay health promoter activity.
❑ Review the database to assure that these outcomes can be tracked.
❑ Schedule regular (twice a year) staff reviews of administrative data to provide input into the planning process.
❑ Establish an advisory council of key constituents. This council should include one or more lay health promoters.

Outcome Evaluation

❑ Include a way of tracking unintended outcomes such as enrollment in a community class, getting a GED, further course work such as nurse's aide certification, or improved employment status.

Step 6: Obtain funding.

❑ Identify possible funding sources and obtain information about funding requirements.
❑ Prepare a proposal using community data, program description and budget.
❑ Obtain letters of support from community providers, agencies, and political entities.
❑ Work with a steering committee to identify in-kind support.

(continued)

Box 22.1 *(continued)*

Step 7: Implement and maintain the program.

❏ Recruit for the first class.
❏ Continue to keep in close contact with representatives of the targeted community.
❏ Continue to look for funding opportunities in the community and at the state and federal levels.
❏ Review program evaluations and continue to revise the program to assure relevance to students.

Step 8: Design and implement alumnae activities.

❏ Survey your graduates on what they would like.
❏ Plan a continuing education program.
❏ Develop a format for a newsletter.
❏ Don't forget that including your graduates in developing these products will help them gain additional skills and confidence.

---

for Hispanics include language, cultural differences, lack of finances, and transportation (Harrisonburg-Rockingham Health and Human Services Planning Council, 1997).

In order to achieve a culturally sensitive project, we invited a collaborative approach with community members to take an active role in its initiation, development, implementation, and evaluation of program activities. This was accomplished through telephone and written surveys and a focus group with persons taking English as second language (ESL) classes. Both quantitative (hospital ED and health Department) and qualitative data (surveys and focus group) frame the curriculum topics and confirm community support.

Program Housing

The health department is frequently a trusted source for health care and information within the local Hispanic community and therefore it seemed a natural home;

however, the physical space was limited. While meeting with representatives from the Hispanic religious congregations the priest at the Catholic church offered the lower level of their education building as a training site. The space offered consists of a classroom with tables, chairs, chalkboard, and TV/VCR and overhead projector; a fully equipped kitchen and nursery; a large separate room to share the noon meal and additional indoor play space as needed for childcare; and a safe grassy area for outside childcare activities.

Community Support

Because health care needs within the Hispanic population have been identified as a local priority (Harrisonburg-Rockingham Health and Human Services Planning Council, 1997), community support exists from local organizations and providers. Many agencies, organizations, or individuals participated in the need-assessment survey conducted in preparation for the

Virginia Health Care Foundation (VHCF) funding proposal. They include the Alliance for Intercultural Action, Hispanic Services Council, Virginia Migrant Education Program, Virginia Council of Churches Refugee Resettlement Program, Harrisonburg-Rockingham County Health Department, Harrisonburg-Rockingham County Free Clinic, Grace Covenant Church, Primera Iglesia Bautista (Augusta Hispanic Mission), Charles L. Buttz (MD), Valley AIDS Network, Dayton Learning Center English as Second Language (ESL) programs. These individuals or groups provided responses to questions about major causes of death and disease in the local Hispanic population, the role of preventive maintenance, the benefit derived from increased health knowledge, areas of health information needs, and acceptance of and obstacles to a LHP program. These organizations recognize the value of an LHP program and either support or represent the community-based referral network that the project will utilize to increase access to health and human services. The James Madison University community of health professions' faculty also recognizes the value of providing service-learning opportunities with diverse populations for their students, the future health care providers.

Program Design

As a replication of a successful lay health-promoter program model for inner city African Americans at Cross-Over Health Center in Richmond, Virginia, this project promotes healthy living within the Hispanic neighborhoods of Harrisonburg-Rockingham County. Because it is a replication model the program design is inherent. Cultural modifications were made as necessary. Health is intimately connected to the way

in which people in a culture construct reality and give and find meaning. Lay health promoters know the population as well as they know their own neighbors, relatives, and friends; they share language, culture, and socioeconomic background and are able to help the community better understand their health problems and the delivery system. Lay health promoters help individuals take greater control of their health and their lives. Objectives of the project are to promote healthy living by (a) identifying, recruiting, training, and supervising 30 LHPs annually; (b) providing 40-hour training curriculum about health promotion, disease and injury prevention, linking to community-based health and social service agencies referral system; and (c) providing LHPs with opportunities for continuing education, recognition, and career advancement. The curriculum for training and educating Hispanic women (the health of the Hispanic family is the mother's domain) to identify health problems, identify local health resources, and help their neighbors access care was designed to meet the particular needs of this community. The needs of trainees were considered in the scheduling of the program (day of week and time). Two classes of trainees were scheduled during the first year of funding. Because the concept of volunteerism is new to the culture, incentives were provided to facilitate the opportunity for training and retention in the program. These incentives include a premium award of $100, childcare, and meals. The LHP training curriculum is based on the most prevalent problems seen in the hospital emergency department, the health department, and those described by LHP trainees. Each training module topic for women and children is organized to include Hispanic American health statistics, basic information, accessing resources, questions, homework assignments, and references. Over the course of 40 hours, specific topics include an overview of the LHP program, the role of LHP, basic concepts of health and wellness, introductory disease and injury prevention, dental care, nutrition, women's health, infant- and child-care guide, and mental health with an emphasis on substance abuse, domestic violence, and depression. Every attempt has been made to integrate cultural influences on health throughout all topics. In addition to cognitive information, special skills are taught to assess health and illness; for example, effective hand-washing, temperature-taking, and blood pressure measurement (see Figure 22.1).

Program Evaluation

Evaluation is multidimensional and may be driven by the program funding source and outcome design. Our funding source evaluates the project by utilizing several instruments. These include progress reports, site visits, client satisfaction surveys, and partner assessment surveys. These instruments are used to determine:

- the extent to which the program has met its objectives
- progress in generating or attracting resources to sustain the program
- the extent of community commitment and support for the program
- the cost-effectiveness of the program's approach
- the overall value of the program's approach to delivering primary health care.

The overall anticipated impact of the project on the Hispanic community is (a) an increased knowledge of the importance of health and healthy behaviors, (b) a more appropriate utilization of resources, and (c) increased multilingual, multicultural

representation in the local health care community. Program monitoring of the first objective occurs through testing at course onset and at conclusion. The program evaluation (classes, teachers, and materials) is reviewed at the conclusion of each session with appropriate revisions to ensure relevance to the participants. Measurement of the second objective is achieved through the development of a computerized database to track LHP reported service outcomes on an annual basis. This includes increased health department and free clinic visits, referrals to physicians, and decreased ED level 1 nonemergency visits (those diagnoses that could be treated more effectively by a primary care physician in an office or clinic setting). Program monitoring for the final objective tracks indicators such as enrollment in a community class (GED, ESL, etc.), completion of GED, further health-related course work such as nurse's aide certification, and improved employment status.

Budget Preparation and Funding

Once the program was designed, we looked at the personnel and other project costs required to implement the program. Our year-one budget totaled $78,296.38 but included $19,191 cash from a private/state foundation; $3,153 from the sponsoring agency; and $55,953 in-kind contributions. Cash personnel real-time costs were underestimated at $14,839 but the in-kind personnel contributions of $44,978 helped meet the deficits. Other nonpersonnel project costs were $7,505 (see sample budget income and expenditures for year one at Figure 22.2). We did not anticipate the high cost of the lesson plans translation. In addition to writing a competitive foundation grant proposal, a "Gift Opportunities

Blue Ridge Area Health Education Center (AHEC)
Agreement Between Promotoras de Salud Program
and
Promotora

Purpose

The Promotora volunteer is dedicated to promoting health care and health education in her community. This agreement between the Blue Ridge AHEC's Promotoras de Salud Program and the Promotora establishes program expectations about the activities and responsibilities of both parties. Each party shall hold harmless the other from and against loss, damage, and expense as a result of a breach of the agreement. Any program questions or concerns should be directed to the Project Director or Training Coordinator.

General Agreements

1. Stipends—$100—half to be paid at graduation and the remainder upon successful completion of the program. Social Security #_____

2. Class Attendance—80% attendance at classes mandatory to meet graduation requirement (two class days can be excused for emergencies). Promotoras are expected to do any homework assignments or reading for missed classes. Arrange to talk with the health educator facilitator for any questions about missed classes. If critical skill content, e.g., B/P or thermometer use, is missed a make-up session will be required.

3. Course Incompletion—if unable to complete the course materials and/or equipment should be returned.

4. Childcare—Free babysitting services available at class location site(s). The Promotora is responsible for providing infant meals or children's snacks during the training period. Please let the training coordinator know on a weekly basis if there are any changes in the number and ages of children attending so that we may provide adequate coverage.

5. Meals—The program will provide one free meal each week of classes.

6. Equipment—The program will furnish each Promotora a blood pressure cuff and stethoscope to use in the assessment of blood pressure. Also oral and rectal thermometers are provided.

7. Continuing Education—Participate in a minimum of one continuing education activity per year.

8. Documentation of Health Contacts—As a grant requirement the health contacts you will be making are to be recorded. If they are not recorded, it is as though they have not been done and so cannot be counted. Forms are provided for this documentation and as well as an explanation on how to complete them.

In Testimony whereof, Witness the duly authorized signatures of the parties hereto:

Blue Ridge AHEC   **Promotora**
Promotoras de Salud

_____   _____
Sandra K. Hopper   Date   Date

FIGURE 22.1 Agreement between Promotora and Promotoras de Salud Program.

Project Budget: Expenditures
Organization: Blue Ridge AHEC at JMU   Grant YTD: Jan 1, 1999 - Dec 31, 1999
531037 Promotoras De Salud: Hispanic Lay Health Promoter Program

	Salary		% of Time	VHCF Grant	Other Project Costs		Total Expenditures
		Hours			Cash	In-Kind*	
1. PERSONNEL							
Paid Staff							
Project Director	$36,183.04		60%			$36,183.04	$36,183.04
Training Coordinator	$11,232.00		15%	$10,741.50			$10,741.50
Social Security				$821.48			$821.48
Health Educator Facilitator	$3,000.00			$497.00	$2,653.00		$3,150.00
Social Security				$126.23	$--		$126.23
Administrative Assistant			11%			$1,315.00	$1,315.00
Volunteer Providers (a)	Number	Hours	Hourly Rate				
Registered Dietician	1	25.5	22.5			$573.75	$573.75
Domestic Abuse Worker	1	7.5	11			$82.50	$82.50
Nurse	1	47	22.5			$1,057.50	$1,057.50
Dental Assistant	1	5	11			$55.00	$55.00
Health Educator	1	13	22.5			$292.50	$292.50
Social Worker	1	4.5	11			$49.50	$49.50
Childcare Coordinator	1	25.5	7			$178.50	$178.50
Students	51	807.25	6.43			$5,190.62	$5,190.62
(ed act, childcare, meals)							
I. SUB-TOTAL		935.25		$12,186.21	$2,653.00	$44,977.91	$59,817.12
II. Other Project Costs							
Free/Reduced Rate Medical Care (c)	# Providers		#Visits				
*Office Visit-Generalist							$-
*Office Visit-Specialist							$-
*Office Visit-Dentist							$-
*Managed Care Coverage (d)							$-
Medications							$-

FIGURE 22.2   Sample year 1 budget income and expenditures.

Medical/Dental Supplies				$-
Lab/Diagnostic Services				$-
Health Education Materials				$-
Lay Health Promoter Stipends	$1,500.00			$1,500.00
Medical Equipment	$600.00			$600.00
Membership in COSSMHO			$100.00	$100.00
Rent			$6,300.00	$6,300.00
Utilities				$-
Transportation	$81.00			$81.00
Office Supplies				$-
Classified Ad for Hth Ed Fac			$504.18	$504.18
Class & Graduation Support	$1,916.18		$82.00	$1,998.18
Curriculum Materials	$2,907.50	$500.00		$3,407.50
Overhead: Project Director			$2,894.64	$2,894.64
Overhead: Trng Coordinator			$898.56	$898.56
Overhead: Admin. Assistant			$105.20	$105.20
Copying			$90.00	$90.00
II. SUB-TOTAL	$7,004.68	$500.00	$10,974.58	$18,479.26
TOTAL PROJECT COSTS	$19,190.89	$3,153.00	$55,952.49	$78,296.38
% OF PROJECT COSTS	24.51%	4.03%	71.46%	100.00%

(a), (b), (c), (d), See Attached Reference Sheet
*All amounts in the in-kind column must also appear in the in-kind column on the income page.

FIGURE 22.2 *(continued)*

SOURCE OF INCOME	CASH	IN-KIND	TOTAL
PROJECT BUDGET: INCOME (Jan 1, 1999-Dec 31, 1999)			
I. VHCF GRANT	$14,727.00		$14,727.00
II. LOCAL PRIVATE SOURCES			
Blue Ridge AHEC	$3,153.00	$604.18	$3,757.18
Catholic Church of Blessed Sacrament		$6,300.00	$6,300.00
$300/day X 21 days			
Project Director		$36,183.04	$36,183.04
Administrative Assistant		$1,315.00	$1,315.00
Registered Dietician		$573.75	$573.75
Domestic Abuse Worker		$82.50	$82.50
Nurse		$1,057.50	$1,057.50
Dental Assistant		$55.00	$55.00
Health Educator		$292.50	$292.50
Social Worker		$49.50	$49.50
Childcare Coordinator		$178.50	$178.50
Students		$5,190.62	$5,190.62
ROCCO		$82.00	$82.00
Overhead: Project Director		$2,894.64	$2,894.64
Overhead: Training Coordinator		$898.56	$898.56
Overhead: Admin. Assistant		$105.20	$105.20
Copying		$90.00	$90.00
III. LOCAL GOVERNMENT FUNDING			
IV. STATE GOVERNMENT FUNDING			
V. FEDERAL GOVERNMENT FUNDING			
VI. FOUNDATION GRANTS			
VII. REIMBURSEMENT:			
Medicaid			
Medicare			
Third Party Insurance			
Capitation			
Self-Pay/Sliding Fee			
VIII. OTHER			
Donations:			
First Presbyterian Church	$1,405.73		$1,405.73
Nancy Farrar	$10.00		$10.00
Kathryn Suyes	$50.00		$50.00
ROCCO, Inc.	$435.00		$435.00
Westside Baptist Church	$58.00		$58.00
WLR Foods	$200.00		$200.00
Bridgewater Church of the Brethren	$325.00		$225.00
Trinity Presbyterian Church	$250.00		$250.00
VIII. SUB-TOTAL	$2,733.73		$2,733.73
TOTAL INCOME	$20,613.73	$55,952.49	$76,466.22

FIGURE 22.2   *(continued)*

List" was distributed to community businesses and selected church congregations that identified specific program costs from which donors could choose to contribute. We initiated an "Adopt a Promotora" campaign that yielded individual and group support to sponsor all or a portion of individual LHP training expenses.

Implement and Maintain Your Lay Health Promoter Program

Identification, recruitment, and training module development activities occurred during the first 4 1/2 months of the project. Every attempt was made to ensure that materials were at an acceptable reading level and were culturally sensitive. Because sensitivity to cultural differences and a degree of flexibility must be applied in recruitment, training, and supervision, the project links to an existing bilingual outreach worker employed part-time at the health department. Twelve hours per week of her time were contracted to coordinate the identification and recruitment of trainees and coordination of training activities. Additional sources of trainee referral came from Hispanic support organizations such as the Hispanic Services Council, churches, and Virginia Migrant Education. Trainee selection incorporated the following criteria: (a) they must reflect the ethnic composition of their neighborhoods; (b) selection is based on their reputation for being natural helpers; and (c) they must have a minimum of a sixth-grade education. Both during and after the training, trainees and graduates are expected to make and document "health education" visits to friends and neighbors to share their knowledge by disseminating Spanish-language health materials and conducting health screenings (e.g., high blood pressure, safety in the en-

vironment) and informal classes like breast self-exam. These activities focus on building the desire, resources, and mechanisms to promote healthy behaviors and environments within Hispanic neighborhoods.

Mechanisms to Keep Your Program Graduates Involved and Connected

The program cosponsored a booth at the Second Annual International Festival as a way of advertising the program and promoting heath, and presented a workshop at the Substance Abuse Awareness Day that was sponsored by a local mental health coalition. The health education facilitator supervises the activities of trainees on an ongoing basis. The project recognizes the importance of continuing education activities by offering one class (Breast Self-Exam Certification) during the first year with a plan to increase to one class every other month in the second year of funding. Health care career advancement opportunities to include both educational and employment tracts and financial assistance are communicated to graduates. A newsletter features post-graduation activities and graduate updates (Figure 22.3). Nursing student and other health care professional guest speakers serve as positive health-career role models with participants. Graduation ceremonies honor the trainees' commitment to the program and community-wide recognition is achieved through local press releases.

SUMMARY

This chapter illustrates how one community developed an approach to health care that is grounded in the community context, specifically, a lay health promoter program. It is essential to recognize that individuals

conexíónes

Volume 1, Issue 1

A newsletter for the Promotoras de Salud

Fall 1999

If You Can Dream it, You Can Do it

Dear Friends,

I wonder sometimes, what does it mean to prepare myself in order to improve myself? Some people understand very well the meaning of these words but others never understand it; some never have the opportunity to improve themselves, but there are many who struggle to go beyond their limitations. Sometimes those who have such an opportunity don't take advantage of it. This is something difficult to understand, but what I do know is that *if you can dream it, you can do it*. I've stopped to consider this and to realize how beautiful it is to be whom you want and can be. There are no barriers to stop you when you fight to achieve.

It's nice when I have someone to translate for me when I need it. When someone can give me a ride when I need to go somewhere I can depend on that person. However, I've also thought "What will happen when I really need help and there's no one around to help me? It would be terrible, and I think about how the people on whom I depend have been able to prepare me. Is there something I can do on my own to help myself reach my goals? In these moments I remember years ago when I wanted to teach people from ages 30 to 50 how to read and write. They often said to me "I'm old and I will never learn." I remember I said to them that it is never too late to learn. *If you can dream it, you can do it,* and the truth is that some of them did learn.

Several years ago when I was in high school, I saw an elderly woman who had just graduated from high school at age 90. I didn't know her, but I knew that her goal was to graduate and that she probably had barriers to break, but at last her dream became a reality. I've also known people who had to work instead of going to school but they continue working on their goals, returning to school with their grandchildren; they break the barriers and somehow make it to graduation. I have participated with them so I know that it's true; *if you can dream it, you can do it*.

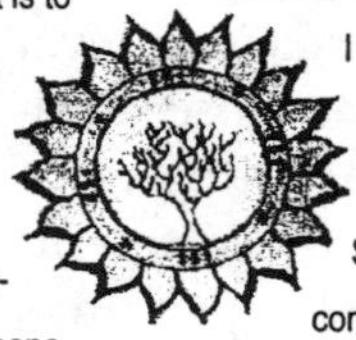

If I had been able to reach the height of my dreams, I would have been a nurse or a doctor. I always liked to be involved in the area of health but for economic reasons I couldn't. With the Promotoras de Salud program, my dreams continue to come true. For me, promoting health is very important. How wonderful it is when someone recognizes you as a Promotora. At the same time, it is my responsibility to be prepared. This is why I will continue to study my notes and any information that was given to me as a Promotora to be the best I can be.

I continue to work toward my dreams and goals as I volunteer two days a week at the Health Department. I get closer to realizing them and I want to become a nurse's aid someday. I invite you all who have had the privilege of being chosen for the Promotora de Salud program to keep on going, preparing yourselves, and studying your materials. Remember that *if you can dream it, you can do it*. For me, helping out my community is a pleasure.

Blessings,
Fernanda Carbajal.

1

FIGURE 22.3　Newsletter cover page.

and communities are complex actors in their own health care and in the health of the larger community. Lay health workers educate individuals and communities, and facilitate access to needed services. They also educate providers and health care systems and help craft services that are more responsive to the communities being served, thereby providing a vital link between communities and health care providers.

REFERENCES

Barnes, M. D., & Fairbanks, J. (1997). Problem-based strategies promoting community transformation: Implications for the community health worker model. *Family Community Health, 20*(1), 54–65.

Centers for Disease Control and Prevention. (1994). *Community health advisors: Programs in the United States. Vol. II*. Atlanta, GA: Centers for Disease Control and Prevention, National Center for Chronic Disease Prevention and Health Promotion.

Centers for Disease Control and Prevention. (1998). *Community health advisors/workers. Selected annotations—programs in the United States, Vol. III*. Atlanta, GA: Centers for Disease Control and Prevention, National Center for Chronic Disease Prevention and Health Promotion.

Furino, A., & Munoz, E. (1991). Health status among Hispanics: Major themes and new priorities. *Journal of the American Medical Association, 265*, 255–257.

Giblin, P. T. (1989). Effective utilization and evaluation of indigenous health care workers. *Public Health Report, 104*(4), 361–368.

Harrisonburg-Rockingham Health and Human Services Planning Council. (1997). *Investing in our community for a future of opportunities: Our community profile*. Unpublished manuscript.

Hoff, W. (1969). Role of the community health aide in public health programs. *Public Health Report, 84*(11), 998–1102.

Leutz, W. (1976). The informal community caregiver: A link between the health care system and local residents. *American Journal of Orthopsychiatry, 46*(4), 676–688.

Love, M. B., Gardner, K., & Legion, V. (1997). Community health workers: Who they are and what they do. *Health Education and Behavior, 8*(1), 15–19.

National Center for Chronic Disease Prevention and Health Promotion of the Centers for Disease Control and Prevention. (1998). *National Community Health Advisor Study*.

Pew Health Professions Commission. (1994). *Community health workers: Integral yet often overlooked members of the health care workforce*. San Francisco: University of California, San Francisco Center for the Health Professions.

Skeet, M. (1985). Community health workers: Promoters or inhibitors of primary health care? *International Nursing Review, 33*(2), 55–58.

U.S. Department of Health and Human Services (1994). *Community health advisors: Models, research, and practice. Selected annotations—programs in the United States, Vol II*. Washington, DC: Author.

U.S. Department of Health and Human Services. (January, 2000). Health People 2010 (Conference Edition in 2 volumes). Washington, DC.

Zarrugh, L. (1997). *Report of subcommittee on immigrant focus groups*. Unpublished manuscript.

Wallerstein, N. (1992). Powerlessness, empowerment, and health: Implications for health promotion programs. *American Journal of Health Promotion, 6*(3), 197–205.

CHAPTER 23

Diabetes Programs in Hawaii

Chen-Yen Wang

I n this chapter, you will learn about the elements of effective community-based programs through case presentations and analysis. Refer to Figure 23.1 throughout for elements of the program development process.

BACKGROUND

Hospitals focus on treating illness, rather than on promoting wellness. Traditionally they may have no partnerships with community leaders. Knowledge and technology are exploding and there must be a shift of health care system from the traditional hospitals to collaboration between hospitals or health centers of communities (Faller, Dowell, & Jackson, 1995). Management of chronic illness such as diabetes mellitus requires prevention of long-term medical complications and health centers or resources based in communities will play increasingly important roles in providing knowledge and resources to the individuals. As a professor at the University of Hawaii, I hoped to bridge the gap between community needs and available resources.

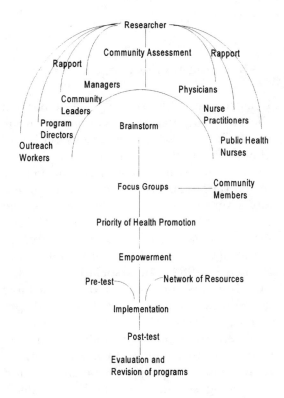

FIGURE 23.1 A proposed model for developing a community-based project.

Before I intervened in a community, I had to know what bound these individuals together. The commonality could be race, ethnicity, age, beliefs, values, illness, geography, economic, occupation, religion, sources of support, or sources of seeking health care. "Who should I develop relationships with?" I had to ask. The answer depended on what benefits I had to bring to this specific community. Would I represent the needs and rights of the community members? If so, I had to let community members know my capability of advocacy in a subtle way.

For example, I told the leader of the Golden Ager Association of Hawaii that I was working on a project with the Community Health Nursing Division in the State Department of Health. Then I waited for the leader's expression of community needs.

One Community Program Process

In December 1995, a colleague told me that she knew volunteers in a Chinese community called the Golden Ager Association of Hawaii and that she could introduce me to them. I met with the volunteers and established rapport by asking about their needs and offering my services. We brainstormed about ways to work together. The Golden Ager Association of Hawaii, a nonprofit community service organization, was formed in 1984. The association is staffed by volunteers and supported by charitable contributions from individuals and private organization.

To ensure success for the health promotion activities I had to involve community members in the project by facilitating and enhancing community members' abilities (Price & Cordell, 1997). Using community volunteers is one way to accomplish this

goal. The Golden Ager Association seemed to be the perfect vehicle. This effort meant empowering the community to meet their own needs. *Empowerment* includes strengthening and support the ability of the community to grow and change. In a study by Voyle and Simmons (1999), their primary aim was to develop a continuing program that community members would eventually run for themselves. Their findings demonstrated that the devolution of power is a key aspect of organizational process involving professional groups and indigenous people. Findings indicated building partnerships for a program included:

- preparatory steps;
- the formation of a partnership committee;
- program planning and development;
- the appointment of a liaison worker.

When training staff for a community project, be sure to consider individual empowerment. Their findings gave me ideas about how to develop my research project just as I did. An example of this is to include volunteers as well as paid workers in training opportunities. Another important element in the development of a community-based project is "collective action" (Moyer et al., 1999). Essential functions of changes must be agreed upon among key community members including leaders, outreach workers, managers, and directors. A collective action means a equal contribution of these members through interactions among them. At the beginning of project, you as a health care provider or a researcher are one of the important contributors in the collective action, just as I was with the Golden Ager Association.

Golden Age members are over 55 years of age who pay a $2 annual fee or $20 for a lifetime membership. This association

---

Box 23.1   Wisdom Box

Collective action is a loose collection of people with creative and technical skills volunteering time to create a program. You may achieve collective action by: (1) inviting leaders, outreach workers, managers, and directors to a meeting to brainstorm; (2) distributing survey items to the above mentioned people; (3) interview them with open-ended questions.

---

provides assistance for needy older adults to obtain proper care and support from government and private agencies, such as welfare (adult education, meal site, food stamps, housing, Medicaid, Medicare, Social Security/SSI), professional and legal services, and employment assistance.

In 1996, after collecting together all ideas garnered from my discussion with Golden Ager community volunteers, I applied for a $700 grant from Sigma Theta Tau International Nursing Honor Society, Gamma Psi Chapter, to examine the impact of the ethnic diversity on the self-care behaviors of Chinese American adults with type II diabetes. The objective was to examine the diabetic self-care among different ethnic groups.

Methods of identifying values, needs, strengths, and resiliences of communities that I used include observation, questionnaire survey by face to face interview or by telephone interview, outreach strategies, and focus groups. Whenever you can, involve community outreach workers in your project. For example, you may train outreach workers to recruit subjects or to administer questionnaires as I did.

Community members may not become involve in assessment if they are not aware of the importance of prevention. I had to deliver the message of prevention to community people by pamphlets and mouth-to-mouth and invite them to an open house community-based activity. I found out that the best location for these activities is the community center or the health center within the community. Community people will come to you when they feel your spirit and nature of caring, not your goal or projects.

Community people may recognize the importance of health promotion, but not connect the events to themselves. In this instance, I had to provide evidence of the connection by going to where they were.

For the Golden Agers project among Chinese-Americans, I developed a questionnaire based on my knowledge of the community. I used the instrument to obtain demographic data including gender, living environment, marital status, occupation, education, duration of diabetes, race, and daily physical activities. Data pertaining to social interaction and decision-making processes were obtained by a questionnaire used in a previous study (Wang & Fenske, 1996). HDSC was measured by the modified diabetic self-care practice instrument (DiSCPI). The DiSCPI, developed by Frey and Denyes (Frey & Denyes, 1989) measured health-deviation requisites: (a) awareness and prevention of effects and results of the diabetes; and (b) adherence to prescribed therapeutic measures. The modified DiSCPI instrument contains 22 statements scored on a scale of 1 to 5. The modified DiSCPI instrument was translated from English into Chinese, then translated back to English to confirm the meaning of questions. Cronbach alphas were 0.85 for Chinese.

Health was measured by the Denyes health status instrument (DHSI-90). The DHSI-90, a 10-item instrument, measures one's perceived general state of health and specific dimensions of health. The score for each item ranged from 0 to 100. DHSI-90 was translated into Chinese, then translated back to confirm the original meaning of questions. Cronbach's alpha coefficients ranged from 0.79 to 0.88. The assessment of the ethnic and cultural diversity, including religious preference, dietary practice, and beliefs and practices related to health and illness, was measured using one demographic data form.

In January 1996, I negotiated with the leader of the Golden Ager Association to teach community members about blood pressure and glucose monitoring without charge in exchange for collecting research data. During 1996, the staff I assembled for this program consisted of one public health nurse, two graduate students, and several undergraduate students. Some students spoke fluent Cantonese, which had been the major language within the Chinese community in Hawaii. Students were involved in health promotion activities (e.g., client education on self-breast examination, pneumonia vaccine, flu vaccine, healthy diet). I interviewed community members using a questionnaire. Community volunteers were paid through the grant to be interpreters. When we worked together, I shared my knowledge of health promotion and pathophysiology with community volunteers and they shared their knowledge of and connections with the community.

The public health nurse provided external resources for this community. She assessed individuals' needs and referred one client to the meals-on-wheels program. She also made home visits with me.

My work in the community included facilitating community leaders to recognize the community's ability to address its community wide problems, to develop its own capacity for action, and to establish connections with external resources. You can assist in this process by offering technical support and information regarding community leadership development, including collaborating with key community members to offer vision workshops, conduct key informant interviews, surveys, and focus group interviews, and to create supportive environments for health.

Eng's model (1993) or theory of community partnerships guided the research process. It includes three stages of network formation. These stages include: (1) exchange network, (2) coalition as an action network, and (3) network formation. In the stage of exchange network, community people do not have common goal yet. Information is traded within the network and among community people who communicate with one another on a as needed basis. In the stage of coalition, community people have a common goal that they work together to achieve. This common goal usually focuses on community needs. The involvement of time and resources are still limited at this stage. The third stage of network formation is a systemic network in which communities have made joint policies to integrate their missions and divide the tasks required. The goal of this systemic network is to meet the needs of a community.

I examined ways to strengthen connectedness with community people through face-to-face engagements, printed materials, telecommunication with ideas, people, events, and visions (Pinfold, 1999). Through written materials, you and community leaders can network to develop a common goal to meet your needs and community needs. In summary, you develop community partnerships by involving community people in the process of program design with a common goal to achieve health promotion within the community.

One of my clients in this Chinese community owned the only Chinese TV broadcast station in Hawaii. Using Eng's model

I asked him to partner with this project. He made announcement of our services and research on TV free of charge. When I completed my project at the end of 1996, the leader of volunteers asked me if I was willing to expand services to a clinic. These actions show how a network was built and diffused to a larger population.

Focus Groups

In 1998, Kalihi-Palama Health Center received a grant to develop community projects and asked me to coordinate two focus groups in Chinatown to collect information about diabetes issues and hypertension issues. Focus group strategy is to use pre-specified open-ended questions to lead discussion among 8–15 participants. I focused on cultural values and preferences. Focus group sessions lasted about 60 minutes for the Mandarin group and about 75 minutes for the Cantonese group, ten participants per group. The following open-ended questions were used to guide the discussions:

1. What does diabetes mean to you?
2. What do you think diabetes means to your family or friends?
3. What do you like to eat every day?
4. How do you feel about having high blood sugar?
5. What makes it hard to stay on the diet?
6. If you could plan activities for this community, what activities would you like to see and participate in?

I facilitated these focus groups for Kalihi-Palama Health Center and the findings are confidential. However, you will read the findings of focus groups among the Pacific Islanders.

At the annual luncheon party of the association, I participated in organization and services and acted as liaison. I coordinated the presentations regarding health promotion at the party. Presenters included a physician, graduate students, and myself. Topics included diet and hypertension, diabetes management, and cholesterol and stroke. Members of the Golden Ager Association in Hawaii participated in the process by suggesting topics of interest. We did not use an evaluation tool to evaluate the community reaction to the presentation, but I obtained feedback by asking community people to discuss their interests with me when they visited the clinic.

I held the health clinic within the association every Tuesday from 8:30 a.m. to 11:30 a.m. using a walk-in and first-come first-served system. By the end of 1997, the average number of clients each time was in the twenties. In 1997, we asked for client input; they suggested paying for our services. From January 1998, clients were charged for the test strips of the glucose test and cholesterol test. The number of walk-in clients every Tuesday morning remained in the twenties. The membership of the association has increased from 1,500 to 2,200 since the health clinic started. The total number of clients in the health clinic was over 400 at the end of September 1999.

Besides direct services, I translated existing pamphlets published by the Hawaii Diabetes Control Group and compiled and translated existing documentation regarding the management of diabetes, hypertension, and cholesterol into Mandarin. The Golden Ager Association of Hawaii pays all expenses related to health promotion. Volunteers of the association also input their suggestions and vision about the delivery of health education.

Focus Groups Among Pacific Islanders in a Low-Income Housing Project

In 1997, I received $9,420 from the Clinical Research Center at the Kapi'olani Medical

Center in Hawaii. This project was supported by a Research Centers in Minority Institutions award, P20RR/A1 11091, from the National Center for Research Resources, National Institutes of Health. The purpose of this study was to examine the perception of diabetes among a sample of Pacific Islanders in a low-income housing project, to develop a community-based diabetes management program for them, and to examine the perception of health status, ideal body image, diabetes knowledge, and support system in this community.

In my research, four focus groups were held with 23 Pacific Islanders (10 Samoans, 6 Hawaiians/part Hawaiians, and 7 Micronesians) who were diagnosed with type II diabetes. Findings were published in the Diabetes Educator (Wang, Abbott, Goodbody, Hui, & Rausch, 1999). The same open-ended questions were used in the focus groups, and focus groups were held in English with translation. Findings were divided into (a) participants' feelings about being diagnosed with diabetes; (b) family members' and friends' perceptions; (c) themes pertinent to barriers to exercise and diet, and themes pertinent to a community diabetes-management program. Participants' perceptions of diabetes included symptoms such as sugar in the blood, weakness, fatigue, pain, thirst, and feeling isolated from friends. The associated loss of control triggered feelings of fear, anxiety, and anger and changes in their own and their family members' lifestyles, including eating and exercise.

Barriers to exercise and diet that were identified included social values such as pressure to eat at social or family visits, cultural values associating weight with wealth or happiness and ideal body image, poverty or lack of employment opportunity to make money to buy appropriate food, and lack of motivation for exercise. Support groups, "talk story" groups, craft classes, bake sales,

walking groups, cooking classes, bingo games, and a community-based health-food store were suggested for the development of a community-based diabetes program.

Based on the input from the initial focus groups (brainstorm and empower phases), I developed a diabetes management program for the Pacific Islanders at the low-income project. This study examined the effectiveness of a diabetes program among Pacific Islanders in Honolulu, Hawaii who were diagnosed with type II diabetes. Of 23 subjects 16 had completed the intervention program. Glycosylated hemoglobin (HA1c) levels ranged from 5.8% to 13.9% (mean = 9.26, SD = 2.05) before intervention and from 5.7% to 10.7% (mean = 7.83, SD = 1.45) after intervention. Emerged themes of focus groups after intervention were confirmed by the co-moderators and participants. An SF-36 questionnaire was repeated and each of the items were analyzed.

Results indicated that participants made changes in eating habits (type, amount, and preparation of food), foot care, medication, and exercise regimen for up to 6 months. Participants perceived support from family and friends and an exercise group as essential elements of keeping them on the right track. Participants also perceived temptation as the biggest hindrance to compliance. There was a significant difference in the mean scores of the SF-36 before and after the interventions indicating the improvement of physical functioning.

Intracommunity Support

Support from existing organizations or programs within the community has been perceived as an essential strategy of developing community-based health promotion program (Berman, Grosser, & Gritz, 1998). To introduce the elements of obtaining intra-community support I will compare my experiences with leaders in community. In 1996, I visited a physician in his clinic, which was located near the housing project for low-income people. The physician and one nurse practitioner see patients at the clinic within the housing project every Tuesday and Thursday. The nurse practitioner introduced me and briefly described my project to the doctor. He refused to support the project. Realizing an alternative population was necessary, I discussed my project with public health nurses who visited clients within this housing project and obtained their support. My students and I visited families with the public health nurses. Later on, I recruited outreach workers within the community. These outreach workers were paid by grant to invite households to participate in my projects. I brought small gifts to the outreach workers and answered their questions regarding diabetes, hypertension, and other health issues. I taught them about patient education on diabetes self-care, helped them to develop a pocket book of pictorial educational materials and to set up bulletin boards on the topic of diabetes awareness. In addition, I discussed my project with an indigenous community health care worker of Ke Ola Mano, Urban Honolulu Project. We planned an exercise program, cooking classes, and educational sessions together. I also invited the worker to participate in the annual health fair held by the School of Nursing, University of Hawaii at Manoa. The public health nurses and I also provided free hypertension and diabetes screening in KPT Family Center's Volunteer Information Person's (VIP) Training. I also participated in the Thanksgiving and Christmas parties held by the outreach workers and health care providers at the clinic center of the community. This project demonstrates how important it is to communicate and forge professional relationships with leaders of different programs and organizations within the community.

REFERENCES

Berman, B. A., Grosser, S. C., & Gritz, E. R. (1998). Recruitment to a school-based adult smoking-cessation program: Do gender and race/ethnicity make a difference? *Journal of Cancer Education, 13*(4), 220–225.

Eng, E. (1993). Partnership theory. In *Nurse Leadership Caring for the emerging majority: Empowering nurses through partnerships & coalitions* (pp. 27–34). Washington, DC: U.S. Department of Education.

Faller, H. S., Dowell, M. A., & Jackson, M. A. (1995). Bridge to the future: Nontraditional clinical settings, concepts and issues. *Journal of Nursing Education, 34*(8), 344–349.

Frey, M. A., & Denyes, M. J. (1989). Health and illness self-care in adolescents with IDDM: A test of Orem's theory. *Advances in Nursing Science, 12*(1), 67–75.

Iso, H., Shimamoto, T., Naito, Y., Sato, S., Kitamura, A., Iida, M., Konishi, M., Jacobs, D. R., Jr., & Komachi, Y. (1998). Effects of a long-term hypertension control program on stroke incidence and prevalence in a rural community in northeastern Japan. *Stroke, 29*(8), 1510–18.

Moyer, A., Coristine, M., MacLean, L., & Meyer, M. (1999). A model for building collective capacity in community-based programs: the elderly in need project. *Public Health Nursing, 16*(3), 205–214.

Pinfold, J. V. (1999). Analysis of different communication channels for promoting hygiene behavior. *Health Education Research, 14*(5), 629–639.

Price, J. L., & Cordell, B. (1997). Empowerment as a source of healing: Redefining the art of nursing management. *Revolution, 7*(2), 45–5.

Voyle, J. A., & Simmons, D. (1999). Community development through partnership: Promoting health in an urban indigenous com-

munity in New Zealand. *Social Science &
Medicine, 49,* 1035–1050.
Wang, C. Y., Abbott, L., Goodbody, A. K., Hui,
W. T. Y., & Rausch, C. (1999). Development
of a community-based diabetes manage-
ment program for Pacific Islanders. *Diabetes
Educator, 25*(5), 738–746.

Wang, C. Y., & Fenske, M. (1996). Self-care of
adults with non-insulin-dependent diabetes
mellitus: Influence of family and friends.
Diabetes Educator, 22(5), 465–470.

CHAPTER 24

Parish Nursing

Susan MacLeod Dyess

HEALTH AND WELLNESS PROMOTION IN THE PARISH

As you ought not to attempt to cure the eyes without the head, or the head without the body, so neither ought you to attempt to cure the body without the soul . . . for the part will never be well unless the whole is well.

—Plato

A holistic caring approach is natural and implicit to parish practice. The holistic wellness model fundamentally embraces whole person health, utilizes minimal technological intervention, and maximizes noninvasive techniques. Parish practice combines elements of primary prevention and the holistic model in community organizations known as faith communities. The client is the faith community (McDermott & Burke, 1993). Faith communities include the congregation members of churches, mosques, and synagogues. The concept of parish practice encourages you to join with communities of faith in efforts to promote the whole-person health of their members. Central to the practice of whole-person health promotion is the spiritual dimen-

sion, but parish approaches also incorporate the psychological, physical and social dimensions of care (Solari-Twadell, McDermott, Ryan, & Djupe, 1994).

Whole-person health promotion in the faith community is a strong area of interest nationally and internationally. It has a longstanding history in Europe, Australia, New Zealand, and it is now being investigated in Korea (Simmington, Olson, & Douglass, 1996, p. 20). Parish practice is being considered as one of several strategies to reform health care in Canada (Martin, 1996; Simmington, Olson, & Douglass, 1996). In America, the parish practice delivery model places emphasis on holistic health care, wellness promotion, and preventive intervention. It has emerged as a noninvasive, nurturing practice in which creative approaches to whole-person health may be unfolded (Solari-Twadell, McDermott, & Matheus, 1997; Weis, Matheus, & Schank, 1997; Schank, Weis, & Matheus, 1996; Miskelly, 1995).

History

Parish practice is not original to this country nor to this century. Conceptually, it can be traced to Judeo-Christian beliefs and actions such as the expressions of health and healing in the Hebrew and Christian scriptures. For the church, the service of health care was a caring expression of the love of God (or Christ) through His dedicated servants. "From the earliest point in its history, the Christian church assumed the care of the sick, the poor and the helpless" (Donahue, 1985, p. 102). In church history the deacons and deaconesses performed services of health care and healing as acts of worship. Zersen (1994) recounts how the early Christian deaconesses and the German deaconesses of the 1800s addressed the diverse concerns of the church members.

Recent History

Four factors have fueled the interest and growth of modern parish practice over the last two decades. In the late 1970s, a shift of focus occurred in the national and international model of health care. The shift from disease care and illness care toward preventive and promotional health care began. In the 1980s, efforts were made to accommodate the transformation of health care focus; but in 1990 *Healthy People 2000* was established as a national initiative and cooperative effort among government organizations, businesses, individuals, professional and voluntary groups in pursuit of improved health for all Americans (U.S. Department of Health and Human Services [DHHS], 1991). Now, *Healthy People 2010* has been set up. It builds on the framework and initiatives of *Healthy People 2000*. Parish practice embodies a position to facilitate the actualization of the whole-person health objectives found in these initiatives. Marty (1990) believes it is obvious to include faith communities in the solutions

for health and healing found in *Healthy People 2010*.

A second factor in the late 1970s was Reverend Granger Westberg. He was a hospital chaplain and medical school professor who contemplated the collaboration of congregations and health care. Westberg worked with several nurses and other health care professionals in whole-person care clinics, a holistic health care project in the Chicago area. He recognized the value of the whole-person approach (Westberg, 1989).

The recognition of the value of having a whole-person approach and Westberg's theological training spawned an idea to promote whole-person attentiveness within a project that united a church, a hospital, and professional nurses (Westberg, 1987). In the early 1980s, Westberg developed and gave leadership to the first American hospital-based parish nurse project, which included six nurses (Holst, 1987; Westberg, 1987, 1989). The modern resurgence of the concept of parish nursing began.

A third factor in the growth of modern parish practice is the National Parish Nurse Resource Center, currently identified as the International Parish Nurse Resource Center (IPNRC). It was established in 1986 with the principal intent of storing and sharing information regarding activities of nursing in congregations across the country. (Solari-Twadell, 1998). The IPNRC has continued to be responsible for the resourcing of parish nursing knowledge and has taken an active role in the education and curriculum development for the parish nurse. Their contributions to modern parish practice are invaluable. They also host and organize the Westberg symposium, which is the annual gathering of professional parish nurses.

Another factor responsible for the momentum of the modern parish nursing movement is its establishment as a specialty practice. The Scope and Standards of Parish Nursing Practice were approved March 1998 by the American Nurses Association (ANA, 1998). These standards "describe the minimum level of professional care and professional performance common to all nurses engaged in clinical practice" (Small, 1997, p. 62). Although the scope and standards are not comprehensive in their description and account of parish nurse practice, they do provide an element of professional grounding and accountability.

MODELS OF ADMINISTRATION

Continued evolution and development of parish practice within individual parishes has occurred across America, but essential generalities remain unchanged. The whole-person practice continues to combine the skill and knowledge of nursing, ministry, sciences, and humanities to facilitate, support, sustain, and strengthen congregations. From the beginning, four basic conceptual administrative models of parish nursing were identified in the literature. These models are organizational frameworks upon which parish programs might be constructed. The models may serve to guide administrative development of parish practice within a community. The four models include:

1. Based from a hospital and salaried: You are salaried by the institution, and an agreement or covenant is made between the faith community and the hospital. This model can serve a single or multiple congregations within the larger community. The hospital can provide professional support and referrals, supplies, and continuing education.

2. Based from a hospital and volunteer: You and others are volunteers identified within various faith communities and are sponsored by the institution. This model can serve multiple congregations based on the volunteer/congregational interest. Again in this model, the hospital can provide professional support and referrals, supplies and continuing education for the participating nurses.

3. Based from a congregation and salaried: You are salaried by the congregation, and an agreement is made between the congregation and the practitioner. This model serves the population of the congregation. The professional support, referrals, supplies, and continuing education are not linked to an institution, nor are they preestablished.

4. Based from a congregation and volunteer: You and others are volunteers, agreeing to serve the congregation's identified needs. This model serves the population of the congregation. Again in this faith community-based model, no institutional link is preestablished.

Modifications in the original four administrative models are seen throughout the literature, such as volunteers receiving a stipend for their efforts or hospitals and faith communities sharing the financial responsibility. No one model has been identified in the literature as the one to emulate (Solari-Twadell & McDermott, 1999; Schank, Weis, & Matheus, 1996).

PARISH PRACTICE FUNCTIONS

An assumption made in the whole-person wellness model found in chapter 1 is that a health-promotion practitioner can facilitate a higher level of wellness. The functions include but are not limited to health educator, health counselor, referral source, and facilitator (Westberg, 1987). These functions actually describe the ongoing activities of the parish practitioner. Striepe,

King, and Scott (1993) offer the acronym HEALTH to denote the varied services of the parish practitioner: Health counselor, Educator, Advocate, Liaison to the community, Teacher, and Health promoter.

As a health counselor, you collaborate with the client regarding health issues and concerns and make home or hospital visits as needed. The health educator duty supports individuals through numerous instructional activities. As a referral source, you are the liaison to the greater community resources. The facilitator function coordinates, role-models, provides leadership, and recruits others for various support activities identified. More recently a fifth function has been defined as interpreter of the relationship between faith and health. This fifth function is described as an ongoing activity that overlaps the other four to promote an understanding of the correlation among well-being, beliefs, values, and behaviors (Noble, Redmond, Williams, & Langley, 1996; Schank, Weis, & Matheus, 1996; Armmer & Humbles, 1995; McDermott & Burke, 1993). It is important to remember, however, that the suggested functions are not an exhaustive nor exclusive list to hinder practice. Rather, the functions may serve to guide you as your practice. Box 24.1 shows an adapted version of the acronym HEALTH first coined by Striepe, King, and Scott (1993).

PRACTICE POSSIBILITIES

The possibilities for parish practice are bountiful. The global makeup of the congregation, who is your client, and the community at large should determine your directional focus. Your practice should not duplicate community services but rather address the unmet needs identified by a thorough community assessment. There is

opportunity for creativity and utilization of your specific talents. Your practice can provide an opportunity for services to transcend a traditional health care role and the traditional boundaries of health care institutions. The practice mandates that you be responsive to the trends and changes in health care. Furthermore, your practice has the freedom to support the spiritual dimension of the clients' faith fellowship. Hilsman (1997) contends that parish practice provides key interdisciplinary links as it addresses the clients' spiritual issues by utilizing the assimilated proficiency of technical and physical knowledge, interpersonal skills, compassion, and ministry awareness. The possibilities for practice are truly endless. See Box 24.2 for ideas for parish practice.

Exemplars

Within the nursing literature there are numerous descriptive reports of how these whole-person health programs have influenced their communities. Four examples highlight the vast primary, promotional, and supportive care possibilities within a faith community.

Exemplar 1: Use of a Church Newsletter

In their discussion of parish nursing, Schank, Weis, and Matheus (1996) relay an experience of health education resulting in a specific positive health outcome. The blend of assessing and anticipating the diversity of the congregation, providing accurate and appropriate information, and using a familiar, friendly church communication impacted a woman as she was experiencing the classic signs and symptoms of a heart attack. Previously, during National Heart Month, the parish nurse disclosed the early warning signs of a heart attack in

---

Box 24.1   Parish Practitioner Functions

Health counselor
   Discusses client health issues, reassures and supports during times of crisis or concerns about illness, medication, and well-being. A parish nurse deals with diverse health issues and makes home or hospital visits as needed.

Educator
   Promotes and sustains the understanding of the relationship between faith, health, attitudes, and lifestyle choices through numerous instructional activities.

Advocate
   Identifies the medically underinsured, indigent, or abandoned members of the faith community who need support and nurturance. Co-narrates the health perspective with the faith community.

Liaison
   Acts as a liaison to a variety of faith community resources and links the faith community members to the services of the greater community.

Trainer/teacher
   Recruits, supervises, and strengthens unpaid workers for health ministry. Provides formation and education to assist them in their role.

Healer/health promoter
   Facilitates whole-person approach through caring Promotes and sustains an understanding of the relatedness of wholeness, beliefs, values, and lifestyle practices.

Box 24.2   Possibilities for Parish Practice

- Personal health counseling
- Comprehensive health screening
- Blood pressure screening
- Weight monitoring
- Stress monitoring
- Homebound screening
- Referral and resource information
- Home and hospital visits
- Educational classes

a church newsletter. Feeling poorly a few weeks later, the woman from the congregation recalled the helpful information. Because she remembered those early warning signals and notified her physician, medical intervention was possible. The woman credits the church newsletter with saving her life.

Exemplar 2: Wellness Practice in an African American Church Community

Armmer and Humbles (1995) developed a parish nursing project they established with a 1-year grant entitled the Christian Nurses Preventive Health Project. The aim of the project was to have a wellness focus on an underserved urban, mainly African American church community. Blood pressure monitoring, breast health education, and wellness counseling were the three primary objectives of the project. Their efforts fostered an arena of trust for dialogue and expression of concerns. They met their objectives as measured by congregation reports of increased self-confidence and the members' willingness to take part in their own health. The 1-year project was deemed successful by both parish practitioners and the faith community participating in the program

Exemplar 3: Parish Practice After a Summer Flood Disaster

Monaco (1990) recounted her experience within a suburban faith community. Initially a health fair inspired congregation members to become interested in the program. The screenings and referrals of the fair revealed three silent, but life-threatening conditions that were not known to the individuals. Thereafter, Monaco's health promotion role became flexible, responding to faith community needs as they developed, including during a summer flood.

Her work as a parish practitioner was to match the strengths and gifts of each volunteer with the needs of the community. Efforts included coordinating clean-up teams, providing a tetanus inoculation center, feeding over 500 families for 2 weeks, assisting the Red Cross with on-site management of aid provision to flood victims, and making referrals to posttrauma counseling services when necessary. Success was measured by the diverse support provided through her efforts.

Exemplar 4: A Rural Parish Practice

A rural experience is highlighted from northwest Iowa (Striepe, 1990). A network of several nurses served a 9,000-square-mile zone. It was noted that many were already serving as informal parish nurses and had already established the trust and acceptance of their clients. Home visits, support groups, exercise classes, and transportation assistance occupied the activities of the professionals. Although some of the parishes wanted the focus to be on physical care, the emphasis on whole-person health and wellness continues to be and should be the focus in the rural experience.

SELF CARE FOR THE PARISH PRACTITIONER

An important part of a holistic wellness model is self care. Self care or self nurturance is discussed by holistic scholars (Dossey, Keegan, Guzzetta, & Kolkmeir, 1995). Because the most important tool within the holistic caring relationship is you, your personal readiness to connect with another is considered a phase of preparation. Spiritual maturity for the professional is implied within the literature as a point of preparation for practice, but specifics of preparation are rarely mentioned. Personal readiness is difficult to quantify. Many times it requires introspection and personal reflection.

Specific self-care practices for the parish nurse are not evident in the literature. Self care of the body is obvious to most of us as a priority. What may not be as obvious is the self care of the spirit. Your spiritual self-care practice must incorporate the spiritual disciplines highlighted by Foster (1978). He discusses the disciplines of spiritual growth. Each section of his book explores instruction and convincing arguments for practicing and celebrating the spiritual journey in the context of human action. It is a clearly articulated guide that humbly suggests the pathway to greater spiritual intimacy.

PARISH PRACTICE THEORY AND RESEARCH

Research in parish practice is limited (Ryan, 1997). A few have considered parish nursing within the framework of applied nursing theory (Berquist & King, 1994; Gustafson, 1993; Schmidt-Bunkers, Michales, & Ethridge, 1997). The theory of nursing as caring (Boykin & Schoenhofer, 1993) is quite appropriate to parish practice. As a grand or meta-theory for nursing, nursing as caring (NAC) encompasses all aspects of wellness and health promotion. NAC is unique as it reframes health promotion within the context of caring and wholeness. The theory describes the focus for nursing as "coming to know person(s) in the moment" and "nurturing wholeness through caring" (p. 3). Wholeness acknowledges the interrelatedness and inseparable nature of the physiological, psychological, social, and spiritual aspects of persons. You may have a selected a theory that resonates with you.

DEVELOPING A PARISH PRACTICE

Exploring how a whole-person health and wellness promotion program can fit into your overall faith community should occur as a parallel and collaborative process between the you, the pastor, a health ministry task force or committee, the greater community, and possibly a specific health care organization. The deliberate involvement of the pastor and a health ministry task force or committee establishes a solid foundation and understanding of the value of a whole-person health within the faith community. From the time of conception until your implementation as a staff or volunteer, many important steps can be taken to prepare your faith community. Often the process takes 6 to 18 months.

Suggested steps in this process include the determination of an administrative model; appraisal of the faith community; education of the faith community; and collaboration with others.

One of the first steps you need to consider is the selection of a model of administration that you will implement. There are pros and cons with each model. Your greater community health care climate may determine this for you. Hidden in the selection process of the model of administration is the obstacle of funding. Once you select a model of administration you can proceed.

Education of your faith community, your client, is also a priority. It is important for the client to understand that your practice will be a noninvasive, community, caring approach to whole-person health. Explain that the practice is grounded in the tenets of primary health care, community nursing, and holistic philosophy. You may want to highlight that you will work within the values, context, and practices of the denomination and that scope and standards for practice exist.

A community appraisal is strongly encouraged and should include a thorough community assessment and focus group interviews. After the analysis of the community appraisal you can then design your unique supportive responses for your faith community. Your ongoing presence will enable the members of your faith community to partake in the continued development and refinement of the responses. Remember client reactions and use them to build your practice in collaboration with the client.

A final suggested step to develop a whole-person health practice in your faith community is to utilize the gifts and talents of others. Involving congregation members—your clients—and empowering them to participate can be accomplished with the help of the health ministry task force or committee. It is suggested that the task force be comprised of several members of the congregation to ensure diverse input in the planning (Westberg, 1990). Creative avenues for utilizing all members of your faith community should be explored to support the practice. Furthermore, collaboration with community service organizations is essential for community partnerships to thrive (Anderson & Mcfarlane, 1998).

SUMMARY

Parish nursing is a newly recognized specialty practice for professional nursing. It is fundamentally linked to Judeo-Christian traditions, the tenets of primary health care, community nursing, and holistic wellness philosophy. It is whole-person focused and is noninvasive. Central to the practice is the awareness of the relationship between lifestyle, faith, personal habits, attitudes, and wholeness. The current health care climate demands that nursing refocus on its ability to provide health care services by nontraditional methods (Oesterle & O'Callaghan, 1996). Faith communities of America can now reclaim their historical role of providing health care ministries in conjunction with local resources. Utilizing your skills, you can be a powerful catalyst within a faith community to bring an assertive and creative approach to wellness and wholeness.

REFERENCES

American Nurses Association. 1998. *Scope and standards of parish nursing practice.* Washington, DC: American Nurses Association.

Armmer, F. A., & Humbles, P. (1995). Parish nursing: Extending health care to urban African-Americans. *Nursing and Health Care: Perspectives on Community, 16*(2), 64–68.

Anderson, E. T., & McFarlane, J. (1998). *Community as partner: Theory and practice in nursing.* New York: Lippincott.

Berquist, S., & King, J. (1994). Parish nursing: A conceptual framework. *Journal of Holistic Nursing, 12*(2), 155–170.

Boykin, A., & Schoenhofer, S. (1993). *Nursing as caring: A model for transforming nursing practice.* New York: National League for Nursing Press.

Donahue, M. P. (1985). *Nursing: The finest art.* St. Louis, MO: Mosby.

Dossey, B. M., Keegan, L., Guzzetta, C. E., & Kolkmeir, L. G. (1995). *Holistic nursing: A handbook for practice* (2nd ed.). Gaithersburg, MD: Aspen.

Foster, R. J. (1978). *Celebration of discipline: The pathway to spiritual growth.* San Francisco: Harper-Collins.

Gustafson, W. (1993). Application of Newman's theory of health: Pattern recognition as nursing practice. In M. Parker (Ed.), *Patterns of nursing theory in practice.* New York: National League for Nursing Press.

Hilsman, G. J. (1997, June). Spiritual pathways: One response to the current standards challenge. *Vision,* 8–12.

Holst, L. E. (1987). The parish nurse. *Chronicle of Pastoral Care, 7*(1), 13–17.

Martin, L. B. (1996, January). Parish nursing: Keeping body and soul together. *The Canadian Nurse,* 25–28.

Marty, M. E. (1990). Health, medicine, and the faith traditions. In *Healthy People 2000: A role for America's religious communities* (pp. 11–14). A joint publication of the Carter Center, Atlanta, GA; and the Park Ridge Center, Chicago.

McDermmott, M. A., & Burke, J. (1993). When the population is a congregation: The emerging role of the parish nurse. *Journal of Community Health Nursing, 10*(3), 179–190.

Miskelly, S. A. (1995). Parish nursing model: Applying the community health nursing process in church community. *Journal of Community Health Nursing, 12*(1), 1–14.

Monaco, S. (1990). The developing practice of the parish nurse: A suburban experience. In P. A. Solari-Twadell, A. M. Djupe, & M. A. McDermott (Eds.), *Parish nursing: The developing practice.* Park Ridge, IL: The National Parish Nurse Resource Center.

Noble, M. A., Redmond, G. M., Williams, J. K., & Langley, C. (1996). A community focused curriculum. *Nursing and Health Care: Perspectives on Community, 17*(2), 66–71.

Oesterle, M., & O'Callaghan, D. (1996). The changing health care environment. *Nursing and Health Care: Perspectives on Community, 17*(2), 78–81.

Ryan, J. (1997). Assuring the future quality of parish nursing practice. *Perspectives, 5*(3), 4.

Schank, M. J., Weis, D., & Matheus, R. (1996). Parish nursing: Ministry of healing. *Geriatric Nursing, 17*(1), 11–13.

Schmidt-Bunkers, S., Michaels, C., & Ethridge, P. (1997). Advanced practice nursing in community: Nursing's opportunity. *Advanced Practice Nursing Quarterly, 2*(4), 79–84.

Simmington, J., Olson, J., & Douglass, L. (1996, January). Promoting well-being within a parish. *The Canadian Nurse,* 20–24.

Small, N. C. (1997). The 5 "w's" of standards of practice; what, why, who, when, where. Abstract presented at the eighth annual conference. Health Ministries Association, Inc., pp. 61–73.

Solari-Twadell, P. A. (1998). [Editorial.] *Perspectives, 6*(3), 2.

Solari-Twadell, P. A., & McDermott, M. A. (Eds.). (1999). *Parish nursing: Promoting whole person health in faith communities.* Thousand Oaks: Sage.

Solari-Twadell, P. A., McDermott, M. A., & Matheus, R. (1997). Education for parish nursing: Assuring congregational health and wholeness for the twenty-first century. *Perspectives, 5*(3), 1–3.

Solari-Twadell, P. A., McDermott, M. A., Ryan, J. A., & Djupe, A. M. (1994). Assuring viability for the future. *Guideline development for parish nurse education programs.* Park Ridge, IL: Luthern General Health System.

Striepe, J. (1990). The developing practice of the parish nurse: A rural experience. In P. A. Solari-Twadell, A. M. Djupe, & M. A. McDermott (Eds.), *Parish nursing: The developing practice.* Park Ridge, IL: The National Parish Nurse Resource Center.

Striepe, J., King, J. M., & Scott, L. (1993, Winter). Nurses in the church: Profiles in caring. *Journal of Christian Nursing,* 8–10.

U.S. Department of Health and Human Services. (1991). *Healthy people 2000: National health promotion and disease preventive objectives.* (DHHS Publication No. (PHS) 91-50213). Washington, DC: U.S. Government Printing Office.

Weis, D., Matheus, R., & Schank, M. J. (1997). Health care delivery in faith communities: The parish nurse model. *Public Health Nursing, 14*(6), 368–372.

Westberg, G. (1987) *The parish nurse: How to start a parish nurse program in your church.* Park Ridge, IL: National Parish Nurse Resource Center.

Westberg, G. (1989). Parish nursing pioneer. *Journal of Christian Nursing, 6*(1), 26–29.

Westberg, G. (1990). *The parish nurse.* Minneapolis, MN: Augsberg Press.

Zersen, D. (1994). Parish nursing: 20th century fad? *Journal of Christian Nursing, 11*(2), 19–21 & 45.

PART VI

Lessons From Sample Health Promotion Programs

CHAPTER 25

Conducting a Survey: The Example of a Youth Service Organization

Robert W. Strack

ELEMENTS OF THE MARS PROJECT

This chapter is based on a project conducted in Maryland that has endeavored to assess the health risks of youth residing in group homes and shelters throughout the state. Through the Monitoring Adolescents in Risky Situations (MARS) Project, a survey was developed and administered to youth that have been historically shown to be at high risk for HIV and other health problems. You might find it helpful to think about how the steps outlined in this chapter might be applied to surveying a population that you are interested in working with. Although not all surveillance efforts are identical, there are commonalties of process and standard protocols that need to be followed when conducting a survey. One of the first steps in the process is to establish the need for finding out more about the population you or your organization is interested in.

Establishing Need for the Surveillance Effort

For the MARS project to get off the ground the case was made that nationally and in the state of Maryland, nearly one fifth of AIDS cases are reported among young adults (Centers for Disease Control [CDC], 1994). Because many of these individuals are likely to have been infected during their teenage years, surveillance of adolescent risk-taking and protective behaviors is vital to prevention. Currently many states collect annual behavioral risk data on adolescents using the Youth Risk Behavior Survey (Kolbe, Kahn, & Collins, 1993; Kann et al., 1998); however, this survey is not designed to capture the high-risk circumstances of "out-of-home" youth (runaway, homeless, and street). Other out-of-home youth include youths living in group homes and shelters (systems youth), many of whom have experienced runaway and homeless episodes (Ensign & Santelli, 1997). Studies have shown that these youth are among the populations at greatest risk for HIV (Slonim-Nevo, Ozawa, & Auslander, 1991) and other health problems. The lives of many of these youth are characterized by lack of family support, poverty, physical and emotional abuse, drug use, and unsafe sexual behaviors. In response to the health risks faced by this population of youth, the Centers for Disease Control and Prevention supported the Maryland AIDS Administration and the Center for Adolescent Health Promotion and Disease Prevention at Johns Hopkins University to assess the risks faced by a portion of out-of-home youth in the state of Maryland.

Setting up a Steering Committee

When conducting a study or survey there is no reason to go it alone. In fact, if you look around you will find there are others who are interested in the same questions, issues, and people that you are. You should consider the possibility of setting up a steering committee to help in guiding your study. A *steering committee* is a group of individuals, typically from external organizations or areas, who can provide guidance to an endeavor, or in this case, a research study. Not only is a steering committee often a prerequisite for funders, but setting up a steering committee is also a great mechanism for gaining valuable insight, direction, and support for your survey efforts. In addition, much of the research being conducted in the name of addressing the public's health is being challenged and encouraged to be inclusive of the professionals and individuals within the community being served. The steering committee for the MARS project included directors and staff members from youth group homes, state health department representatives, and a representative from a national orga-

nization that advocates on behalf of youth. A steering committee is a simple first step in engaging vested interests within the community surrounding your population of interest.

There are some of critical components to keep in mind when forming a steering committee for your study. You should make a list of organizations that would benefit from the results of your survey as well as those that have insights to the population being surveyed. From this list you should establish those who are likely to be available to guide your project as it is developed and carried out. You should also consider how organizations might benefit from their involvement with your project. Might new relationships be formed as a result of their talking and listening to each other through their steering committee capacity? Might new funding opportunities arise from these budding relationships or from the results of your survey? There is no reason a steering committee should be any less useful to its members or to their organizations than it is to the project or study itself.

Reporting of Results to Project Constituents

If your are entering a community to conduct a survey or targeting a particular population in order to determine a question of interest, you are likely to be a visitor within someone else's domain or world. As a visitor you have the foremost responsibility to give before you have the right to take. In this spirit, you should enter your study or survey with the intention of giving, or benefiting, the group you are surveying and the professional community that supports this population. You should determine in advance what information is to be collected, with whom the information will be shared, and in what forms. Answers to these questions will guide the formation of your project and will provide direction as to how the results of your survey should be shared. The results and lessons learned from the MARS project is being shared with state and local agencies in an effort to promote communication and collaboration between organizations for the benefit of out-of-home youth.

STEPS TO CARRYING OUT A SURVEY PROJECT

Before you begin your project you should have some idea of the sequence of events that will take place as your project progresses. The *principal investigator* (PI) is the lead researcher, manager, and responsible agent of a research study. It is the responsibility of the principal investigator to establish the grand plan for conducting the survey, which includes establishing and monitoring the study's activities and progress and adherence to quality standards. A significant component of this responsibility is establishing a sensible timeline, gaining organizational approval for the survey or study, hiring, training, and monitoring data collectors, and carrying out the actual steps of the data collection effort.

Establishing a Timeline for Project Activities

Establishing a timeline for project activities will likely be a requirement for securing funding to get your data collection effort going. In order to undertake this task you will need to have an idea of the major events or milestones your project will face. One of the first will be the task of gaining approval from one or more institutional review boards (IRBs), which is needed before a study can be carried out. Time will also

need to be budgeted for preparation and planning of the surveying process in addition to the actual time needed for collecting data. Including your steering committee in this process will assist you in your planning by offering insights to the workings of the organizations with which you will be collaborating to collect data. Mapping out how long the data collection process will take will be dictated by the data collection methods employed and the limitations of you and your team's ability to complete the process. Box 25.1 provides a simplified timeline for the MARS study.

Gaining Approval from Institutional Review Boards

An *institutional review board* (IRB) is the governing body of an institution that provides initial and continuing reviews of research being undertaken by and through the institution. IRBs carry the primary function of assuring the protection of the rights, welfare, and personal privacy of human subjects who participate in study activities. Your institution's review committee has the responsibility to make an independent determination of whether your study poses any possible risks and whether the study's procedures offer protections for study participants. Because the process of gaining approval can often be a lengthy one, potentially involving multiple IRBs and review meetings, you should familiarize yourself with the process required within your organization and within the organizations with which you will be working. This process should take 1 to 3 months, but could take much longer. In the case of the MARS project, approval from several review boards was required before a single youth could be contacted. This involved preparing documents for the review boards of the univer-

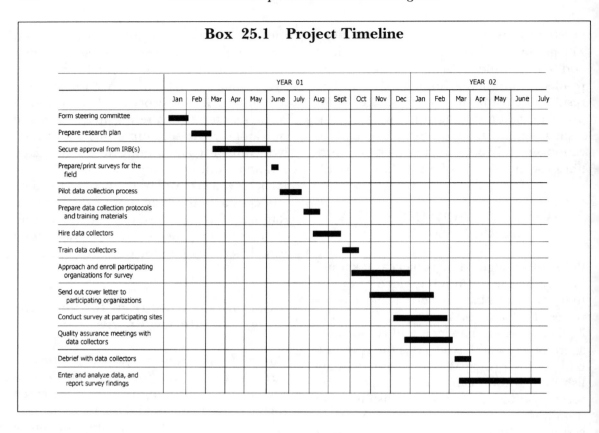

Box 25.1   Project Timeline

	YEAR 01												YEAR 02						
	Jan	Feb	Mar	Apr	May	June	July	Aug	Sept	Oct	Nov	Dec	Jan	Feb	Mar	Apr	May	June	July
Form steering committee	■																		
Prepare research plan		■																	
Secure approval from IRB(s)			■■■■																
Prepare/print surveys for the field						■													
Pilot data collection process							■■												
Prepare data collection protocols and training materials								■											
Hire data collectors									■										
Train data collectors										■									
Approach and enroll participating organizations for survey											■■■								
Send out cover letter to participating organizations												■■■							
Conduct survey at participating sites												■■■							
Quality assurance meetings with data collectors													■■						
Debrief with data collectors															■				
Enter and analyze data, and report survey findings														■■■■				

sity, the state department of health, the Centers for Disease Control, and the state agencies that oversee the welfare of youth in group homes and shelters. Because of the sensitive nature of the questions being asked, the age of the survey's respondents, and the number of institutions from which approval for the study was needed, the MARS project required a very lengthy review process. The principal investigator should be prepared to carefully shepherd the project through this process. Allowing for adequate to time navigate the IRB process should be a critical component of any project plan.

Gaining IRB approval from the organizations relevant to your survey effort will likely be the first major milestone in your planning process. To navigate the IRB process

you will need to prepare a study protocol, participant assent/consent forms, parental consent forms, and provide any instruments you will be using as part of your study or survey. For more information on institutional review boards, you can access the home page for the Office for Protection from Research Risks (OPRR) (*http://www.nih.gov/grants/oprr/oprr.htm*). It is OPRR responsibility to monitor compliance with the Code of Federal Regulations, Title 45, Part 46–Protection of Human Subjects, which is used to inform and monitor federally funded domestic and international research involving human research participants. The 45 CFR 46 federal code can be accessed at *http://www.nih.gov:80/grants/oprr/humansubjects/45cfr46.htm*. OPRR is currently housed in the National

Institutes of Health (NIH) within the U.S. Department of Health and Human Services.

The Research Protocol

Most IRBs will need a research protocol that outlines the study or survey you are proposing to carry out. The *research protocol* is a concise report of a proposed research study that highlights the information necessary for an institutional review board to understand a study's purpose and impact on study participants. Box 25.2 contains the necessary components of a research protocol; however, the review board of your institution should be consulted to ensure that the research protocol follows its required format and content.

The Informed Consent Process

The *informed consent process* is the written and oral explanation of a research study that a potential participant will need for determining whether or not they would like to become involved voluntarily in the research study. An informed consent process is needed any time a study involves the participation of human subjects such as the MARS project with its survey of youth in group homes and shelters. The consent process should be given a very high priority by the principal investigator because the protection of human participants in a research study is an ethical imperative. It requires that researchers present in written form and oral explanation the necessary information that a potential participant will need for determining whether they would like to become involved in a research study. It should be stressed that the informed consent process is designed to ensure the voluntary nature of participation. There are

some basic principles of informed consent that need to be adhered to:

1.   No research study may involve human beings as participants without effective informed consent of the participants or their legally authorized representative.

2.   The conditions under which consent is sought should provide potential participants with sufficient opportunity to decide whether to participate and should minimize the possibility of coercion.

3.   The information that is given should be in language that is understandable to potential participants or their representative.

4.   No informed consent should include language whereby potential participants are made to waive their legal rights or that releases the investigator, study sponsor, or institution from liability for negligence (DHHS, 1991).

Consent/Assent Forms

The central components of the informed consent process are the consent and youth assent forms used to describe the study to participants. Because the MARS study involved participants under the age of 18, parental consent and youth assent were required for youth participation. Similar to the research protocol, consent forms should address a number of required elements before it can be approved for use in a research study. For more information on institutional review boards, you can access the home page for the Office for Human Research Protections (OHRP) (*http://ohrp.osophs.dhhs.gov/*). It is OHRP's responsibility to monitor compliance with the Code of Federal Regulations, Title 45, Part 46—Protections of Humans Subjects, which

Box 25.2 Writing the IRB Research Plan

- Name of research study
- Purpose of research study
  What are the research questions being addressed by the proposed study?
- Rationale for the research
  What is the related research that provides justification for the study, and why is the proposed study important?
- Study methods
  What is the study's design? What is the sample size or particulars of the study's participants? How will participants be recruited and involved with the research project? What instruments will be used in carrying out the study? Are procedures in place for dealing with illegal or adverse events? (In the case of the MARS project, procedures needed to be established if youth revealed that they were currently being abused. This was established due to the fact that state law dictates that any adult with knowledge of a child's being abused is required to report such abuse to the legal system.)
- Risks and benefits of the study
  What are the risks that your participants are exposed to from their involvement? What steps are being taken to minimize risk to participants? How many burdens does your study place on participants? Do the participants gain any benefit from participation? Will the research study and its results benefit others?
- Study disclosure and consent processes
  How will the study be disclosed or presented to potential participants? Does the process allow for participants to decline to participate comfortably and easily? Are participants coerced to participate in any way? Do participants have the opportunity to ask questions and get clarification on their questions? Is the consent form easy to read and understand? Are participants given ample time to think about whether they would like to participate? Are the proper procedures being followed for the assent/consent of minors?
- Assurances of confidentiality
  Are procedures in place for ensuring the confidentiality of the study's data and for protecting the anonymity of study participants? Who will have access to the study's data?
- Collaborative agreements and IRB approvals with other organizations
  Is the study being conducted in collaboration with other organizations? Do the organizations you are working with have a study review process or IRB?

Box 25.3   Elements of an Informed Consent Form

An informed consent must include:

1. The purpose and procedures of the research study
2. A description of any risks or discomforts to the participant
3. A description of any benefits for the participant or for others
4. A statement informing individuals of the available alternatives to their participation
5. An explanation of the level of confidentiality
6. A statement disclosing any greater than minimal risks (minimal risk is the probability and magnitude that any harm from the study is not greater than those ordinarily encountered in daily life)
7. The listing of a contact person who can be called if the participant has any questions
8. A statement that emphasizes the voluntary nature of participation and that the participant may refuse to participate or withdraw from the study at any time without penalty

---

is used to inform and monitor federally funded domestic and international research involving human research participants. The 45 CFR 46 federal code can be accessed at *http://ohrp.osophs.dhhs.gov/humansubjects/guidance/45cfr46.htm.* OHRP is located in the Office of Public Health and Science within the Office of the Secretary of the Department of Health and Human Services. Additional information on consent forms can also be found at the OHRP site (*http://ohrp.osophs.dhhs.gov/humansubjects/guidance/ictip.htm*).

Box 25.3 provides a summary of the necessary elements for a consent form.

Keeping the IRB Informed through Amendments and the Annual Review

Once your study has been approved by the relevant IRBs you will need to keep them up-to-date on any changes that you make to your study's procedures or instruments. Through the use of amendments, you will be able to modify your file with the respective IRBs. If the changes are relatively minor, your study may be reviewed again by a subcommittee of the IRB, at which point it will either be accepted or recommended for review by the full committee. The activity of your research study will also need to be reviewed at least annually by each IRB for the duration of the study. This annual review will incorporate any changes in the IRBs' policies on protecting human subjects as well as address any changes your study protocol has undergone since the last full committee review.

The review processes that have been established are designed to ensure that human subjects are protected and are based on previous research experiences. Although it may seem onerous at times, one should never minimize the importance of the charge of protecting study participants. Once the principal investigator has successfully navigated this process, he or she can move on to the task of collecting data.

Preparing and Carrying Out the Data Collection Process

Once the necessary review boards have approved your study, there are plenty of preparatory steps that will need to take place before the actual collection of data can begin. The survey instrument will need to be prepared and copies made ready for administration. Field testing of the survey administration process should be conducted in order to determine whether changes to the data collection protocols are needed. Data collectors will need to be hired and trained prior to going out into the field. Organizations that are participating in the administration of the survey will need to be informed of the study, and plans will need to be worked out for administering the survey at their site. With the proper planning and preparation you will hopefully be able to collect your data in an efficient manner.

Conducting a Field Test of the Survey Administration Protocols

Writing up a protocol for the administration of the survey will better ensure that your survey is administered in a standardized manner by the data collection team. To better anticipate the issues that will arise during the data collection process, you should field test the survey administration protocols that you have established. If you have established that the data collectors should call the site the day before the survey is to be administered and that they should talk to a predetermined individual, you should do the same during your field test. If you have scripted a text that data collectors should read or discuss with potential participants, you should follow it exactly as you have planned it. By following the same steps that you are expecting your data collectors to follow, you will gain an understanding of the limitations of your survey administration protocols and will be able to make the necessary adjustments before the larger data collection effort is underway.

With the MARS project, we realized during the field testing of our survey administration protocols that we needed to add instructions for separating individuals during the administration of the survey in order to eliminate the temptation for participants to distract one another. We also realized that site visits should be timed so as not to interfere with other potential distractions for the youth such as a daily basketball game, recreational time slot, or favorite television show. Based on field testing experience, an outline or script of events was drawn up to help guide and prepare data collectors. Although it is difficult to anticipate all of the potential issues that will arise, it is important to provide data collectors with a realistic prediction of what they will likely encounter. An example of a portion of the data collection guide used by the MARS project is provided in Box 25.4.

Hiring and Training Data Collectors

The data collectors hired to carry out your survey may very well be the only contact that participants will have with your study. For this reason it is important to consider how participants will react to the individuals you hired to garner their trust and cooperation. You should consider whether or not the data collector could relate to and communicate with the survey's respondents. This will involve consideration of a data collector's age, race, sex, and demeanor in relation to those being surveyed. How will participants feel about asking questions of a particular person? Is the data collector considered a good communicator? Is the data collector intimidating? For

---

Box 25.4   Data Collection Protocol for Youth Meeting

- Confirm that no one has taken the survey in recent weeks.
- Set out **snacks**.
- Introduce self to youth, briefly why you're there (to *invite* them to participate in taking a survey).
- During the pilot work, we found it helpful to take time to chat with the youth about themselves: give them a chance to feel you out before jumping into the survey.
- Encourage them to help themselves to refreshments.
- Impress upon them that the purpose of the study is to help set up programs to help youth like themselves. Emphasize that they are the experts on their own health and that they can help others by participating in the study and taking the survey.
- Make it clear that the survey is NOT A TEST, but a survey about their own personal experiences.
- Pass out **survey packets** *(minus the survey)* that contain a consent form and sharpened pencil.
- Ask them to pull the **consent form** from the envelope. Tell them that the consent form is your way of making sure that they are willing to take the survey and that you will be reading through it with them. Read through **consent form**.
  This is often a tedious process for youth because of the 'official' and scary nature of the consent process. Try to make it interesting and fun. We found from our interviews that this portion of the process can influence how completely and honestly youth fill out the surveys.
- Briefly talk through **example survey** table question emphasizing that all lines should be answered unless indicated otherwise.
- Field questions.
- **Collect consent forms** and give them a blank copy for themselves; point out the phone numbers on the consent form that they can call with questions after completing the survey.
- Let them know that you have **educational materials** dealing with some of the issues addressed in the survey. They are welcome to take any of the materials after completing the survey.
- Instruct them to take the envelope with them and to put their completed survey in the envelope and to seal it.
- Pass out 1999 **Out-of-Home Youth Survey** and ask them to find a private place to take it. Let them know they can ask questions while taking the survey.
- While the youth are taking the survey, fill out **participant log** by printing each youth's name and date of birth.
- Upon completion, have them place their survey in their envelope and seal it.
- As you collect surveys, one by one, pass out **gift certificates** as each youth signs the **Participant and Receipt of Gift Certificate Log.**
- Pass out and leave behind the **educational materials.**

surveys containing sensitive questions, participants may feel more comfortable asking clarification questions of someone of the same race and sex. It is additionally important for data collectors to have a non-judgmental approach to their task. Survey respondents are providing a reflection of themselves through the survey and should not be the target of on-the-spot interventions by data collectors. Data collectors who are not able to curb their desire to influence or offer guidance to survey respondents will not be effective survey data collectors. The task of hiring qualified data collectors is only the first step; the appropriate training and monitoring of data collectors will be critical for ensure the quality and consistency of the data collection effort.

Careful thought should be given to the training of data collectors. How should data collectors represent themselves and the purposes of the study? What are some approaches or techniques that can be use to gain early acceptance by survey participants? How much assistance should data collectors offer when asked questions about survey items? Understanding the potential issues that might arise during the administration of the survey will assist greatly in the training effort. The training sessions for data collectors should cover a thorough background of the study, including discussion of its purpose, methods, and anticipated utility. Adequate time should be spent on discussion of the consent process and the required consent forms. Each data collector should become very familiar with the survey instrument before going into the field. You might find it useful to have the data collectors take the survey with the same level of introduction and support that will be given during the later administrations of the survey. This will allow data collectors to experience the survey in the same manner as the participants. Time should

also be allotted for a discussion of the ethics of administering a survey, covering topics such as confidentiality, anonymity, respondent bias, and appropriate boundaries between data collectors and survey participants.

Contacting Organizations

Organizations should have advance notification of the survey, its purpose, and what to expect once they agree to participate. This notification can be conducted through the mail, by phone, or by personal visit. Organizations will tend to be more supportive of your data collection efforts if they are well informed in advance of the data collector's coming to their organization. Because the MARS study needed to screen potential group homes and shelters based on whether the homes fit a predetermined criteria, each home was contacted more than once prior to data collection. By the time the MARS data collectors arrived at a home, the site had received a minimum of three calls and one formal survey announcement via mail.

Carrying Out the Final Data Collection Process

By the time you get the point where you are ready to begin the data collection phase, you will have gone through a number of preliminary steps. The data collection phase may very well be the shortest of the entire surveying process. Establishing a data collection schedule for you and your data collection team will increase the likelihood that the process will be carried out expeditiously. Consideration should be given to the length of time that will be allocated to the actual collection of data. In the case of the MARS project, a relatively short time frame was established due to the fact that youth were often shuffled from one group home to another. A short data collection time frame limited the potential for youth to be selected more than once as survey participants. It is the responsibility of the principal investigator to ensure that data is being collected in a timely and efficient manner. To aid in this process, procedures should be in place that will allow for the tracking of the data collection effort.

Tracking the Data Collection Process

Along with careful planning prior to data collection, you will need to establish procedures for monitoring the data collection process. This is especially true in situations in which hired data collectors are being used. Monitoring whether scheduled site visits are kept, whether surveys are completed, and ensuring that the survey administration protocols are followed is a fundamental responsibility of the principal investigator. Depending upon the complexity of the survey process, quality control checks by means of observing data collectors in the field may be warranted. You should also plan a mechanism for data collectors to relay information back to the principal investigator. This can take the form of weekly meetings or post-site-visit debriefings. If careful planning and field testing of the survey and administration protocols is completed prior to survey administration, then only minor issues should arise during the final data collection phase.

SUMMARY

The process of conducting surveys has been a fundamental building block for assessing and addressing the health issues of populations. Without the knowledge of those we are serving, we are limited in our ability to direct our intervention and policy initiatives. At the same time, we must always be diligent in our efforts to ensure that the collection of survey data actually serves a purpose for our population of interest. To this end, we should involve within the process those who would most benefit from the survey's results whenever possible. This can encompass anything from including organizations and individuals on a steering committee to sending out reports of survey results to relevant organizations and individuals.

During the surveying process, surveyors would be wise to always remember that they are guests within someone else's realm, and that youth should be viewed as volitional individuals and not as potential sources of data. The experience with the MARS project revealed that youth are more than willing to advance the state of knowledge and to better the lot of others by sharing what they know. The youth often probed and asked questions regarding the purpose of the MARS study and expressed an interest in knowing how the collected information was going to be used. Many stated that the reason they agreed to participate was their desire to help others.

Conducting a survey in youth organizations requires careful planning and project management. This includes preparing a detailed research plan, gaining approval for the survey effort from the relevant institutional review boards, and carefully carrying out and monitoring the data collection process. It is the responsibility of the principal investigator to monitor and manage all phased of the data collection effort. There is much more to learn about the administration of surveys than this chapter can provide. For further information on survey design and administration consult Aday (1996) and the Survey Kit (1995).

REFERENCES

Aday, L. A. (1996). *Designing and conducting health surveys* (2nd ed.). San Francisco: Jossey-Bass.

Centers for Disease Control. (1994). Health risk behaviors among adolescents who do and do not attend school—United States, 1992. *Morbidity and Mortality Weekly, 43,* 129–132.

Ellis, G. B. (1999). Keeping research subjects out of harm's way. *Journal of the American Medical Association, 282,* 1963–1965.

Ensign, J., & Santelli, J. (1997). Shelter-based homeless youth. *Archives of Pediatric and Adolescent Medicine, 151,* 817–823.

Kann, L., Kinchen, S. A., Williams, B. I., Ross, J. G., Lowry, R., Hill, C. V., Grunbaum, J. A., Blumson, P. S., Collins, J. L., Kolbe, L. J., & State and Local YRBSS Coordinators. (1998). Youth risk behavior surveillance—United States. In CDC Surveillance Summaries. *Morbidity and Mortality Weekly, 47*(SS-3), 1–89.

Kolbe, L. J., Kahn, L., & Collins, J. (1993). Overview of the youth risk behavior surveillance system. *Public Health Reports 108*(Suppl.), 47–55.

Slonim-Nevo, V., Ozawa, M., & Auslander, W. (1991). Knowledge, attitudes and behaviors related to AIDS among youth in residential centers: Results from an exploratory study. *Journal of Adolescence, 14,* 17–33.

The Survey Kit. (1995). (Vols. 1–9). Thousand Oaks, CA: Sage.

U.S. Department of Health and Human Services. (1991). Federal policy for the protection of human subjects, Title 45, Pt. 46. [On-line]. Available: *http://www.nih.gov:80/grants/oprr/humansubjects/45cfr46.htm.*

CHAPTER 26

Violence Prevention in Schools: A Model Violence-Prevention Center

Pamela P. DiNapoli

April 20 , 1999

■ **ABCNEWS.com**

It started just before lunchtime. Two young men cloaked in long trench coats and armed with guns and pipe bombs began what would end up being nearly five hours of mayhem and terror.

■ **Littleton, Colorado (CNN)**

At least two heavily armed young men opened fire and tossed explosives Tuesday at an affluent suburban Denver high school, killing students and possibly faculty members, authorities said. Sheriff John Stone said as many as 25 people were killed, including two suspects found dead in the library.

Recent incidents of violence by adolescents, like those in Jonesboro, Arkansas (March 1998), and more recently in Littleton, Colorado (April 1999), have refocused the nation's attention on a public health epidemic—adolescent violence. Unfortunately, school violence is becoming an all too familiar media event. Box 26.1 summarizes the extent to which violence has become a public health epidemic among our nation's youth.

This chapter will introduce you to one health promotion intervention designed to reduce violence in the future—School-Based Violence-Prevention Center. The necessary elements of a violence-prevention center will be reviewed, as well as the pitfalls and lessons learned from the development and implementation of such a center in one rural community.

PURPOSE

The most direct link between families and communities is currently found in schools. Measured purely in terms of available time to reduce risk factors for crime, schools

---

Box 26.1 Violence Among Adolescents

- Homicide rates are dropping among all groups, but the decrease is not as dramatic among youth who already exhibit the highest rates.
- Homicide is the second leading cause of death for young people aged 15 to 24 and the leading cause of death for African American and Hispanic youth in this age group.
- In 1995, 7,284 young people between 15 and 24 years old were victims of homicide, amounting to almost 19 youth homicide victims per day in the U.S. Of all homicide victims in 1994, 38% were younger than 24 years old (*Healthy People 2010*, DHHS, 2000).

Box 26.2 *Healthy People 2010 National Health Promotion Objectives: Adolescent Violence*

Reduce to 16% the proportion of people living in homes with firearms that are loaded and unlocked (baseline: 20% in 1994)

Enact laws in 50 states and the District of Columbia requiring that firearms be properly stored to minimize access and the likelihood of discharge by minors (baseline: 15 in 1994)

- referring those students defined as high risk to appropriate health promotion resources.

The goals of this proactive violence prevention approach are consistent with *Healthy People 2010* (DHHS, 2000) objectives relative to adolescent violence (Box 26.2).

COMPONENTS OF A SUCCESSFUL VIOLENCE-PREVENTION CENTER

Education

This successful violence-prevention center began with the design of an education component to provide training to faculty and staff. This education component must include factors that help to identify students who may be potentially at risk for violence either as perpetrators or as victims. While there is still a great deal of research to be done to identify the root causes of adolescent violence, the risk factors have been narrowed down for the purposes of education and training and are included in Box 26.3.

have more opportunity to accomplish national violence-reduction objectives than any other agency of government (U.S. Department of Health and Human Services [DHHS], 2000). The school-based violence-prevention center is designed to assist the school community in preventing violence. For purposes of this center, violence has been defined as causing harm to others as a result of an individual's personal history and the circumstances currently faced (Earls, 1994). Components of this health promotion initiative include:

- educating community members regarding both individual and community-based risk factors for violence;
- identifying and screening those students whom the community identifies as at-risk;

Box 26.3   Assessment of Risk Factors for Violence

- Is the student socially isolated?
- Has the student experienced recent situational stressors?
- Is the student a product of a disrupted upbringing?
- What is the student's socioeconomic status? Measures may include parents' income; free/low-cost lunches; access to health care; disparity in resources.
- Has the student been a witness or victim of previous violence or suicide?

In addition to these factors, faculty and staff were advised that students who are identified through routine health-risk appraisals should be referred for a comprehensive violence risk assessment. Following the design of this education component it became evident that because of both vulnerability and responsibility the school needed a vehicle for violence prevention.

Training

The Violence-Prevention Center staff conducted a series of initial in-service training sessions for the school related to the risk identification, prevention, and postvention of adolescent violence. This training then extended to the community via the parent-teacher organization. Training was individualized to the group and limited in size to 10 to 15 participants. A true/false pretest evaluation of existing knowledge was the framework for training. Core concepts including risk identification, resource identification, and crisis intervention were designated as "essential knowledge," and

each group was required to demonstrate competency in these areas on a posttest evaluation. These core concepts, including risk identification and available support services, are distributed annually in faculty and student handbooks. No further formal training was conducted (see "Pitfalls and Lessons Learned" section of this chapter).

Resource Identification and Referral

The nature of violence by adolescents—associated with a constellation of individual, social, and environmental factors—requires a diverse team to ensure successful intervention. Following these training sessions, an advisory board of faculty, staff, parents, and students was identified to be the backbone of the School-Based Violence-Prevention Center led by a designated "gatekeeper" (see Box 26.4). These designees meet on an ongoing basis to discuss the school climate, to study the elements of risk, and to use their expertise to design a prevention strategy and make suggestions for future programming with the Violence-Prevention Center gatekeeper.

With the input of the advisory board, the gatekeeper is charged with making recommendations based on lethality in risk situations and implementing prevention initiatives. Community practitioners with a broad multidisciplinary education and a holistic view of health are well suited for this role. One major premise is that while

Box 26.4   Wisdom Box

The critical element for the success of any prevention or policy initiative is to bring adolescents to the decision-making table

---

Box 26.5   Wisdom Box

The central thread linking the internal and external factors consistently associated with violent behavior is the adolescents' need to belong.

---

all cases of potential violence must be treated as emergent, not all require emergency mental-health referral. Developmental science perspectives of violence would suggest that violent behaviors are choices made as a result of a normal developmental progression toward resolving conflict (Hoff, 1995). As such, the Violence-Prevention Center subscribes to interventions that enable students to overcome the adversity prompting these "bad choices." Such resiliency-based strategies include mentoring, referral, and networking with existing in-school support groups such as Students Against Destructive Decision Making (SADD) and the Alliance for Gay and Lesbian Youth.

Internal factors including physical differences and biases and external factors such as lack of peer and family support prompt students to act violently (Catalano & Hawkins, 1996). The single greatest influence on the behavior of an adolescent is his peers. A successful violence-prevention center acknowledges this by offering opportunities for successful relationships with peers. It should be recognized that violent behavior often does not occur in isolation; usually there are other comorbid behaviors (such as smoking, drinking, and drug use) that may serve as entree into the health promotion system. The gatekeeper must be proactive in encouraging students who are experimenting in comorbid behaviors to become involved in these groups. Intensive marketing of the groups encourages membership. With support of the school admin-

istration peer leaders who exert their influence by focusing on the positive aspects of group involvement encourages membership. Strategies for encouraging involvement include:

- allowing for peer leadership of the groups—do not impose your agenda!
- offering the violence-prevention center as a confidential meeting place
- reducing barriers by offering refreshments and transportation
- membership cannot be punitive

Information related to peer-support-group networks is available on the World Wide Web. It is essential, however, that the gatekeeper know what is right and for whom. For example, if there is an identified interest in Latin American dancing, start a club. Encourage high school students to be peer counselors and mentors of middle-school students as part of a community service requirement, giving students opportunities to fulfill graduation requirements through their community service. In other words, step out of the box.

Finally, the Violence-Prevention Center encourages students to involve themselves in traditional in-school activities (music, drama, athletics) to increase their sense of support and connection within the school community. Remember that the interventions should be holistic and enlist the support of your community stakeholders. The rewards that come from a health connection between the community and the school are reciprocal.

Responding to Violent Incidents

While the ultimate goal is violence prevention, a successful violence-prevention center must also be prepared with an effective response plan to maintain school functioning and prevent contagion in the wake of violent incidents. A coordinated and planned response to violent incidents is essential. This role again falls to the gatekeeper of the violence-prevention center. Immediate issues to be addressed in the aftermath of such a school crisis may include:

- media issues and the need to set media policy
- clear definition of roles delegated to administration, faculty, and staff
- maintenance of order in the school and accountability of the students
- plan for meeting the needs of students most affected by the incident
- outreach to parents to notify them of the incidents and its possible effects

Media Issues

The media wants the story and will get the story. Before a violent incident occurs at the school it is essential to identify (a) who will be the point person who talks to the media (it should not be the principal or the superintendent, as these individuals have too many other related roles); and (b) which media outlets will be given the story. The community should have an idea of where they will be able to get accurate school sanctioned information rather than rumor. Remember rumors are contagious.

Administrative Issues

Within a school, individuals have clear roles, and these roles must be maintained during a crisis. For example:

- the nurse takes care of health issues
- guidance counselors must establish control using their understanding of group dynamics

- teachers must be accountable for students—count your students.

Follow-up

Students need to return to their school after an incident. The violence-prevention center should make immediate plans to supervise this return. In situations of criminal activity like a pervasive violent act, the gatekeeper should maintain communication with the criminal justice investigators to ensure that students return safely and quickly. Preparation for the aftermath of a crisis is of equal importance to the prevention strategies employed on a daily basis. Postvention planning cannot be completed and relegated to a policy manual; regular review of these plans is essential to the smooth handling of a crisis situation. Keep everyone informed.

Pitfalls and Lessons Learned

The greatest lessons we have learned from the development of this center is as "scientists in health promotion," that is, mental health professionals, nurses, educators and parents, we should not respond to the media adapting the role of "scientist." The center was driven by the need to respond to media attention surrounding adolescent violence rather than by scientific evidence supporting its concept. In this respect major pitfalls have been:

- The education component was done in a single training session with no provisions made for ongoing awareness to the issue.
- A lack of resources limits our ability to do individual health risk appraisals.
- Dissemination of the information to the community was done through the

parent-teacher group, where there is a very small audience.

You can avoid these pitfalls. When involving the community in a violence prevention initiative such as this, keep in mind that the essential element is training, training, and more training. Today's problem will also be tomorrow's problem.

FUTURE RESEARCH

The development of an entity called a violence-prevention center deludes us into thinking we are combating this national epidemic, yet concerted health promotion and health policy initiatives must be undertaken to find adequate, sustainable solutions. These initiatives must consider the issues of poverty, discrimination, and lack of education and employment opportunities as important risk factors for violence. Second, strategies for reducing violence should begin early in life, before violent beliefs and behavioral patterns can be adopted. Finally, there needs to be ongoing evaluation of programs to help identify effective approaches for violence prevention. Such violence-prevention initiatives are crucial to promote the healthy development of youth in our society. While the violence-prevention center outlined here is in a high-school, initiatives must begin before the initiation of problem behaviors. Health promotion initiatives require coalition-building with the school as the core and with a mechanism for ongoing evaluation. It is not enough to adopt a cookie-cutter approach to health promotion. Violence-prevention initiatives require a introspective look at the community, its resources and its problems. From this assessment will come developmentally appropriate solutions and with it advocacy for promoting our youth.

REFERENCES

Earls, F. (1994). Violence and today's youth. *Critical Health Issues for Children and Youth, 4*(3), 11–30.

Catalano, R. F., & Hawkins, J. D. (1996). The social development model: A theory of antisocial behavior. In J. D. Hawkins (Ed.), *Delinquency and crime: Current theories* (pp. 149–197). New York: Cambridge University Press.

Hoff, L. A. (1995). *People in crisis: Understanding and helping* (4th ed., rev.). San Francisco: Jossey-Bass.

U.S. Department of Health and Human Services. (January, 2000). *Healthy people 2010 (Conference edition in two volumes)*. Washington, DC: Author.

CHAPTER 27

Evaluating Small Community-Based Health Promotion Programs: Lessons Learned from Colorado Health Promotion Initiatives

Kathryn A. Judge, Deborah S. Main, Carolyn Tressler, Douglas Fernald, Jill Parker, Kitty Corbett, and Jennifer Horton

D uring the past decade, communities have received increased recognition as leaders and participants in promoting the health and well-being of citizens. Communities have tackled a variety of health issues ranging from heart disease to HIV infection to teenage pregnancy. The potential impacts of the largest, federally funded community-based health promotion programs are widely known, but we continue to know very little about what some of the smaller community-based health promotion projects accomplish, even though these more modest programs are far more common in communities where resources are scarce.

The purpose of this chapter is to describe the journey of four evaluators working as a team to capture the key impacts of relatively small community-based health promotion projects that received funding through a statewide initiative—the Community Action for Health Promotion Initiative. The initiative was purposefully designed to build capacity for health promotion through locally initiated activities, ideally creating a web or system of efforts to support the health and well-being of citizens across the state of Colorado. Understanding the story of the evaluation of these community-based health promotion projects requires some background on the initiative itself and an introduction to some of the challenges of this type of work.

BACKGROUND

The Community Action for Health Promotion Initiative (CAHPI) is a 5-year $5.2-million initiative designed to increase local health promotion activities in Colorado and to build the capacity of Colorado communities to identify and address preventable health problems. The initiative is funded by the Colorado Trust, a local philanthropic foundation, and administered by Colorado Action for Healthy People (the management agency). Each year, the management agency announced requests for proposals (RFPs) addressing one or two health promotion issues. We present the specific health issues addressed by the initiative in Box 27.1, below. Importantly, these targeted areas reflect the health priorities identified for Colorado during the mid-1980s, as well as Healthy People 2000 priority areas. For more information about *Healthy People 2000* priority areas, please see the *Healthy People 2000* homepage at *http:// odphp.osophs.dhhs.gov/pubs/hp2000/ prior.htm.*

The management agency established the guidelines for the grants: proposals should demonstrate the use of multiple strategies, collaboration, and a commitment to capacity building. If funded, grantees could expect to receive up to $10,000 per year for a maximum of 3 years and technical assis-

tance delivered by the management agency and its network of consultants.

Since August 1995, the management agency has funded 48 local health promotion projects, distributed among 29 of Colorado's 64 counties. While most projects were funded for the full duration allowed under the guidelines of the grants—3 years in most cases—two projects terminated their participation in the initiative after 1 year, and one project terminated its participation after 2 years.

More than anything else, diversity defines these CAHPI projects. Some projects stem from the efforts of strong grassroots groups or loose networks of organizations, while other projects grow out of the efforts of structured and sophisticated agencies. The 48 projects represent a variety of nonprofit entities, including:

- churches
- community service organizations
- community health centers
- cooperative extension offices
- family resource centers
- hospitals
- libraries
- nursing services
- regional health departments
- schools

The organizations are based in a variety of settings, as well, from the mountains of western Colorado to the Denver metro area to the eastern plains.

Because there is no uniform planning process required for CAHPI projects, each community creates its own project and processes. Within the general requirements of the RFP, each site selects its own director or coordinator, devises its own strategies for implementing programs, and defines its own target population(s). Among project directors and coordinators, experience in

---

Box 27.1 Specific Health Issues Addressed by the Initiative

- Physical activity and fitness
- Diet and nutrition
- Tobacco use prevention
- Substance abuse prevention
- Violence prevention
- Child injury prevention
- Heart disease prevention
- Diabetes prevention
- Healthy habits for children and adolescents
- Adult wellness

health promotion, in general, and project and grant management, more specifically, varies a great deal. Strategies for promoting health include the delivery of individual education and instruction, general education and awareness raising (outreach), participatory events or activities, and products or services. Finally, target populations range from infants to seniors, from the residents of neighborhoods to counties.

The Challenges

Perhaps the most important thing to remember when designing any evaluation is that "evaluation follows program." What this means is that the scope and focus of evaluation activities are dependent upon the intent of a program (in other words, what it seeks to accomplish), as well as its organizational framework and design. Given the goals of CAHPI, for example, we did not set out to measure health outcomes. Rather, we focused primarily on capacity building and its effect on increasing and enhancing health promotion activities across Colorado. The overall objective to determine what effect the initiative has on a community's capacity to plan and implement health promotion activities has guided our evaluation efforts.

Perhaps the most important thing to remember when designing any evaluation is that "evaluation follows program." What this means is that the scope and focus of evaluation activities are dependent upon the intent of a program, as well as its organizational framework and design.

At the outset, we assumed that funded projects would act like complex and dynamic systems with different variables having diverse (and sometimes unexpected and unmeasurable) effects at different levels. To reflect this fluid, ecological (i.e., context-dependent) approach, we conceptualized the evaluation as a study of the "natural history" of how diverse communities mobilize to plan, develop, implement, and sustain health promotion programs. We designed the evaluation as a series of case studies and planned to use multiple methods to collect both qualitative and quantitative information to tell the story of how each project unfolded in communities across Colorado.

Comprehensive, intensive, and ambitious, our initial evaluation proposal reflected our eagerness to capture all the potential learnings the initiative would offer. On paper this sounded fine, but had we actually completed all that we initially planned, legions of additional personnel would have been necessary, not to mention years added to the time frame. Given the structure, scope, and duration of the initiative, coupled with project diversity—differing health issues, organizations, target populations, project directors, planning processes, and implementation strategies—we faced some daunting challenges. As a practical matter, we wondered how we could

- keep track of all the projects and their important details
- keep up with all the data that needed to be collected
- standardize and simplify data collection
- make sense of (process and analyze) all the data

We needed strategies for collecting different pieces of data systematically in order to form ultimately a comprehensive picture of what was occurring. We also needed tools that were flexible and easy to use.

These concerns and needs, as well as our desire to find solutions, helped shape the evaluation process over time. We describe the story below of our journey to address these challenges through a cyclic process of communicating, planning, implementing, reflecting, and revising. Importantly, the process involved all the key *stakeholders* in the initiative—funders, management agency staff, and representatives from the projects and their communities. To this day, this inclusive, iterative process is shaping how, when, and why we collect and analyze data.

EVALUATION OF SMALL COMMUNITY-BASED HEALTH PROMOTION PROJECTS

The evaluation design for CAHPI had to be innovative. We could borrow only minimally from the existing literature, which primarily reported on larger community-based studies with highly defined programs and intended outcomes. With little literature available on which to base our evaluation design, we recognized the need to employ processes that would allow us to:

1. immediately begin learning "what happens" in these smaller projects
2. continually refine our approaches to data collection
3. efficiently analyze data to ensure that we were capturing what is important about these projects.

These processes allowed us to learn and change with the initiative, and the evolution of the evaluation over time reflects this learning and flexibility. The journey from our initial evaluation plan to our final evaluation design may be divided into three major stages or phases, which we call *scouting, locating the trail,* and *sharing the journey with others* to reflect our sense that this evalua-

tion process was truly an exploration of relatively uncharted territory.

Phase I: Scouting

During the first stage of the evaluation we felt like explorers in a new land. We knew very little about what to expect from these projects beyond what we read in the original proposals. (And as many of us have experienced, what we propose in grants and what we eventually end up doing are often very different things.) There was so much we needed to learn before we could identify what we should measure across all community-based projects. We needed to cast a broad net to capture what was happening in these projects, their communities, and with their project leaders. This necessitated using qualitative methods that would allow us to ask more general questions, but ones that would generate a great deal of detailed information. (We describe the benefits of starting out broadly and then narrowing the focus as you become more familiar with the subject matter you want to understand in Box 27.2.)

As a first step in our exploration, we conducted interviews with project directors and other key staff, community leaders, project officers from the management agency, and program participants to learn more about the inner workings of these community-based projects. Often we started with project directors and coordinators; our list of key informants grew from there as we asked, "Who else should we talk with to learn more about your project?" Like any good scout, we visited the actual project sites to observe program activities, talk with people, and generally get a feel for each project and the community context within which it resided. Figure 27.1 presents the contact summary form we use to document, in a standardized way, the learn-

Box 27.2   Be an Anthropologist

In the evaluation of CAHPI, we started out big in terms of what we set out to learn from the Initiative and our data collection efforts. We soon realized that we needed to be more realistic about what we could expect from the project staff, other community representatives, and ourselves. But we want to emphasize that there is nothing wrong with starting out broadly. Ultimately this might help you hone in on what you really want to learn and prevent you from making ungrounded assumptions about what is important to communities of people and their health. This was certainly our experience.

The technique of starting out broadly, absorbing what is happening, where, when, and how, and later focusing your efforts with a keener sense of this context is a method that anthropologists use. This technique is called ethnography. Entering a community as an anthropologist—as an outside observer—allows you to assume an appropriate level of naivete, while it places those familiar with what you want to learn about in the role of local experts.

site-visit summary notes, and other qualitative methodologies quickly accumulated in hundreds and hundreds of pages of textual data. We present the full range of qualitative methods we use to learn about these community-based projects in Box 27.3. The rate of accumulation would only accelerate in years to come as new projects entered the initiative each year and the funding cycle for grants increased from 1 to 3 years. Though our tools and data seemed to be providing us with an adequate assessment of the landscape of community-based health promotion (i.e., the key features of communities, projects, and leaders that facilitated or detracted from project implementation), we began to realize that our exploration could be expedited if we had some sort of a map to help us navigate through waves of data collection. In order to develop such a map, we first needed to reflect on our field notes to determine exactly what we knew and did not know about the terrain before us. Because each member of the evaluation team knew some community projects better than others, we used a team-based approach to examine critically all of the information we had gathered about each health promotion project. Figure 27.2 describes and illustrates how our team used a dynamic, iterative process for reviewing information.

This process confirmed that our qualitative information was useful and necessary to capture characteristics both unique to and common across projects. But we recognized the need to revise our qualitative data collection instruments to be more sensitive to the changes going on within projects across 3 years of funding. This team-based approach also led us to identify other salient aspects of the experiences of these health promotion projects that we were not fully capturing with our qualitative methods. This map or guide provided a distinct direction for our exploration, purposefully

ings, impressions, and questions generated primarily through interviews and site visits. Whether you are serving in the role of evaluator or project coordinator, we recommend that you consider using a similar tool that not only allows you to document important information, but also to process it (that is, make sense of it and determine its larger relevance and connections to other data).

The information generated through interview transcripts, detailed interview and

---

CAHPI CONTACT SUMMARY FORM

Site: **Date:**
Type: **Length of time:**
(Interviewee):   **(Interviewer):**

1. **What were the main issues or themes that struck you in this contact/document?**
   •

2. **What new (or remaining) target questions do you have in considering the next contact or in pursuing other documents with this site?**
   •

3. **Other impressions, concerns, ideas or reflections** (what is the informant/document really saying, doubts about the quality of some data, new hypotheses about puzzling observations, personal reactions):
   •

4. **Force-field analysis**

   Positive influences:
   •

   Negative influences:
   •

5. **Project director and/or coordinator checkpoints**
   • **Personality characteristics** (personable, energetic, confident):
     •

   • **Charisma** (thrives in the spotlight, confident, personal conviction, praises contributions of others, celebrates accomplishments):
     •

   • **Leadership skills** (articulate, assertive, asks for what s/he needs, creates system for accountability, good listener, elicits ideas from others, puts people on the defensive, savvy):
     •

   • **Facilitation skills** (encourages participation from everyone, talks about "we" and not "I," makes eye contact with everyone, shares vision, seeks to fully understand others, looks to others for answers and guidance, negotiates well, pushes her/his ideas on others, control freak):
     •

FIGURE 27.1   Contact summary form.

We adapted this instrument from Miles, Matthew B. and Huberman, Michael A. *Qualitative Data Analysis*, 2nd edition. Sage Publications: Thousand Oaks, CA. 1994.

Box 27.3 Qualitative Methods Used in the CAHPI Evaluation

- **In-depth interviews** with project directors/coordinators, key informants, and management agency staff (recorded and transcribed; standardized contact summary form completed after each)
- **Site visits** (direct observation of project activities, impromptu interviews with key staff and program participants; standardized contact summary form completed after each)
- Biannual **grantees' meetings** (direct observation of project staff interaction and leadership styles; note-taking during project updates)
- Periodic **telephone contact** with project directors/coordinators and management agency staff (standardized contact summary form completed after each)
- Biannual **project progress reports** (detailed summary notes developed from each)
- **Focused discussions** with management agency staff (recorded and transcribed; standardized contact summary form completed after each)

ultimately gave rise to two important changes in our evaluation. First, we modified our qualitative instruments to capture the life cycle of these types of projects from the start-up phase through implementation and maintenance to sustainability. When the funding cycle of grants increased from 1 year to 3, we needed to adapt our instruments and methodologies so that we could take advantage of the opportunity to follow and learn from each project over a longer period of time. This is another implication of "evaluation follows program." Any changes in a program (or, in this case, an initiative) mean that corresponding changes need to occur in the evaluation.

Second, through the team-based approach we discovered new quantitative pathways for exploring different elements of the terrain and developing a fuller perspective of hard-to-get-at (i.e., complex) features of the landscape. We learned that we needed to add more detailed information to our map about:

- the history of health promotion in communities and settings (i.e., what existed before)
- leadership development
- the delivery of technical assistance by the management agency
- the dynamics of working with others to implement programs

With respect to leadership development (more broadly, skill and knowledge development), technical assistance, and collaboration, we developed three written surveys to measure each of these important aspects of CAHPI projects quantitatively. Specifically, we developed the self-assessment survey, the technical assistance survey, and the working with others survey.

We designed the self-assessment survey to assist with the systematic and longitudi-

leading us to new vantage points from which to view community-based health promotion.

Phase II: Locating the Trail

We spent nearly two years in the scouting phase—time well invested as these efforts

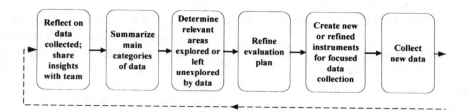

FIGURE 27.2 Iterative process employed to focus and guide data collection efforts.

Although we depict this as a linear process here, we did not always go through every step of the process or in this order, and, often, these steps overlapped.

nal tracking of project director and coordinator growth and development in relevant skills and knowledge. We administer the survey annually each fall to all project directors or coordinators. We use three versions of this survey. Incoming and outgoing versions are administered to project directors or coordinators just beginning or just ending their funding with the initiative. (The initiative funding cycle begins and ends in October.) We also administer a current self-assessment survey to project directors or coordinators who just received renewal funding with the initiative. We present an abbreviated version of this survey in Figure 27.3 to provide a sense of the general format used, as well as the types of skills and knowledge that we feel are important to developing, implementing, and sustaining a community-based health promotion project.

In order to track the types of technical assistance provided by the management agency and other sources, we developed the technical assistance survey. This survey also helps us document whether project directors' and coordinators' perceived needs for technical assistance are met consistently. Additionally, we ask about the project staff's anticipated future technical assistance needs and request that they specify whether they would like for us to pass this information on to staff at the management agency. The technical assistance survey is

the survey that we administer most frequently, once every 4 months or three times a year. We also use a special version of the survey to capture technical assistance delivered during the application (i.e., concept letter and grant-writing) phase of the initiative. We present sample items from the regular, periodic survey in Figure 27.4.

Finally, the working-with-others survey helps us track the degree to which project staff works with others to implement community-based health promotion projects. Because we administer the survey every spring, this tool allows us to document the sustainability of collaborative relationships over time, as well as how the initiative affects these relationships (for example, whether the initiative reportedly strengthens or weakens relationships with contributors). We also ask about what a given entity (i.e., an individual or organization) contributed to a project in terms of ideas, time, money, or supplies; the frequency of the contribution; and the relative helpfulness of the contribution to project implementation. We present sample items from this survey in Figure 27.5 to illustrate what features of collaborative efforts might be important to consider when developing or evaluating a community-based health promotion project.

The overall goal of developing these surveys was to collect information in an efficient and standardized manner that would

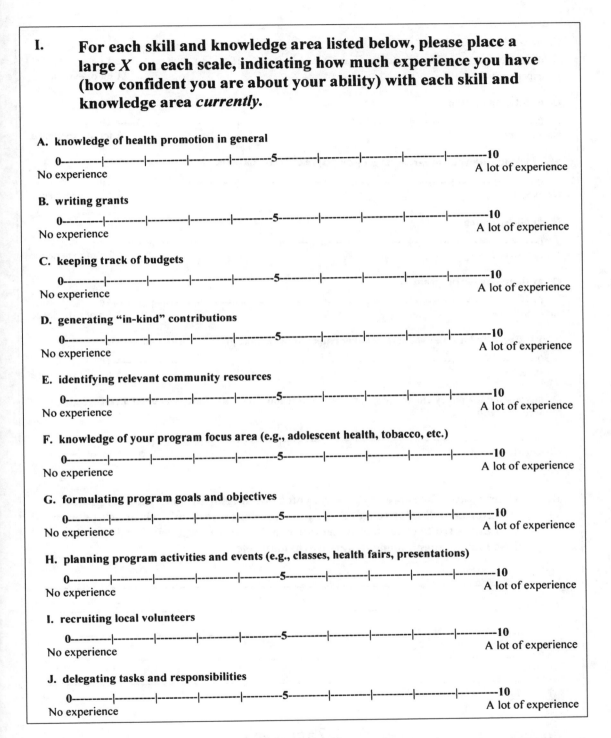

I. For each skill and knowledge area listed below, please place a large *X* on each scale, indicating how much experience you have (how confident you are about your ability) with each skill and knowledge area *currently*.

A. knowledge of health promotion in general

0----------|----------|----------|----------|----------5----------|----------|----------|----------|----------10
No experience   A lot of experience

B. writing grants

0----------|----------|----------|----------|----------5----------|----------|----------|----------|----------10
No experience   A lot of experience

C. keeping track of budgets

0----------|----------|----------|----------|----------5----------|----------|----------|----------|----------10
No experience   A lot of experience

D. generating "in-kind" contributions

0----------|----------|----------|----------|----------5----------|----------|----------|----------|----------10
No experience   A lot of experience

E. identifying relevant community resources

0----------|----------|----------|----------|----------5----------|----------|----------|----------|----------10
No experience   A lot of experience

F. knowledge of your program focus area (e.g., adolescent health, tobacco, etc.)

0----------|----------|----------|----------|----------5----------|----------|----------|----------|----------10
No experience   A lot of experience

G. formulating program goals and objectives

0----------|----------|----------|----------|----------5----------|----------|----------|----------|----------10
No experience   A lot of experience

H. planning program activities and events (e.g., classes, health fairs, presentations)

0----------|----------|----------|----------|----------5----------|----------|----------|----------|----------10
No experience   A lot of experience

I. recruiting local volunteers

0----------|----------|----------|----------|----------5----------|----------|----------|----------|----------10
No experience   A lot of experience

J. delegating tasks and responsibilities

0----------|----------|----------|----------|----------5----------|----------|----------|----------|----------10
No experience   A lot of experience

FIGURE 27.3 Items from the annual CAHPI project director/coordinator self-assessment survey. *(continued)*

K. networking

0----------|----------|----------|----------|----------|----------5----------|----------|----------|----------|----------10
No experience   A lot of experience

L. facilitating meetings

0----------|----------|----------|----------|----------|----------5----------|----------|----------|----------|----------10
No experience   A lot of experience

M. working with your program target group(s) (e.g., teens, parents, etc.)

0----------|----------|----------|----------|----------|----------5----------|----------|----------|----------|----------10
No experience   A lot of experience

N. public speaking

0----------|----------|----------|----------|----------|----------5----------|----------|----------|----------|----------10
No experience   A lot of experience

O. evaluating your program

0----------|----------|----------|----------|----------|----------5----------|----------|----------|----------|----------10
No experience   A lot of experience

P. working with local newspapers; writing letters to the editor, press releases, and articles

0----------|----------|----------|----------|----------|----------5----------|----------|----------|----------|----------10
No experience   A lot of experience

Q. advocating for policy change (e.g., presenting to school board and/or city council members about tobacco-free campuses)

0----------|----------|----------|----------|----------|----------5----------|----------|----------|----------|----------10
No experience   A lot of experience

II.   **Briefly describe some of the ways you have developed your skills as project director/coordinator (e.g., on-the-job experience, through relationships with and exposure to other health service providers, through relationships with [the management agency] staff/workshops, etc.).**

_____

_____

_____

_____

_____

Thank you!

FIGURE 27.3   *(continued)*

1. For each of the following types of technical assistance:
   a. please check whether each was received during the past 4 months (specify months)
   b. *if received*, please indicate if it was received from [the management agency] and/or other source(s);
   c. *if not*, please indicate whether it *would* have been helpful to have received each type of technical assistance during the **past 4 months**.

Types of Technical Assistance		
Budget issues (e.g., planning your budget, managing grant money, documenting in-kind contributions, etc.)	**Did you get it in the last four months?** ❑ Yes → ❑ No ↓ **If *no*, would it have been helpful?** ❑ Yes ❑ No	**If *yes*, did you get it from** *(please check all that apply)*: ❑ CAHP staff ❑ Some other source(s); **please specify:** _____ _____
Obtaining program materials (e.g., books, posters, pamphlets, etc.)	**Did you get it in the last four months?** ❑ Yes → ❑ No ↓ **If *no*, would it have been helpful?** ❑ Yes ❑ No	**If *yes*, did you get it from** *(please check all that apply)*: ❑ CAHP staff ❑ Some other source(s); **please specify:** _____ _____
Learning about program topic area (e.g., smoking cessation, other successful programs related to my own, etc.)	**Did you get it in the last four months?** ❑ Yes → ❑ No ↓ **If *no*, would it have been helpful?** ❑ Yes ❑ No	**If *yes*, did you get it from** *(please check all that apply)*: ❑ CAHP staff ❑ Some other source(s); **please specify:** _____ _____

FIGURE 27.4 Items from the periodic CAHPI technical assistance survey. *(continued)*

| Program management skill building (leadership, collaboration, etc.) | Did you get it in the last four months?

☐ Yes →
☐ No
↓
If *no*, would it have been helpful?
☐ Yes

☐ No | If *yes*, did you get it from *(please check all that apply)*:

☐ CAHP staff
☐ Some other source(s);

please specify:

_____

_____ |
| Evaluating your project (e.g., brainstorming evaluation possibilities, designing surveys and/or other instruments, analyzing data, presenting information to community members) | Did you get it in the last four months?

☐ Yes →
☐ No
↓
If *no*, would it have been helpful?
☐ Yes

☐ No | If *yes*, did you get it from *(please check all that apply)*:

☐ CAHP staff
☐ Some other source(s);

please specify:

_____

_____ |

*Other types of technical assistance that we ask about include planning program activities, fundraising/grant writing, revising CAHPI program objectives, facilitating relationships/communications with others, and media relations.

2. **Please list and describe any types of technical assistance that might be helpful to receive from [the management agency] and/or other sources during the _next_ 4 months (specify months).**

_____

_____

_____

_____

_____

Would you like us to share your response(s) to question #2 (above) with CAHP staff?

☐   Yes
☐   No

Thank you

FIGURE 27.4   *(continued)*

allow us to monitor changes in these important features systematically across the life of community-based projects. In this way, the second phase of our evaluation brought a more narrow, well-defined focus to our data collection efforts. We purposefully employed quantitative methods to improve the quality of the data we were collecting and, simultaneously, to scale down the quantity of information generated. Throughout this transition, we never lost sight of the fact that this quantitative data still needed to be supplemented with more contextual information. During this phase, the reason for applying qualitative methods simply shifted from their usefulness as tools for exploration to tools for triangulation. Rather than serving as primary data sources, qualitative methods assumed a more supportive, but no less important role in providing supplemental information to complement that which we were collecting with survey instruments.

To maximize the usefulness of both the qualitative and quantitative data, we need to administer surveys and conduct interviews and site visits on a consistent basis according to our data collection timelines. We also need to maintain a consistent commitment to data analysis. Specifically with respect to the survey data, to facilitate ongoing and timely data analysis, we work as a team to enter these data into established databases as we receive completed surveys. (See Box 27.4 for more information about how we work together to coordinate survey mailings and follow-up with project staff.) Because we enter all data as soon as we receive surveys, this information is immediately ready for quantitative analysis.

While we adhere to a rigid timeline for data collection, the schedule that guides data analysis is much more fluid. Several factors serve as the impetus for the analysis of data at particular points in time. Often, during our regular team meetings, our dis-

---

Box 27.4 Periodic Mailings—A Special Case of Teamwork

Although we share the responsibility for entering data into established databases, and even take turns "cleaning the data" (that is, making sure that it is consistently and accurately entered), one person on the team is primarily responsible for overseeing mailings and providing a gentle reminder when we have not yet received a completed survey from a project director/coordinator. We have found this to be an efficient way to keep track of when mailings need to go out, as well as which projects still need to return a survey. This arrangement also minimizes confusion on the part of project staff who have a single "point of contact" when negotiating who on their project staff is the most appropriate person to complete a survey, when they have questions about how to complete a survey, or when they need extra time for returning a survey.

---

cussions will lead to the development of some hypothesis about what is occurring with respect to CAHPI projects. (The contact summary form assists with hypothesis-generation outside team meetings; see, for example, item #3 in Figure 27.1.) Examples of hypotheses that we have formulated include educated guesses about the leadership styles or contextual factors that facilitate project implementation; hypotheses have also concerned the impacts on project integrity of project staff turnover. These hypotheses serve as a framework for generating questions that lead us to explore the data in novel ways. The longitudinal and systematic collection of standard types of data has facilitated testing such hypothe-

	Is this contributor still involved with your project at some level? (check one)	Did you or your organization work with this person or group before the CAHPI grant? (check one)	How has the CAHPI grant influenced the working relationship? (check one)	How do/did they contribute to your CAHPI project? (check all that apply)	How often do/did they contribute to your CAHPI project? (check one)	How helpful are/were their contributions to the project? (check one)	What do you think about the level of their contributions to the project? (check one)	Do you think this contributor will be involved with your project in the future?
Contributor Name 1	□ yes □ no □ not sure	□ yes, often □ yes, not often □ no □ don't know	□ initiated □ helped sustain □ strengthened □ weakened □ no influence	□ money □ ideas □ goods □ services □ time □ people □ space □ other____ □ nothing, yet	□ always □ very often □ fairly often □ sometimes □ almost never □ one time only □ never	□ very helpful □ somewhat helpful □ neither helpful nor unhelpful □ somewhat unhelpful □ very unhelpful	□ I wish they would do *more* □ I think they do about the *right amount* □ I wish they would do *less*	...in 6 months? □ yes □ no □ not sure ...in a year? □ yes □ no □ not sure
Contributor Name 2	□ yes □ no □ not sure	□ yes, often □ yes, not often □ no □ don't know	□ initiated □ helped sustain □ strengthened □ weakened □ no influence	□ money □ ideas □ goods □ services □ time □ people □ space □ other____ □ nothing, yet	□ always □ very often □ fairly often □ sometimes □ almost never □ one time only □ never	□ very helpful □ somewhat helpful □ neither helpful nor unhelpful □ somewhat unhelpful □ very unhelpful	□ I wish they would do *more* □ I think they do about the *right amount* □ I wish they would do *less*	...in 6 months? □ yes □ no □ not sure ...in a year? □ yes □ no □ not sure
Contributor Name 3	□ yes □ no □ not sure	□ yes, often □ yes, not often □ no □ don't know	□ initiated □ helped sustain □ strengthened □ weakened □ no influence	□ money □ ideas □ goods □ services □ time □ people □ space □ other____ □ nothing, yet	□ always □ very often □ fairly often □ sometimes □ almost never □ one time only □ never	□ very helpful □ somewhat helpful □ neither helpful nor unhelpful □ somewhat unhelpful □ very unhelpful	□ I wish they would do *more* □ I think they do about the *right amount* □ I wish they would do *less*	...in 6 months? □ yes □ no □ not sure ...in a year? □ yes □ no □ not sure

FIGURE 27.5 Items from the annual CAHPI Working with Others survey.

What else should we know about how others contribute to your project?

_____
_____
_____
_____
_____
_____
_____
_____
_____

Briefly describe any <u>challenges</u> you experienced working with others on your project:

_____
_____
_____
_____
_____
_____
_____
_____
_____

Who else should be involved in your project?

_____
_____
_____
_____
_____
_____
_____
_____
_____

Thank You !

FIGURE 27.5 *(continued)*

ses by allowing us to identify confirmatory, as well as disconfirming, cases.

Importantly, because we enter the information provided by project directors and coordinators ourselves, we know the data intimately. This familiarity or immersion enriches our discussions and facilitates the articulation of hypotheses that help us return to the data with fresh insights. This cyclic process of gathering information, processing it individually and collectively, asking questions, and returning to the data has no true beginning or end, yet it keeps us on a path that is leading to an in-depth understanding of community-based health promotion.

We are also challenged to keep up with data analysis due to commitments to provide biannual progress reports and presentations as part of our grant contract with the funding agency. Progress reports give us an opportunity to document where we are on this journey of understanding community-based health promotion. Subsequent meetings provide an opportunity to share what we are learning in a more interactive forum, involving members of the funding agency who are professionally and financially invested in understanding how such work can be conducted successfully in communities across Colorado.

We have found that project staff always appreciate hearing how the information that they provide contributes to a larger understanding of community-based health promotion. They also want to hear what others like them are thinking, feeling, and experiencing. These realizations, and the acknowledgement that we would have very little data if it were not for the efforts of these project directors and coordinators, serves as an additional impetus to reciprocate by analyzing the data in a timely manner. In sharing the data with project staff, we always attempt to do so in creative and easily accessible ways that do not require

busy project directors and coordinators to wade through dense technical jargon.

Phase III: Sharing the Journey with Others

In this final year of the initiative, we are approaching the end of the trail and a wide valley has opened up before us. From this vantage point, we can see vividly the paths we have traveled. We see how we retraced our own footsteps at certain points. The ongoing process of finding our way meant that we needed to continue checking and rechecking to ensure that we were on the path that would lead us to most adequately and accurately depict the richness of what these community-based health promotion projects accomplish.

As we begin to test our assumptions about processes such as sustainability, we want to continue to seek out the perspectives of project directors and other key staff to help us to fill in the picture of what is happening within and across these small community-based health promotion projects. After having narrowed the focus of our data collection efforts, we want to ensure that we do not lose the flavor of each project's unique experience with respect to leadership, the project's own growth and development, working with others, and needs for and satisfaction with technical assistance. As indicated above, part of this process also involves dissemination— sharing with others our journey, the challenges and successes, as well as what we have learned along the way.

Lessons Learned

Our story documents the dynamic journey of evaluating small community-based health promotion projects. This journey is punctuated by milestones of trial and error, by periods of stability, and by spurts of activity and learning. While lessons more specific to certain types of data collection efforts emerged during the course of telling our story, in this section we present some broader, more general lessons from our experience. In Box 27.5, we present these "pearls of wisdom" that we would like to share with others who are or potentially will be embarking on similar evaluations.

Be Open to What Else Is Going On

We anticipated early on that if we just looked at project-specific goals and objectives, we would miss much of "what else" these community-based health-promotion projects accomplish. We also knew that one of the fundamental goals of the initiative was to build the capacity at the local level for developing and implementing health promotion activities. As a result, we needed to examine the various indicators of community capacity-building that emerged throughout the initiative and that were supported theoretically in the literature. Specific indicators of capacity-building (that is, success in the context of this initiative) include leadership development; the development of other skill and knowledge areas important to community-based health promotion work; mobilization (getting others involved); and self- and collective efficacy (or the confidence to take action at the individual and community level, respectively).

We measure skill and knowledge development, including leadership, in project directors or coordinators directly through the standardized self-assessment survey, but are also able to document such development anecdotally and through direct observation at site visits. By being active in state public-health associations ourselves, we have additional opportunities to observe project staff assume leadership positions, network with professionals focusing on similar health issues, and actively seek new ideas and resources to enhance their projects. Our presence at important project events and organizational meetings also provides us with key insights about the networking that occurs within a community or region to mobilize local resources and effectively leverage the seed money granted through the initiative. We document these observations carefully using the contact summary form and track the degree to which these projects work with others through the standardized Working with Others Survey. Together, various data

---

Box 27.5   Lessons Learned through the Evaluation of a Statewide Initiative

1. **Be open to what else is going on.** Small community-based health promotion projects may be shortchanged if evaluators only look at project goals and objectives.
2. **Strike a balance between staying out of the way and staying in touch** with project staff.
3. **Be reflective** about what types of methods are most appropriate for different stages/phases of the evaluation process.
4. **Develop relationships** among and between key stakeholders. Relationships are critically important to conducting a successful evaluation that generates meaningful and relevant knowledge that will contribute to an understanding of community-based health promotion.

sources and data types help to formulate a picture of self- and collective-efficacy, as well as the resiliency of projects to bounce back through the ups and downs characteristic of project development. By being open to what else is going on with these projects, we have gained a much broader perspective of what constitutes project success within the context of this initiative.

Strike a Balance Between Staying in Touch and Staying out of the Way

Throughout the initiative, we have struggled to strike a balance between collecting comprehensive data (in order to learn as much as we could about the important work being done in communities across the state) and being realistic in terms of the time and energy available to project staff to devote toward these efforts. In the forefront of our minds have been the conditions under which many project directors or coordinators work. First, project staff receive $10,000 a year to implement a community-based health-promotion project. They receive no monetary compensation for answering questions appearing on a survey or posed during a telephone interview; yet, completing a survey or a telephone interview can be draining and time-consuming. Second, few project directors and coordinators have the luxury of paid support staff. Consequently, the time they devote to data collection activities detracts from the time that these project directors and coordinators have for the work that keeps their projects going. Third, many of these project directors and coordinators already work overtime and serve multiple roles at work and in their communities. All these factors together make these project directors and coordinators vulnerable to burnout. We certainly do not want to intensify these pressures.

In order to minimize the imposition of data collection efforts, we have taken advantage of documents and presentations that grantees are already required to provide as part of their funding. For example, we develop detailed summaries of each 6-month progress report that project directors and coordinators are required to write according to the conditions of the CAHPI grants. (Figure 27.6 presents components of the standardized form we use to develop these detailed summaries). We also take copious notes at grantees' meetings, the biannual meetings at which project directors and coordinators give project updates. These updates typically consist of information about various activities that have been carried out in recent months, as well as the number of participants and volunteers who took part; any new programs, activities, or relationships that have developed as a result of these activities; and information about facilitators and barriers to accomplishing project goals and objectives. In addition to taking advantage of existing data sources to minimize the burden of data collection on project staff, we attempt to make our survey instruments as succinct and straightforward as possible, making as few revisions as possible to the general format, so that project directors and coordinators do not have to spend valuable time figuring out how to complete our surveys. We administer two out of the three standard surveys only once a year, and we stagger them 6 months apart to minimize the burden of data completion at given points in time.

To strike a balance between staying in touch and staying out of the way, we attempt to make data collection efforts as meaningful as possible for project staff as a way to reciprocate their contributions to these efforts. As mentioned above, we complete a detailed summary of what we have learned following each site visit and interview. In

Site: **Completed by:**
Date completed: **Period covered by report:**

PART I: Project Summary Report Contents

1. Objectives and action steps

    Objective #: [*Type out the objective here*]
       a. Progress and accomplishments
       b. Barriers
       c. Important Objective or Alternatives for Consideration
       d. Action Step Changes
       e. Frustrations
       f. Rewards

2. Volunteer and staff time
       a. How time was spent
       b. Changes

3. Collaboration
       a. Additions/deletions
       b. Any other information, resources, or support

4. Community climate

5. Anything else?

PART II: Other Information Reported

Based on what you know from this 6-Month Report,

	NO	YES →	Specify
1. Was the target population exposed to the project?	☐	☐	Numbers, description, etc.
2. Were policy changes or new policies implemented?	☐	☐	Type, content, etc.
3. Was there publicity or media coverage?	☐	☐	Type, content, etc.
4. Is there other funding?	☐	☐	Type, amount, etc.
5. Is there a plan for continuation funding?	☐	☐	Type, amount, etc.
6. Is there an internal evaluation in place?	☐	☐	Methods, findings, etc.
7. Are there any spin-offs?	☐	☐	Type, purpose, etc.
8. Any other pertinent information from the past 6 months?	☐	☐	

PART III: Speculations and Impressions from the Report

1. What can you say about the impact or effect of the project's last 6 months?

2. What were the main issues or themes that struck you in this contact/document?

FIGURE 27.6 Components of the 6-month report summary form.

some cases, we share these summaries with project directors and coordinators, as well as with management agency staff, to facilitate ongoing discussions and brainstorming about particular issues or challenges that have emerged for a project. Such information-sharing is particularly important in connecting project staff with information and people resources. We hope that project directors and coordinators are able to use these summaries as a data source when developing their required 6-month progress reports.

Through site visits and interviews, we also attempt to share any ideas or technical assistance we think might be useful based on what we are observing or hearing. During the course of an interview, we often ask about any challenges project directors and coordinators experience as they carry out a community-based health-promotion project. During one interview, for example, a project director talked about her struggles with program evaluation. What she is actually doing to learn about her program and its impacts, we learned, is quite sophisticated and impressive given the resources available for local evaluation. This project director conducts and oversees a telephone survey of families in a three-county region who receive child safety kits and education through the project. As a result of these local evaluation efforts, she has received important feedback about the contents of the kits such as the relative usefulness of certain items and what items would also be helpful to include. These follow-up calls serve as both a prompt, reminding parents to use the contents of the kits, as well as a way for the project director to collect anecdotal information about the impact of the child safety kits and education on how parents talk with their children about safety issues and institute safety measures in their home.

Because this project relies extensively on in-kind contributions, the interviewer (one of the evaluation team members) suggested that the project director share some of this positive feedback with the business contributors to her project. This feedback will help these partners know that their contributions really are making a difference in the community, as well as serve as way to give something back to these valuable project partners. Such feedback serves as an incentive for continuing to contribute to a project. Our evaluation team knows firsthand the magic of incentives. We include prepaid phone cards with the Working with Others Survey, which is our longest and most detailed survey. These phone cards are very popular with project directors and coordinators, and perhaps these incentives facilitate networking. Such reciprocity is an important feature of partnerships that are meaningfully sustained, and we hope that through these deliberate efforts to provide feedback and suggestions (as well as incentives) we have reciprocated and truly collaborated with project staff in data collection.

. . . Reciprocity is an important feature of partnerships that are meaningfully sustained . . .

Be reflective about what methods are most appropriate for different stages and phases. Different stages or phases of a process will have different information needs. This is as true of the process of evaluating an entire initiative as it is for implementing the individual community-based health promotion projects that received funding through the initiative. In the beginning, we had relatively little literature available to us that documented the evaluation of multiple, small, community-based health promotion projects over as much as a 5-year period and that went beyond measuring specific project goals and objectives. As a result, and given that we had 5 years available to us, our initial strategy was to use qualitative methods to simply explore and document what occurred. When the bulk of data generated through these efforts started to feel overwhelming, we recognized the need to identify a few key elements that seemed to be important mediators of how these projects are implemented and sustained over time. Through this process, we developed a strategy for narrowing the scope of data collection. Subsequently, we began to use quantitative methods to collect data on these identified factors in a more systematic fashion. We did not abandon qualitative methods such as site visits and telephone interviews, as we recognized the value of these methods as a primary source for contextual information that supplemented the data collected through regularly administered surveys. Such triangulation provides a more complete picture of what is occurring and is an especially important strategy when the phenomena being considered are poorly understood. Because community-based health promotion is such a dynamic process, we have relied on more flexible qualitative methods throughout the evaluation process in order to capture and document those dynamics adequately.

The old adage "Don't throw the baby out with the bathwater" is relevant to developing data collection strategies. When there is a need to make a shift methodologically, it is important not to disregard the methods used previously; consider, rather, how these same methods can supplement or complement newly applied data collection strategies for triangulation.

Relationships Are Critically Important to Conducting Successful Evaluation

Our journey illustrates why evaluation entails flexibility, reflectiveness, and openness to learning. Evaluation is a dynamic process that must adapt and change as the projects and initiative change. If evaluation efforts do not respond to the evolving, iterative (or trial and error) nature of community-based health-promotion work, evaluation instruments will be less sensitive, and the data collected with these tools will fail to adequately capture what happens. Ultimately, the products of the evaluation will be less relevant and meaningful to the intended audiences.

It follows that successful (that is, meaningful and relevant) evaluation is conducted within the context of partnerships (or collaborative working relationships) among and between key stakeholders such as evaluators, staff representing the management agency, and project directors and coordinators. Figure 27.7 illustrates how such partnering facilitates learning, innovation, and responsiveness through reciprocal information-sharing that augments data

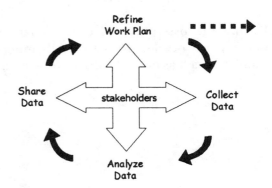

FIGURE 27.7 Stakeholders as the pivotal point for information sharing that drives the iterative evaluation process.

Funders, members of the management agency and representatives from local projects and communities should be central to the evaluation process as each stakeholder group possesses expert knowledge that will provide important insights about the data that have been collected and that need to be collected in the future.

collection and enhances the ability of both evaluators and management agency staff to stay abreast of what is occurring, what new challenges are emerging, and what new successes should be celebrated.

Barriers to forming and sustaining partnerships may take the form of issues over territory and authority. Such barriers may be overcome if the parties involved keep the bigger picture in mind: the cause or mission of facilitating and promoting health in community-based settings. For their part, staff of the management agency and the evaluation team should prioritize assisting with and learning from the important work of local experts, that is, the project directors and coordinators. Our own experience has taught us that relationships, even in the working world, take time to develop. Trust, in particular, must be deliberately and diligently attended to and nurtured to facilitate openness, sharing, and learning.

SUMMARY

During the first phase of our evaluation journey, we needed to learn and understand as much as possible about these community-based projects. In the second phase, we needed to narrow our focus to understanding those things that seemed more important or salient to the health promotion work being conducted within the context of these smaller projects. And now, in the final year of the initiative, we are again expanding our focus to ensure that our understanding of specific aspects fits within the broader context of what we learned during the initial phase. In reflecting on our evaluation journey, we have realized that the shifting scope of our focus at different points resembles the shape of an hourglass: broad in the beginning and end and narrower in the middle.

While the findings generated through this evaluation may not be generalized to other contexts, the processes used to generate these findings are germane to other domains of study and exploration. We hope that the description of our journey and the lessons we have learned along the way will be useful to you as you undertake your own exciting journey into community-based health promotion. The journey may be difficult and strenuous at times, but always filled with the rewards of new adventures and discoveries.

CHAPTER 28

Health Promotion in a Homeless Center

Carl O. Helvie

This chapter describes the experience of the Old Dominion University nursing center and its health promotion program for the homeless.

NURSING CENTERS DEFINED

Nursing centers are centers that are nurse-managed; where nurses are accountable and responsible for client care and professional practice; and where nurses are the primary provider of care and the practitioner most often seen by clients (Riesch, 1992).

BACKGROUND OF ODU NURSING CENTER

The ODU Nursing Center opened in March 1997 and was funded by a grant from the Department of Health and Human Services, Division of Nursing. The three major goals for the center are (a) improving the health of the homeless and low-income populations by better access to care and the provision of quality primary care including health promotion; (b) providing a variety of experiences for nursing and other students; and (c) developing, implementing, analyzing, and reporting on health care needs and practices of the homeless and low-income populations and the attitudes of students toward these populations.

Access is increased by the location of the center at a homeless shelter that provides an evening meal to anyone who is in need, by providing outreach services to a local day center, and when hours for care are in the afternoon and evening when most clients are available to attend the center.

All homeless clients in the community and low-income clients in census tracts surrounding the center (lowest average income of the community) are eligible for care at the center and about 120 to 150 people are seen monthly. A broad definition of homelessness is used so that those leaving a sheltered situation who are financially precarious will not be denied care when it is needed.

Primary care for acute and chronic conditions is provided by a family nurse practitioner. The most common acute conditions include upper respiratory infections, acute bronchitis, cough, influenza, gastrointestinal problems, dermatitis, elevated blood pressure, sinusitis, and chest pains. For a 1-year period there were 140 patients with 138 different acute conditions, which averaged 2.5 acute conditions per patient. Common chronic conditions include: alcoholism, chemical dependence, asthma, hypertension, depression, allergic rhinitis, obesity, nicotine addiction, migraine headache, low back pain, hypercholesterolemia, and arthritis. Over a 1-year period 99 patients were treated for 250 chronic conditions, which averaged 1.78 chronic conditions per patient.

The nurse practitioner modified the protocols that were published in *Clinical Guidelines in Family Practice* (Uphold & Graham, 1998) so that they were appropriate for the clinic population and setting. These protocols were then approved by the back-up physician who is available by telephone and visits the center monthly to review at least 10% of all records to validate that protocols are being followed and to discuss any concerns and problems. A medical staff meeting is held every 2 months.

The nurse practitioner has prescriptive rights and is supported in her diagnosis and treatment by the following resources: laboratory and X-ray services available by contract with local hospitals; medication orders faxed to local pharmacies, filled, and delivered to the center; dental care provided in local dentists' offices; eyeglasses provided by the Lion's Club; and specialty care provided in the offices of local physician specialists. Records at the center are computerized, and nursing diagnoses, interventions, and outcomes are added to the standardized system of acute and chronic diagnoses. Staff at the center include the family nurse practitioner, a full-time office specialist who serves as part-time secretary-receptionist and a part-time secretary-receptionist. Policies and procedures identify

the role and duties of each staff member. The project director oversees all activities of the center including the budget.

The nursing center currently consists of 700 sq. ft. that includes two examining rooms, a waiting and reception area, a laboratory, bathroom, and an office for the nurse practitioner and for the project director. The project director has worked with a council member from the district for the past year and has obtained funding for an additional 900 sq. ft. that will add two examining rooms, a larger waiting and reception area, a room for educational activities with clients, and an office for the office specialist.

The additional space will allow implementation of a new proposed grant from the division of nursing for expenses of staff and primary care. This grant will provide for care to low-income clients in additional census tracts and add complementary and alternative therapy to the current primary care. New objectives include adding complementary care to primary care; education of students on primary care and health-promotion, including complementary care; and evaluation of primary care including complementary care. A group of health care personnel have agreed to participate in the primary care, including a physician neurologist who is a certified acupuncturist, a chiropractor, massage therapy students, an herbalist, a nurse who practices therapeutic touch and imagery, and others.

Nursing students rotate through the nursing center and provide primary care and health-promotion activities. Graduate students in family nurse practitioner and pediatric nurse practitioner roles provide primary care, and graduate students in administration develop marketing plans, brochures, and administrative policies. Undergraduate nursing students in community-health nursing complete community assessments and present health fairs covering many health promotion activities.

Research is the third objective of the center. The attitudes of nursing students have been evaluated before and after a classroom course on the homeless and before and after a clinical experience with them in the center. Outcomes of nursing interventions have also been evaluated by the nurse practitioner and clients before and after treatment. Results from these ongoing studies have been presented at the American Public Health Association in Indianapolis, Indiana, and in Washington, DC; at Sigma Theta Tau in Amsterdam, Netherlands, and in London, England; and at a family nursing conference in Helsinki, Finland. The efficacy of primary care in a nursing center was discussed in an article that reviews several pieces of research carried out in the center and was published in *Nursing Case Management* in July/August 1999. An article on the homeless and the nursing center also appeared in the *Public Health Nursing Newsletter* of the American Public Health Association (Helvie, 1999).

HEALTH PROMOTION

Health promotion is an important part of care in the ODU nursing center. A review of records for current patients showed the following health promotion activities included in primary care over a 5-month period (April to September 1998) by the nurse practitioner. There were 21 Pap smears, 35 cholesterol tests, 10 prostate cancer tests (PSA), 10 mammograms, and 12 digital rectal exams as part of the complete physical exam. Seventeen school physicals were also completed, and health teaching on prevention was provided as part of all care. Other health promotion activities identified from a recent chart review in-

cluded the teaching of breast self-examination, testicular self-examination, diet and exercise and dental health, immunizations, sex education, and others. For example, obese patients were counseled on nutrition and exercise, and smoking cessation and stress-management techniques were taught to clients who smoke.

In addition, students from community-health nursing assessed the homeless and low-income populations, using secondary data on disease incidence and prevalence and other factors, and also developed an assessment tool to obtain data on what the homeless and low-income populations perceived as their needs for health education. Based upon these assessments the students developed health promotion teaching materials to meet the identified needs. Appropriate educational materials were displayed, and students taught health-promotion activities related to them at a yearly health fair. During the spring of 1998, the following health-promotion areas were implemented: screening and about hypertension and diabetes; foot care and foot examinations; oral hygiene and supplies; breast and testicular self-examination; communicable disease information, including HIV/AIDS, STDs, and free condoms; a resource booth with resources specific to homeless and low-income populations; and an upper-respiratory-infection education booth. Sixty-five homeless and low-income clients visited the booths, and verbal evaluations were very positive. Using an evaluation tool, students gained information on the value of the materials for the population.

During the spring of 1999 the community health nursing students repeated community assessments with the homeless who were living in shelters, with those attending a day center but living in the woods or sleeping in temporary sites, and with a low-income population living near the nursing center. The health fair that was planned by the students displayed teaching materials on the following topics: substance abuse, personal hygiene, nutrition, foot care, skin cancer, oral care, smoking cessation, alcoholism, hypertension, STD prevention, and diabetes. Evaluations of these materials and the teaching that was implemented were rated very highly by those attending.

Registered-nurse students receiving their community-health nursing experience in the nursing center for the summer of 1999 developed videos to be used in the clients' waiting room. Topics developed included stress management, smoking cessation, and proper breathing. This need was identified by assessments of clients' clinic data and by consultation with the nurse practitioner and project director. The videos will be used with appropriate clients while they wait to see the nurse practitioner or upon referral from the nurse practitioner.

SUMMARY

Nurses are adept at providing health promotion activities to homeless clients. This chapter has identified nursing centers as an appropriate site for providing primary care including health promotion to this population.

REFERENCES

Helvie, C. (1999, Spring). Nursing the homeless—A vulnerable population. *Public Health Nursing*, 8–9.

Riesch, S. K. (1992). Nursing centers: An analysis of the anecdotal literature. *Journal of Professional Nursing*, 8(1), 16–25.

Uphold, C., & Graham, M. (1998). *Clinical guidelines in family practice* (3rd ed.). Gainsville, FL: Baramarrae Books.

INDEX

Dr. Clark Wants to Hear From You

Dear Reader:

Please send the following information to me and I will incorporate your suggestions in the next edition:

- other topics/chapters that need to be covered
- other information that needs to be incorporated in current chapters
- information that should be removed from subsequent editions
- names and email addresses of faculty, students, or organizational representatives who wish to contribute information about their community programs in subsequent editions
- other information that should be included in the next edition

Please email this information to me at *cccwellness@earthlink.net.*